NURSING OF THE FAMILY
IN HEALTH AND ILLNESS
A DEVELOPMENTAL APPROACH

Edited By
Martha J. Bradshaw, RN, MSN
Assistant Professor, Parent-Child Nursing
Medical College of Georgia
Augusta, Georgia

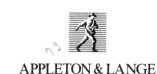

APPLETON & LANGE
Norwalk, Connecticut/San Mateo, California

ISBN: 0-8385-7012-7

88 89 90 91 92 / 10 9 8 7 6 5 4 3 2 1

Prentice-Hall of Australia, Pty. Ltd., *Sydney*
Prentice-Hall Canada, Inc.
Prentice-Hall Hispanoamericana, S.A., *Mexico*
Prentice-Hall of India Private Limited, *New Delhi*
Prentice-Hall International (UK) Limited, *London*
Prentice-Hall of Japan, Inc., *Tokyo*
Prentice-Hall of Southeast Asia (Pte.) Ltd., *Singapore*
Whitehall Books Ltd., Wellington, *New Zealand*
Editora Prentice-Hall do Brasil Ltda., *Rio de Janeiro*

Library of Congress Cataloging-in-Publication Data

Nursing of the family in health and illness.

  Includes index.
  1. Nursing. 2. Family medicine. I. Bradshaw,
Martha J. [DNLM: 1: Family. 2. Nursing Care.
WA 308 N974]
RT42.N867 1988   610.73   88-3495
ISBN 0-8385-7012-7

Acquisitions Editor: Marion K. Welch
Production Editor: Christine Langan
Designer: Steven M. Byrum

PRINTED IN THE UNITED STATES OF AMERICA

I wish to dedicate this book to my beloved son, Carl,
who has shown me the true meaning of parenthood

CONTRIBUTORS

Kitty Bishop, RN, MSN
Albany, Georgia

Martha J. Bradshaw, RN, MSN
Assistant Professor
Parent-Child Nursing
Medical College of Georgia
Augusta, Georgia

Marion Broome, RN, PhD
Associate Professor and Assistant
  Chairperson
Maternal-Child Nursing
Rush-St. Luke's Presbyterian
  Medical Center
Chicago, Illinois

Sandra Dale, RN, MSN, MEd
Doctoral Candidate
Georgia State University
Atlanta, Georgia

Cathryn Glanville, RN, EdD
Associate Professor and
  Chairperson
Department of Parent-Child
  Nursing
Medical College of Georgia
Augusta, Georgia

Lois Hasan, RN, MSN
Clinical Nurse Specialist
Richland Memorial Hospital
Columbia, South Carolina

Vickie A. Lambert, RN, DNSc
Associate Dean
Frances Payne Bolton School of
  Nursing
Case Western Reserve University
Cleveland, Ohio

**Clinton E. Lambert, Jr., RN,
  MSN, CS**
Private Practitioner in
  Psychiatric/Mental Health
  Nursing and Doctoral Student
School of Nursing
University of Maryland
Baltimore, Maryland

Elizabeth Pond, RN, EdD
Assistant Professor
Parent-Child Nursing
Medical College of Georgia
Augusta, Georgia

Mary Ann Rogers, RN, EdD
Assistant Professor
Psychiatric/Mental Health Nursing
Medical College of Georgia
Augusta, Georgia

Thayer Wilson, RN, MN
Doctoral Student
School of Nursing
Medical College of Georgia
Augusta, Georgia

CONTENTS

PREFACE

INTRODUCTION

This book examines a number of factors that are influential to individual and family development. Recognition of these factors is the foundation of nursing interventions with families and family members. The expanding nurse's role, beyond that of caregiver, to include advocacy and collaboration, plus teaching and guidance, warrant the use of the knowledge and principles presented.

The ideal American family consisting of mother, father, 2.2 kids, and a dog does not always match a personal definition of "a family." What was previously more common now shares an almost equal plane with a variety of living patterns—single-parent, all-adult, or homosexual households are but a few examples. While these various family forms are recognized in this text, this book focuses on the regenerating group form as the prevailing family structure. Components of this family structure include a male and female, who have perpetuated themselves by having children. These nuclear family members interact with and are influenced by satellite or extended family members and a support system in society.

The individual striving to establish and maintain him or herself as a family member is also presented from the developmental viewpoint. Whereas each of us may not have our own family of regeneration, we all have, at some time, been a family member during infancy and childhood. Many of us will continue through adulthood, ending our lives during the senescent period. The individual and family adaptation to change brought on by development through the life span carries specific implications for the role of the nurse in caring for a family. We all have, or will have, needs or interruptions in health requiring nursing intervention. The nurse who understands and applies the dynamics of individual and family processes thus will be able to provide quality care and assist the family in optimal functioning.

ORGANIZATION OF TEXT

A special feature of this book is the coverage of the individual from the time of birth until the time of death. Within this "birth to death" review are descriptions of the physical, psychosocial, societal and cultural influences affecting our evolution as human beings. Each chapter identifies those factors that are especially significant to individual development at that particular time of life.

A brief explanation of the structure of this text should provide the reader with continuity from chapter to chapter. Nursing roles and responsibilities are addressed consistently throughout. The chapters are:

Chapter 1. *The Family: An Overview*—This chapter addresses approaches to family assessment, such as systems and developmental theories. Includes a summary of the roles and functions common to families and a description of the key features of family assessment.

Chapter 2. *The Expanding Family: Pregnancy*—This chapter describes significant physical changes and emotional adjustments that occur during the antepartal period. Maternal needs and physical requirements are presented, along with paternal needs and adjustments. This chapter indicates the preparations made by the childbearing couple for family expansion.

Chapter 3. *The Expanding Family: Childbirth*—This chapter examines the developmental tasks, physical concerns and health needs of the immediate childbearing period. Provision of family centered care is a focal point. Components of the normal intrapartal period are discussed. Variations from the norm, along with appropriate nursing interventions are presented.

Chapter 4. *The Family with a Neonate*—This chapter introduces a new family member and the related adjustments are characterized. Individual tasks of the neonate stress the importance of adjustment to extrauterine life. Specific tasks related to parenting are given, along with nursing measures to promote optimal parenting.

Chapter 5. *The Family with an Infant*—This chapter depicts the progress of the new individual, the neonate, into infancy. It gives a broader emphasis on the family developmental tasks at this time period, and indicates how the individual tasks of the infant and the collective tasks of the family may be in conflict. Health stressors not related to birth are introduced.

Chapter 6. *The Family with the Toddler/Preschooler*—This chapter analyzes continued individual and family development, describing early psychosocial components that have a strong influence on the individual's subsequent development. The numerous and rapid changes in the toddler and preschooler also are addressed. It is during this time period that the family may add an additional child, thus increasing the complexity of the family tasks.

Chapter 7. *The Family with the School Age Child*—This chapter presents the individual's expanding world as he or she attends school and broadens the existing social network. Family tasks which deal with adjustments to the child's new world are explained, along with changes occuring simultaneously with other family members. Accidents are a health concern at this time and the nursing activities directed at health promotion by the child are provided.

Chapter 8. *The Family and the Adolescent*—This chapter illustrates how the desire for independence and maturity can have an impact on the individual and family. The psychosocial stressors of this period highlight conflicts between increasing freedom and self-responsibility on the part of the adolescent. Family tasks address coping by family members with the adolescent's search for identity, plus concurrent changes by the other members.

Chapter 9. *The Family and the Young Adult*—the initial focus in the chapter is that of the individual as he or she moves away from the family and begins a separate way of living. Adjustments accompanying these changes include establishing patterns for lifestyle, work, and interpersonal relationships. The young adult also finds him or herself with an affiliation to two families—those of orientation and procreation. Adaptations by the family to the exit of the young adult from the home are described.

Chapter 10. *The Family and the Middlescent*—This chapter deals with the individual in the middle years of adulthood. Significant occurrences during this time period include, changing career responsibilities, new health problems, shrinkage of the original family and expansion of the extended family with the addition of grandchildren.

Chapter 11. *The Family and the Senescent*—In this chapter the final years in the life of an individual are presented. Psychosocial stressors such as loneliness and grief share equal emphasis with physical stressors such as major illness or loss of physical abilities. The role of the extended family members in caring for the senescent adult is described.

STRUCTURE OF EACH CHAPTER

This book presents the concept that individuals and families proceed through life with a predictable amount of conformity from one phase to the next. Consequently, the separate chapters address the same outline:

1. The Family and the individual
    A. Family tasks
    B. Individual tasks
        1. Physical
        2. Personality
        3. Interpersonal relationships
        4. Competency and achievement
        5. Society and culture
2. Potential stressors
    A. Physical
    B. Social/emotional
    C. Conflicts with family tasks
3. Coping mechanisms
    A. Health beliefs and behaviors
    B. Responses to stressors
        1. Adaptive responses
        2. Maladaptive responses

4. Nursing assessment of the family and the individual
   A. Environmental data
   B. Communication patterns
   C. Problem solving skills
   D. Life style
   E. Potential stressors
   F. Family response patterns
5. Alterations in health of the individual
   A. Acute conditions
   B. Chronic conditions
6. Nursing responsibilities
   A. Health promotion
   B. Accident/illness prevention
   C. Caregiver

FEATURES IN EACH CHAPTER

The chapters contain additional material that should guide the reader in obtaining maximum benefit from the text. Such benefits include viewing individual health care clients in the context of their family, increased understanding of factors taking place within a given family at a specific time of life, and the ability to recognize deviations from normal individual and family health.

These features are:

■ **Chapter objectives** presented at the beginning of each chapter for the purpose of orienting the reader to the content of that chapter. The objectives indicate desired learning or increased understanding that will occur upon integration of the chapter material.

■ **Care plan for the individual** based upon a Nursing Diagnosis (NANDA), each care plan addresses a common health problem for the individual in a specific age group. The care plan demonstrates to the reader how to apply the concepts and specific information when developing nursing care for the individual and family at a certain time of life.

■ **Discussion questions** provided at the conclusion of each chapter, the questions can be used both by the single reader or for use in groups. The reader can review the questions in order to conduct a self-evaluation of material learned. The questions can be used in teaching/learning situations to guide learners in applying information they have read. Student clinical groups can use a question from one chapter and apply it to various other situations involving family nursing.

Appendices contain information about the specific theorists whose works appear in this text. Some of the theories are applicable with numerous age groups, such as Evelyn DuVal and Erik Erikson. Others are more applicable to a specific age range, such as Jean Piaget or Lawrence Kohlberg. The appendices provide a summary of the main tenets of the theories and indicate the age range or developmental phase for which they are intended.

It is recognized that the discussion of family and individual health is quite broad. It also is recognized that there are numerous textbooks that provide information about certain aspects of nursing care in clinical settings. In order to present an overview of family development, information on how to implement very specific nursing care was minimized. It is hoped that the reader will find this book useful in providing an understanding of the family and individual at a particular time of life. With that understanding as a foundation, nursing care to meet identified needs can then be derived.

Martha J. Bradshaw

The Family: An Overview

*Sandra E. Dale and
Cathryn Glanville with
Lois Hasan*

OBJECTIVES

Upon completion of this chapter, the student will be able to:

1. Identify and discuss the implication of variations in structure and function of families
2. Discuss the relationship between individual and family development
3. Discuss the differences among a systems perspective, an interactional perspective, and a developmental perspective of the study of families
4. Conduct a systematic family assessment
5. Describe the effects of health beliefs and health behaviors on family health goals
6. Describe the critical elements of a nursing plan that would facilitate the health promotion of the family

CONCEPTS

Assessment: Evaluation or appraisal of the family in a systematic fashion for the purpose of identifying and prioritizing needed areas for intervention. The parameters for family assessment include data about the environment, family roles and relationships, communication patterns, affective patterns, problem-solving skills, behavior control approaches, and the autonomy of individual members.

Development: Growth or expansion of a family which occurs systematically and sequentially.

Developmental task: Tasks determined by the varying developmental stages that

must be completed by the family members for continued growth of the
family and its members.

Family: A group of persons usually related by marriage, birth, or adoption having
a mutual obligation of influencing social and moral values, transmitting
physical characteristics, and contributing to the emotional and psychological
makeup of its individual members.

Family functions: Those functions that reflect the interaction of the family with
other social institutions and include economic, protective, religious,
educational, recreational, affectional, and status giving activities.

Family interaction: The manner in which family members deal with the
environment and each other (role relations), as determined by the family's
power, communication, and affection structures.

Family life cycle: The family's existence from the time of its inception to its
dissolution which consists of distinct and separate stages or divisions.

Family roles: These are based upon the prescribed responsibilities, expectations,
and rights of individual members and are determined through interaction
among individual members over time.

Family structures: Structures are determined by characteristics of the individual
members and can vary from a traditional nuclear family to one loosely
connected.

Health: A state of well-being in which the individual perceives himself to be
functioning normally and free from disease.

Health behaviors: The operationalization of health beliefs and values. Those
actions taken by the family or individual family members that contribute to
illness prevention and health promotion.

Health beliefs: Attitudes arising from the family's mores and culture that
contribute to healthy behaviors.

THE FAMILY

The family, described as the basic unit of society, differs from other social groups
through its modes of communication, living, interaction, and cultural experiences.
As a unit of society, the family influences social and moral values, transmits physical
characteristics, and contributes to the emotional and psychological makeup of the
individual. This ability to influence individual actions suggests that the family has the
potential of being the most powerful societal unit. As an organization, the family has
continuity; a past, present, and future (which provides commonality of behaviors), a
sharing of values and goals, and safety in response behaviors (Messer, 1971).

Historically, the early American family frequently consisted of the immediate
family plus extended-family members who also contributed to the functioning of the
family unit. The role of children in this early family was to provide valuable resources

for the maintenance of the unit through contributing to the work of family survival. Thus, in our preindustrial society, children were considered valuable assets to family wealth and played an active role in family work.

Today's families generally are not the extended work group of our preindustrial relatives. The traditional definition of the family as a unit composed of individuals joined by marriage, blood, or adoption, who live together or separately and enact designated social roles, such as husband, wife, daughter, son, sister, and brother (Burgess, Lock, & Thomas, 1963), does not reflect accurately all of today's families. Families do not necessarily consist of blood relatives, nor do family members always live together. In addition, the designated social roles are rapidly changing within some segments of our society. A critical element in understanding families would appear to be recognition of the obligation of mutuality within the group. Thus, the family group would be defined as a group composed of members who have a mutual obligation to provide a broad range of support, both material and emotional (Dean, Lin, & Ensel, 1981). In addition, families can also be defined as having structure, multiple functions (tasks), roles, interaction styles, resources, a life cycle, and a unique family history as well as a collection of individual histories.

Family Structure

A family's structure is determined by the characteristics of its individual members. Characteristics include gender, age distribution, spacing of children, and the number of family members. The actual family structure can vary from the traditional nuclear family to one consisting of a loosely bound network.

The traditional *nuclear family* is also often called the *conjugal family* and is the family of marriage and procreation. It consists of husband, wife, and their children, living together. Some families may form a part of a large *extended-family* structure. This structure consists of a nuclear family and individuals related by blood and/or marriage (e.g., grandparents, uncles, aunts, cousins). In the United States and Canada, the prevalence of the traditional nuclear family has been influenced by societal changes, such as the woman's movement, employment of mothers, marriage, divorce, and remarriage. This has resulted in greater recognition of other family structures, such as communal families, cohabiting couples, homosexual unions, single-parent families, and blended or reconstituted families.

There are numerous questions and unresolved issues related to the specific effects of different family structures on childrearing and individual growth and development. Single-parent families, blended families, and homosexual families, in particular, pose a challenge to the health care provider. For example, Dokeckie, Dunlap, and Moroney (1980) found that about 42 percent of single-parent families, headed by women, are living below the poverty line. Therefore, nutrition, dental care, and health care are jeopardized. According to Visher and Visher (1979), approximately 250,000 blended families are formed each year. The complexities of this family system are influenced by variables such as acceptance of stepparent/stepchild, past history, differing childrearing patterns and expectations, and conflicts between biological parents. The discrimination experienced by gay families results in social isolation for all family members.

Health providers need to recognize the variations in family structures and the accompanying problems. Nurses must also be knowledgeable about community resources, referral policies and procedures, and availability of specific health care services to effectively assess and provide health care services for today's families.

Family Functions

The many functions performed by a family reflect the relationship of the family with other institutions as well as its contribution to society. Functions may be performed by the family group, by individual members, or may be shared. Broadly defined, these functions include economic, protective, religious, educational, recreational, affectional, and status-giving activities (Ogburn, 1938). Educational functions are currently subsumed under socialization functions, a description more reflective of the informal learning that children receive within the family structure (Nye & Berardo, 1973). Additional activities within the family include sexual and therapeutic functions. Therapeutic functions may include general wellness and minor illness care, while sexual functions include marital relations as well as provision of sex role modeling and development of sexuality. Many family functions are shared by the community. For example, formal education takes place in schools and homes, just as religious training takes place in both the church and home.

Family Roles

The roles of family members are determined through interaction, change over time, and need not be mutually exclusive. They are based upon prescribed responsibilities, expectations, and rights of the individual members. Societal changes have also brought about changes in the traditional roles assumed by family members. Most significant is the assumption by working mothers of a multitude of roles, such as homemaker, caretaker, and wage earner. Smith (1979) has noted that by 1990, one half of all mothers of preschool-age children will be in the work force. Concurrent with this has come a change in role assumption by the adult male family members. More husbands/fathers are assuming homemaking/caretaking responsibilities. Although there has been and will continue to be a shift in roles within families, working mothers continue to carry a major responsibility for household management and child care (Musnik & Bane, 1980). This is a potential source for stress within the family.

Interaction Styles

A variety of interaction styles are adopted by family members to deal with the environment and with one another for problem solving and decision making. The style is dependent on family power structures, communication structures, and affection structures. *Power structures* are activated to accomplish decisions regarding resource allocation and task division. *Communication structures* are activated to provide information, define boundaries, and express feelings. Communication structures may be verbal or nonverbal and vary according to topic and individual families.

Affection structures involve the communication of individual sentiments and the desire to reduce distance between family members. Activation of the family structure will vary according to culture, age, and sex of the family members. The interdependence of these three structures determines the individual family interaction styles (Aldous, 1972).

Resources

Resources are those means available to families to assist with task accomplishment. Examples of needed family resources are individual health, social support, finances, social skills, and personality characteristics. The quality of these resources and the family's ability to utilize them influences the way a family interprets significant events (Hill, 1949).

Family and Individual Histories

Developmental changes and life experiences of individual family members contribute to the development of a unique family history. The family history is a result of interacting individual personalities and responses to the internal and external environments (social and physical). Included within this family history are coping styles and interpretation of previous stressful events. The family history and characteristics such as roles, interaction styles, and resources will influence the manner of response to future stressful events.

THEORETICAL FRAMEWORKS

Theoretical frameworks used in the study of families are highly relevant to nursing care of families. They are of particular assistance in identifying and defining family relationships. Because of the complexity of the family, most practitioners utilize an eclectic approach in analyzing family needs. While there are a number of pertinent frameworks that could be used for this textbook, three appear to have particular relevance: systems, interactional, and developmental.

The family, as a system of interacting individuals, experiences differing tasks and resource needs according to its developmental stage characteristics. The developmental approach is particularly useful in organizing and structuring the study of families and has been chosen as the organizing framework for this text. The developmental stages identified by Evelyn Duvall (1977) are used because they represent the physical, psychological, emotional, and interactional changes that occur in each of us throughout life. Family analysis within the different development stages will be primarily developmental but will utilize an eclectic approach.

Systems Perspective

The application of the systems perspective to the study of families provides the practitioner with an understanding of the family organization and the internal and external family relationships. This approach allows the family to be viewed as a system with multiple related subsystems, or "as a complex of elements or components directly or indirectly related in a causal network, such that each component is related to at least some other in a more or less stable way within any particular period of time" (Buckley, 1967, p. 41). Thus, families and their subsystems (e.g., husband–wife, parent–child dyads) can be viewed as being composed of members related to one another within an interactional network.

While systems may be either open or closed, a family system is usually considered to be open. Openness is dependent on the degree of interaction with the external environment and the various community social systems such as schools, churches, etc. In addition to system openness, family systems are characterized by their complexity and intricate organizational structure, by their homeostatic mechanisms to maintain or restore balance, and by their ability to modify their structure (Hill, 1961; Speer, 1970).

A family is composed of positions that consist of a number of roles. Each role is made up of a set of related norms that are culturally defined or expected. Examples of possible roles within the position of husband-father include those of provider, affection giver, child caretaker, and sexual partner. Family positions are interdependent, with changes in behavior by one family member resulting in a need for change in other family members. This interdependence is noted in both conflict and cooperation situations. The family's emotional interdependence is also shown in both marital and parent–child relationships.

A family identifies itself as a unit through the process of selective boundary maintenance. This allows a family to set itself apart and monitor the outside influences that affect it. Boundaries are encouraged by rituals, separate residences, and shared experiences. The degree of interdependence within the family system will determine the degree of susceptibility to external influences. Families having critical needs that cannot be met within the system will be much more vulnerable to the external environment. An example of this is the unemployed or underemployed single mother who, by necessity, must rely on public financial assistance to meet the basic family needs. The degree of boundary maintenance also determines the ability of the family to acquire and utilize external resources essential for the family's growth.

Another aspect of the family's ability to modify structure is in its use of feedback processes. The complexity of relationships between the family and outsiders as well as the interdependence within the family structure is the source of much feedback regarding the family's status. Patterns of communication develop that not only transmit and receive information but also interpret its significance to the family. These patterns of communication can be either positive or negative in terms of the family's response. A positive feedback process may produce structural modification or goal change through the process of creating or innovating change within the system. Negative feedback processes alert the system to a mismatch and may result in behavioral change to return to the normal level of functioning. The emphasis is on the maintenance of a state of relative stability or homeostasis.

The concept of task performance emphasizes the group aspect in which goals critical for group continuity and maintenance are determined and tasks are performed by the family. The accomplishment of specific tasks enables families to maintain selective boundary maintenance and family or group integrity. Tasks are interrelated, and task completion may be affected by external influences that cross family boundaries. These can facilitate, modify, or hinder task performance. Both internal and external demands on the family system will influence task performance.

Interactional Perspective

An interactional perspective of families emphasizes the active and highly symbolic interactions among the family members and their environment. The underlying assumption is that man lives in a symbolic, as well as a physical, environment where the stimuli for action are symbolic and the individual self is developed through the process of social interaction. According to Hansen and Hill (1964), the basic assumptions in an interaction model are that (1) social conduct is a function of the social environment; (2) humans are independent actors as well as reactors; and (3) the basic unit is the individual. In other words, the family and individual members are active information processors. They seek out and evaluate information or the sources of stress and disruption. They evaluate available resources to respond to the threat. They act on their environment and evaluate the response (Hansen & Hill, 1964; Hill, 1949).

The component parts of an interactional model are the concepts of position, role, reference group, adaptation, and communication. This model highlights the nature of the fit among individual, family, and environmental demands and focuses on the family as a unity of interacting persons, each with a particular position within the family. Stress is the result of a discrepancy between the demands that impinge on the family and/or individual. Within the family, the perceived stressfulness of the event and the resulting coping abilities of the family defines the stress (Hansen & Hill, 1964).

Critical within this approach is the fact that family behaviors tend to be affected more by intrafamilial factors than by social norms. As a unit of interacting persons, each person has positions within the family. Each position has a number of assigned roles, and each role is enacted according to the perception of the role expectations held by the reference group (other family members). Interaction is therefore viewed from the perceptions of the participants within the social setting. It is a dynamic process, and thus a constant state of flux exists within families.

Developmental Perspective

The developmental perspective attempts to synthesize a number of compatible concepts from other theoretical approaches with the goal of viewing family change over time. Concepts considered within this perspective include developmental tasks, positions, roles, and norms. The family, itself, is viewed as a small group system organized into paired positions such as wife-mother and daughter-sister. The nuclear family is considered the primary family unit. Within this semiclosed system, individuals interact as a unit utilizing role behavior prescribed by norms, which direct the maintenance of interpersonal relations or interactions (Burgess, 1926; Rogers, 1973). A family changes in both its internal and external functions with the increasing age and development of its members. Time shifts are described as developmental stages within the family and reflect the family's life cycle or career (Rogers, 1973).

The *family life cycle* refers to the existence of the family as a unit from its inception to its dissolution. The addition of stages within the life cycle allows for divisions that are significantly different and separate periods. Family life cycle stages are defined by the amount of time needed to complete each stage as well as changes in family membership. This approach allows a view of the family over time and provides an understanding of family interaction during the various stages. Hill (1961) has identified three influences on the stages. These are changes of tasks and role expectations of children over time; changes of tasks and role expectations of parents over time; and a variation in family tasks over the family's life because of variation in both cultural expectations and individual developmental needs.

A family life cycle can be viewed as having two primary stages, expansion and contraction. Duvall (1977) has described an eight-stage division that allows for greater differentiation of the family changes over time and a closer analysis of the relationship between the family and the individual's developmental tasks. These cycles are primarily based on the age and/or school placement of the eldest child and begin with the establishment of the marital relationship. Childbearing and childrearing stages are only a part of the family life cycle. Duvall assumes a repetition of family experiences with each successive child, with some modifications. Her eight stages are used to describe age periods in this text. Family expansion begins with pregnancy and childbearing. Specific age periods and related tasks are recognized in the family with a neonate and continue through the family with an adolescent. Family contraction begins with the family with a young adult and proceeds through the family with a senescent.

The *developmental task* concept is critical to a family development framework. The developmental task, according to Havighurst, is a "task which arises at or about a certain period in the life of an individual, successful achievement of which leads to his happiness and to success with later tasks, while failure leads to unhappiness in the individual, disapproval by the society and difficulty with later tasks" (Havighurst, 1953, p. 2). Family developmental tasks differ from those of the individual family member. The family's tasks are generated when the family works together as a unit to assist individual members in their developmental task accomplishment (Friedman, 1986). Applying the individual developmental task concept to the family allows pertinent family content to be defined within each stage of family life.

The family developmental task has been defined by Aldous (1972) as a family function determined by each life cycle stage. As an autonomous unit, the family responds to society and its individual members by accomplishing family functions essential to its survival. The functions essential to family growth are specified by each family developmental stage. The five primary functions of the family as defined by Aldous (1972) are physical maintenance, socialization, motivational maintenance, social control maintenance, and addition of family members. Within each stage,

ASSESSING THE FAMILY

Theoretical and conceptual frameworks for each of the approaches cited offer a particular perspective for studying the family. None, however, is extensive enough to cover all aspects of family life. The primary foci of nursing the family as a client are assessment, health promotion, and accident/illness prevention. Any conceptual framework used must provide broad parameters for family assessment and facilitate implementation of strategies for health promotion and illness/accident prevention.

Epstein and Levine (1973) suggest that the parameters for family assessment should include:

1. Environmental data
2. Family roles and relationships
3. Communication patterns
4. Affective expression and involvement
5. Problem-solving skills
6. Behavior control
7. Autonomy of family members

In addition to these seven, the composition of the family should be identified, including the ages of the individual members.

Environmental data encompasses a description of the family's dwelling and conditions of the home as well as the family members' perceptions of its adequacy. Characteristics of the neighborhood and larger community, as well as the family's interactions with these, are also pertinent data.

Data about *roles and relationships* provide knowledge and understanding of the family's decision-making process. It is important to determine whether the role structure is flexible or rigid. When roles are flexible and changes occur as needed, the family's ability to cope with stressors is much more apparent than in families where roles are rigid and inappropriately assigned to family members. In addition, role conflict is minimized in families where roles are flexible and family members are sensitive to one another's needs. Information about the decision-making process provides insight into the overall family power structure. Usually, families with flexibility in role structure engage in shared or mutual decision making. Suggested questions designed to elicit information about roles and relationships are: How are the household chores divided up? Who makes the decisions regarding chores? How are conflicts between siblings or between parent and child resolved? How does the family member perform the task? How are changes in task/chore assignment made? Do family members contribute equally to family chores? Do family members perceive themselves as contributing equally to family tasks? If there is a discrepancy, how is it resolved?

The nature and types of *communication patterns* utilized by the family will often reveal the most accurate information about family functions. Communication patterns are reciprocal, sequential, and circular. When these are used as a parameter for assessment, suggested questions are: To what extent is there clarity, openness, and congruency in interactions among members? Do family members express their true feelings, elicit and use feedback? Describe the affective expressions used in interac-

family members may be involved in a variety of individual development. addition to the family developmental tasks.

The developmental perspective allows the family to be viewed not task-performance group but also to have specific stage-related behaviors. Su accomplishment of these tasks promotes growth and provides a basis for suc the next developmental stage. Conversely, failure to successfully complete thes may result in unhappiness, societal disapproval, and difficulties in accompli tasks within the next stage.

Physical maintenance is a critical family task and involves the interaction of family with the external environment, particularly the economic system. This par ular task involves the economic systems related to work and wage exchange a includes the provision of food, clothing, and the purchase of goods and services. addition, as family members interact with the external environment, new experi ences contribute to changing expectations within the family. For example, a family member who utilizes the health care system for prenatal care may increase the family's awareness of good nutritional habits, thus promoting and enhancing family health. Inability to perform these tasks satisfactorily may necessitate involvement with other external systems, such as welfare or health systems, to assist in remediation.

Socialization involves the preparation of family members for family roles and roles in other social groups. It is encouraged within the family through the provision of an arena for children to observe and play out adult roles. The performance of roles is assisted by the family's ability to maintain family and individual morale. Role performance is facilitated by praise or affection as well as by the demand for task performance. Socialization responsibilities are most heavy on the family with young children.

Motivational maintenance as a family task is directed toward the individual member's performance of family and individual roles. This can be seen in the family's inclusion of close friends and extended family for role performance. For example, the birth of the first child is a critical role change, and the involvement of experienced extended family members can assist in the development of the role through modeling as well as reassurance and praise. This function can also be seen in the family's preparation of the child for a first school experience. Older siblings and parents provide assurance and support for the individual child's role transition.

The family's *social control* behaviors are important to maintain the comfort and integrity of the family. They also promote socialization of behavior. The discipline and reward behaviors utilized in parenting are examples of this function. Another aspect of this task is how the family resolves conflict and adapts to the changing expectations and demands of individual family members.

The final task of *addition of family members* is somewhat less critical in today's society. Current societal trends, particularly in the Western hemisphere, have shifted the emphasis from the traditional family roles and the heavy emphasis on childbearing. The increased involvement of families with their external environments has also changed the role of the family in the socialization or childrearing tasks. Addition of family members now is more by choice rather than necessity, so effective contraceptive behaviors would provide an example of fulfilling this task.

tions. How is conflict resolved? Describe the family's use of feedback to alter their perceptions of self and others. How are family rules communicated to the individual family members? Describe the effects of communication patterns on the autonomy of individual family members.

Data gathered regarding *affective expression and involvement* should provide an understanding of the family's need-response patterns. Suggested questions include: How frequent is support and encouragement offered among family members? What is the frequency of put-downs? How is anger expressed? To what extent do family members demonstrate empathy toward one another? Are family members interested in and involved with one another's individual activities?

Demonstration of *problem-solving skills* utilized by the family provides clues relative to coping patterns within the family when faced with instrumental and affective threats such as unemployment, illness, death, or divorce. When assessing the family's problem-solving skills, methods used for problem identification and solution should be obtained. Questions to be considered are: Who perceives the problem? Who labels the problem and seeks outside help if needed? Why is the presenting problem perceived as a threat? Are there other problems affecting family functioning? If so, what is the relationship of the presenting problem to any existing problem? Have the family members shared with one another enough information about the problem so that responses will be appropriate? Is there reality distortion associated with the problem? Relative to problem solutions, what positive coping mechanisms exist within the family? Does the family have a repertoire of solutions from past experiences? If so, which ones are being utilized at present? Is the family working together in a concentrated effort to resolve the problem? Do family members freely express their feelings about the existing problem? What is the degree of adaptability and integration exhibited by the family? What types of leadership patterns emerge during problem resolution? Is the extended family being utilized as a support system? What other resources are being utilized for problem resolution?

An exploration of *behavior controls* present in the family provides insight into the family's rationale for what they perceive as acceptable and unacceptable behavior. Possible questions include: What are the standards for governing behavior? Are they clear to each family member? What methods are used for controlling behavior? Are the controls appropriate to the situation? Are the controls applied consistently or on impulse?

The extent to which *autonomy* exists within the family is often an indication of how much the rights of each member are expected and encouraged. Questions for consideration are: In what way is individual autonomy related to that of other family members? Are family members permitted to make separate choices if they are responsible choices? Describe the individual's autonomy outside the home. What are the cultural influences on autonomy of family members? (Epstein & Levine, 1973.)

HEALTH PROMOTION IN FAMILIES

Health promotion by the nurse includes the immediate intervention in acute conditions, maintaining existing functional patterns, enhancing the family's growth potential, and preventing future crisis events. Working from an identified conceptual framework for family assessment, the nurse can identify and prioritize needed areas for intervention. A developmental perspective of the family provides a framework for assessing family changes over time. Thus, the nurse is able to address the ongoing family needs and provide anticipatory guidance for future developmental tasks.

Selection and implementation of strategies for health promotion and prevention are based on outcomes of family assessment and the establishment of a collaborative relationship with the family. The extent of family involvement in meeting its health needs will be influenced by the family's (1) concept of health and illness, (2) health beliefs and values, (3) health behaviors, and (4) utilization of health services.

Concepts of Health and Illness

People have various ways of defining whether they are sick or well. Their perceptions are based on spiritual beliefs, mass media advertisements, folk beliefs, and general interpretation and understanding of scientific medicine. Some persons only feel sick when they can no longer work or perform daily activities of living. Another person may recognize changes in bodily symptoms as an indication of illness.

Bauman (1961) found the public to believe that health and illness are multifaceted concepts that include a feeling-state symptom and performance orientation. Bauman also noted that sociodemographic factors need to be considered when health and illness are defined. For example, persons with more education tend to look at the presence or absence of symptoms as one criterion when defining health or illness. Koos (1954) further demonstrated the influence of the socioeconomic position on an individual's concept of symptoms. Results of this study revealed that the lower socioeconomic group did not perceive the symptoms or seek medical care as early as the higher economic groups.

While there is a general consensus that the family is the major socializing agent of children, the manner in which the family determines the child's definition of health and illness and their health-related beliefs and behaviors has received limited research. Studies of the mother's role in the development of children's health concepts have provided some data on this relationship (Campbell, 1975a, 1975b, 1978; Mechanic, 1964, 1980). These studies showed little or no relationship among maternal education, the mother's interest in the child's symptoms, the mother's judgment of the symptoms, and the child's recognition of symptoms. Campbell (1978) did observe, however, that the combination of mother's educational level and the father's occupation (socioeconomic level) was related to the child's concept of sick role or illness behaviors. In addition, while age and sex did mediate the relationship, as the mother's educational level increased, the child's illness responses became more stoic and less emotional. Only maternal education, therefore, appears to have some predictor ability in determining the child's health concepts.

Health Beliefs and Values

It is within the family system that health beliefs and behaviors based on values are acquired and passed from generation to generation. These values and beliefs are related to health: sleep, food, work, sexuality, procreation, birth, and parenting. Children gradually incorporate the family value system into their own lives and patterns of conduct. The health beliefs and values transmitted by the family are operationalized through health behaviors. These behaviors become indicators of the value and attitudes of individuals and family members toward prevention and health promotion. In addition, utilization of health care services by families will often provide clues relative to health beliefs and values.

Assessments of health beliefs and values are pertinent in that they enable the nurse to determine inappropriate health beliefs or misconceptions about health conditions. Utilization of these data also enables the nurse to develop individualized strategies based upon unique family health beliefs. Families will be more likely to use appropriate health behaviors when they are in keeping with the family mores and culture.

Health Behaviors

Health-related behavior is particularly important for the nurse to understand when assessing families. As noted with health beliefs, if the intervention strategies are individualized according to family definitions, family members are more likely to use appropriate health behaviors in their own care. Health behaviors vary from individual to individual and are dependent on a number of psychosocial variables. It is also important to note that persons engaged in one health behavior may not be so engaged in another. For example, one family may actively use seat belts for all its members, but both adults may continue with the nonhealthy habit of cigarette smoking.

Persons will take preventive action, according to Becker (1974), when they perceive themselves as susceptible to a disease, when they view the disease as serious, when they believe that a particular action will decrease the seriousness or severity of the disease, and when they believe that the benefits of the preventive action are greater than the perceived barriers to care. The individual's perception of susceptibility to and seriousness of the disease are referred to as readiness factors. Several modifying factors and cues for action have also been shown to affect the perceived threat of disease. Modifying factors include age, sex, personality, social class, peer and reference group pressure, and knowledge about the disease. The cues to action include advice from others, newspaper or magazine articles, and mass media campaigns (Rosenstock, 1974).

Langlie's study (1977) of social networks and their effect on health beliefs and preventive health behaviors showed these beliefs and behaviors to be strongly influenced by individual perceptions. The most significant perceptions related to health behavior were control over health status, great benefit at minimal cost, belonging to a social network of middle to high socioeconomic class status, and frequent interaction with nonrelatives (receiving outside information).

Utilization of Health Services

Health behavior and the use of health services is determined, to a large extent, by the developmental stage of the family. Young and healthy childless couples do not use many health services, while families in the childbearing and childrearing stages tend to make frequent hospital and physician visits. These visits are mostly associated with maternal and child care (McEwan, 1971; Bruce, 1973). Demographic variations also affect the use of health services by families. Higher socioeconomic groups are more likely to obtain hospital, medical, and dental services. A much higher utilization rate is also seen in whites as opposed to nonwhites (Freeborn, 1977).

In a study of the factors influencing the use of ambulatory services, Kronenfeld (1978) found that (1) the more health care providers seen, the greater the frequency of visits; (2) the use of health services increased with the number of health conditions present and the days of disability accrued per year related to the health services; (3) those persons with Medicaid or Medicare used ambulatory services more often, and (4) the lower the income level, the greater the use of service.

These results, while appearing to be in conflict with the Freeborn (1977) study, most likely represent a difference in site of service rather than actual utilization differences. Lower socioeconomic groups are more likely to utilize hospital outpatient or health department clinics, while upper socioeconomic groups are more likely to be seen in private doctors' offices. Data from the National Health Interview Survey (U.S. Public Health Service, 1981) shows that as income rises, the frequency of patient visits to hospital outpatient departments or emergency decreases and the frequency of visits to doctor's offices, clinics, or group practices increases. As income decreases, the reverse occurs.

Cultural expectations and values have also been shown to have an impact on the utilization of health services. The decision to seek services is influenced by the expectations and values that have been acquired through the family socialization process (Berkanovic & Reeder, 1974; Hoppe & Heller, 1975).

Value of Assessment to the Nurse and Family

Health beliefs, values, behaviors, and utilization of health services must be considered if successful and realistic nursing actions are to be determined. Health-promoting behaviors manifested by the individual or family must be supported and reinforced for maximum health potential. Health-promoting behaviors as described by Stuart (1971) are (1) a wholesome perspective or attitude toward one's self and life in general, (2) active adjustment to environmental changes, (3) identifying and accepting reality, and (4) taking appropriate responsibility for managing one's own health.

Nursing actions are implemented through teaching, counseling, and referral. Teaching is aimed toward assisting the family to gain accurate information that will enable family members to initiate effective problem-solving approaches to dealing with health issues. Counseling enhances the family's self-confidence as each member participates in the decision-making process about health issues. Sometimes the needs of the family are complex and referrals are necessary. In order to make adequate referrals, the nurse must possess knowledge of available resources and the mechanisms by which the family can access these resources. Briefly stated, then, the successful enactment of the role of the nurse with the family in health promotion, treatment, and prevention requires (1) recognition of cultural differences and how these influence nursing practice; (2) knowledge of health-promoting behaviors; and (3) supportive nursing actions that increase individual health responsibility.

SUMMARY

Some type of family unit exists in all societies, yet there are variations in structure and function. As societal changes occur, changes will also occur within the family in an effort to meet the demands of the environment. The development of appropriate response patterns can be a growth experience for the family and its individual members, provided there is a high degree of adaptability and integration within the family. The ultimate achievement of nursing goals related to health promotion and prevention occurs through recognizing supportive behaviors and reinforcing wellness behaviors demonstrated by individual family members and the family as a whole.

REVIEW QUESTIONS

1. To what extent do the structures and functions of the family affect the reciprocal nature of task achievement of (1) individual development, and (2) the family as a unit?
2. Compare and contrast the three theoretical frameworks discussed in the chapter.
3. Describe the family life cycle and identify the critical influences on the different stages.
4. Discuss the family developmental tasks and describe their relationship to individual development.
5. Discuss the parameters that should be included in a comprehensive assessment of the family.
6. Identify and discuss the factors that will influence the family's involvement in the planning and implementation of health promotion.
7. Describe the relationship of health beliefs and health behaviors in the setting and achieving of family health goals.

REFERENCES

Aldous, J. (1972). *Conceptual framework*, Vol. 1. In Course syllabus, Developmental approach to family analysis, Sociology 5-505, University of Minnesota (unpublished).
Bauman, B. (1961). Diversities in conceptions of health and physical fitness. *Journal of Health and Human Behavior, 2* (1), 40.
Becker, M. H. (Ed.) (1974). The health belief model and personal health behavior. *Health Education Monographs, 2* (4).
Berkanovic, E., & Reeder, L. (1974). Can money buy the appropriate use of services? *Journal of Health and Social Behavior, 15,* 93–98.
Bruce, J. (1973). Family practices and the family: A sociological review. *Journal of Comparative Family Studies, 4,* 10.

Buckley, W. (1967). *Sociology and modern systems theory*. Englewood Cliffs, NJ: Prentice-Hall.

Burgess, E. W. (1926). The family as a unity of interacting personalities. *Family*, 7, 3–9.

Burgess, E. W., Lock, H., & Thomas, M. M. (1963). *The family*. New York: American Book.

Campbell, J. D. (1975a). Attribution of illness: Another double standard. *Journal of Health and Social Behavior*, *16*, 114–126.

Campbell, J. D. (1975b). Illness is a point of view: The development of children's concepts of illness. *Child Development*, *46*, 92–100.

Campbell, J. D. (1978). The child in the sick role: Contribution of age, sex, parental status, and parental values. *Journal of Health and Social Behavior*, *19*, 35–51.

Dean, A., Lin, N., & Ensel, W. M. (1981). The epidemiological significance of social support systems in depression. In R. G. Simmons (Ed.), *Research in community mental health: Vol. 2. A research annual* (pp. 77–109). Greenwich, CT: JAI Press.

Dokeckie, P., Dunlop, K., & Moroney, R. (1980). *The situation of American families*. Working paper, Vanderbilt University, Vanderbilt Institute for Public Policy Studies, Nashville.

Duvall, E. M. (1977). *Marriage and family development*. Philadelphia: Lippincott.

Epstein, N. B., & Levine, S. (1973). Training for family therapy with a faculty of medicine. *Canadian Psychiatric Association Journal*, *18*, 203–208.

Freeborn, D. (1977). Health status, socioeconomic status and utilization of outpatient services for members of a prepaid group practice. *Medical Care*, *15* (2), 115–128.

Friedman, M. (1986). *Family nursing theory and assessment*, 2nd Ed., New York: Appleton-Century-Crofts.

Hansen, D., & Hill, R. L. (1964). Families under stress. In H. Christiansen (Ed.), *Handbook of marriage and the family* (pp. 3–41). Chicago: Rand McNally.

Havighurst, R. J. (1953). *Human development and education*. New York: Longmans, Green and Company.

Hill, R. L. (1949). *Families under stress*. New York: Harper & Row.

Hill, R. L. (1961). Patterns of decision-making and the accumulation of family assets. In N. Foote (Ed.), *Household decision-making*. New York: University Press.

Hoppe, S., & Heller, P. (1975). Alienations, familism and the utilization of health services by Mexican Americans. *Journal of Health and Social Behavior*, *16* (3), 304–314.

Kronenfeld, J. (1978). Provider variables and the utilization of ambulatory care services. *Journal of Community Health*, *19*, 68–76.

Koos, E. (1954). *The health of Regionville*. New York: Columbia University Press.

Langlie, J. (1977). Social networks, health beliefs and preventive health behavior. *Journal of Health and Social Behavior*, *18* (3), 244–260.

McEwan, P. (1971). *The social approach*. Working paper, World Health Organization consultation on statistical aspects of the family as a unit in health studies.

Mechanic, D. (1964). The influence of mothers on their children's health attitudes and behavior. *Pediatrics*, *39*, 444–453.

Mechanic, D. (1980). Education, parental interest, and health perceptions and behavior. *Inquiry*, *17*, 331–338.

Messer, A. (1971). *The individual and his family: An adaptational study*. Springfield, IL: Thomas.

Musnick, G., & Bane, M. J. (1980). *The nation's families: 1960–1990*. Joint Center for Urban Studies of MIT and Harvard University, Cambridge, MA.

Nye, F. I., & Berardo, F. M. (1973). *The family, its structure and interactions*. New York: Macmillan.

Ogburn, W. F. (1938). The changing family. *The Family*, *19*, 139–143.

Rogers, R. H. (1973). *The family, its structure and interactions*. Englewood Cliffs, NJ: Prentice Hall.

Rosenstock, I. (1974). Historical origins of the health-belief model. In M. Becker (Ed.), *The health belief model and personal behavior. Health Education Monographs, 2*(4), 328–335.

Speer, D. C. (1970). Family systems: Morphostasis and morphogenesis or is homeostasis enough? *Family Process, 9* (3), 259–278.

Stuart, R. (1971). Behavioral contracting within the families of delinquents. *Journal of Behavior Therapy and Experimental Psychiatry,* 1.

U.S. Public Health Service. (1981). *Health: United States* (DHHS Publication No. PHS 82-1232). Washington, DC: U.S. Government Printing Office.

Visher, E. B., & Visher, J. S. (1979). *Step-families: Myths and realities.* Secaucus, NJ: Citadel.

The Family During Pregnancy

Kitty P. Bishop

OBJECTIVES

Upon completion of this chapter, the student will be able to:

1. Discuss how the anticipation of a new family member can mark a critical transition point in the life of the family
2. Compare and contrast the developmental tasks of the expectant mother and the expectant father
3. Identify how feelings of ambivalence toward pregnancy could have an effect on the family unit
4. Discuss the implications for nursing actions related to role preparation and adaptations of the family unit to the unborn child
5. Identify potential stressors affecting the mother, father, infant, and siblings during pregnancy
6. Discuss how the well-being of the family unit might affect the well-being of the expectant mother

---

CONCEPTS

Family unit: encompasses not only the pregnant female, husband or baby's father, offspring, and blood relatives, but also those significant others with whom the pregnant woman has a close personal relationship and who form the family's support network

Family developmental framework: an approach based on the observation of families that accounts for change over time and the dynamics of interactions of its members

Pregnancy: the period of time between conception and delivery of the products of conception

---

Pregnancy is an event in the process of life that offers the ideal opportunity for nurses to promote healthy family development. Pregnancy should be seen as an additional stress that is superimposed on the usual life stresses of the family unit. An important, all-prevailing point to consider is that pregnancy and childbearing affect the *total* family unit and not just the expectant female. The previous statements provide justification for the use of a family-centered approach when addressing the issue of pregnancy. Inclusion of the total family unit serves as the basic underlying theme for the direction of this chapter. The physiological, psychological, and social needs that arise during the adaptation of the family unit to the events surrounding the birth of a new family member have stimulated some of the viewpoints expressed by the author of this chapter.

It is the contention of the author that nursing care of the pregnant female should be learned within the context of the family unit. In this respect the needs of the family unit as a whole must be considered, as well as the needs of the individual family members. *The primary goal of health care during pregnancy is to ensure a healthy and happy outcome for the family unit experiencing pregnancy and the events surrounding the birth.* Personal growth of family members may be either enhanced or inhibited by the guidance and support that they receive during this period.

Empirically we realize that the quality of family life is closely associated with the health of the individual family members. Historically society mandates that the family forms the basic unit of our society. The family unit is seen as a social institution that can have a marked effect on its members—so strong an effect as possibly to determine the success or failure of an individual family member's life. As a basic unit in society, the family shapes and is shaped by external forces within the environment. Research seems to indicate that health and illness behavior is learned (Becker, 1974); the family, then, is a primary source of health education within our society.

FAMILY TASKS

In keeping with the philosophy of family-centered care, the *family unit* discussed here encompasses not only the pregnant female, husband or the baby's father, offspring, and blood relatives, but also those significant others with whom the couple has a close personal relationship and who form the family's support network. As the family unit expands, its members are faced with the responsibilities necessary for the continuity, survival, and growth of the family. Duvall (1971) identified these responsibilities and labeled them *family developmental tasks*. Duvall identified the following eight basic family developmental tasks:

1. Physical maintenance
2. Allocation of resources
3. Division of labor
4. Socialization of family members

5. Reproduction, recruitment, and release of family members
6. Maintenance of order
7. Placement of members in society
8. Maintenance of motivation and morale

These basic family developmental tasks must be achieved by a family during each stage of its development (Table 2–1). Internal and external forces shape these tasks by acting on the family unit. The anticipation of a new member may mark one of the first critical transition points in the life of the family.

Childbearing forces a major reorientation of roles and relationships within the family unit, as well as behaviors associated with these roles and relationships. Pregnancy is a time of life when each member of the family unit must begin to prepare for his or her new role. Changing roles can involve assuming new responsi-

TABLE 2–1. THEORISTS

Name	Source	Age Group	Concepts	Remarks
Duvall	*Family Development* (1962, 1971)	Reproductive years	Family life cycle, family developmental tasks, the expectant phase	Just as individuals go through successive stages of growth and development, so do families. Each stage of family development has its own specific developmental tasks. *Family developmental tasks* refer to growth responsibilities that must be achieved by a family during each stage of development so as to meet (1) its biological requirements, (2) its cultural imperatives, and (3) its own aspirations and values. The *expectant phase* is considered to be second within the family life cycle.
Colman & Colman	*Pregnancy: The Psychological Experience* (1971)	Reproductive years	Fundamental tasks of pregnancy 1. Pregnancy validation 2. Fetal embodiment 3. Fetal distinction 4. Role transition	Pregnancy has subtasks to be accomplished in order for the experience to be integrated into the total life process. Successful resolution of each task prepares one for coping with future tasks.

bilities, altering one's self-image, acquiring new skills, shifting priorities in one's life, and experiencing a significant change in relationships with others. A look at each member and some of the role changes afford a glimpse at the multifaceted adaptations surrounding pregnancy.

INDIVIDUAL TASKS

The Expectant Mother

The expectant female must be more than physically capable of conceiving and producing children. She must be emotionally mature enough to have another individual, her child, dependent on her. She must be able to sacrifice her own needs when they conflict with the needs of her child. In following Erikson's (1963) developmental tasks it seems logical that, at the minimum, parents need to have mastered at least the developmental tasks up through identity formation, which usually occurs during adolescence (13 to 18 years). During identity formation one usually steers toward independence from one's parents. During pregnancy the real challenge occurs when a young woman strives to meet each of her individual developmental needs, as well as the family developmental tasks.

The changes that occur during pregnancy will affect the pregnant woman physiologically as well as psychologically. Physiological changes due to endocrine responses to the pregnancy affect the intensity of the psychosocial reactions.

Like other developmental tasks, pregnancy has subtasks to be accomplished in order for the experience to be integrated into the total life process. Successful resolution of each task prepares one for coping with future tasks. The fundamental tasks of pregnancy as identified by Colman and Colman (1971) are:

1. Pregnancy validation
2. Fetal embodiment
3. Fetal distinction
4. Role transition (see Table 2–1)

Pregnancy Validation. The dominant theme implied by researchers of the psychological processes of pregnancy appears to be the development and acceptance of a coherent sense of self as a person, as well as a parent. Colman and Colman (1971) and McCauley (1976) suggest that a primary task of the first trimester of pregnancy is *pregnancy validation*. During this period the expectant female attempts to ascertain if the pregnancy is a reality and incorporates the pregnancy into her life-style. Some typical responses by the pregnant female might include:

1. Shock at the possibility of having conceived
2. Decreased activity due to the physiological responses accompanying pregnancy
3. Fantasies and dreams about the yet unforeseen organism she has conceived
4. Seeking prenatal care to validate her pregnancy
5. Deciding with whom she will share the news of the pregnancy

During this time when the woman is seeking validation of her pregnancy, the nurse can help to set the stage for incorporating the pregnancy into the expectant mother's life-style. Assessing the meaning of this pregnancy to her and her family assists the expectant mother in continuing pregnancy validation. This inquiry should encourage expression of both positive and negative feelings toward the pregnancy. Initially, even if the pregnancy is planned, there is an element of ambivalence. The ambivalence experienced may be due to job commitments and the need to modify career plans, interpersonal relationships, excitement, as well as fear of assuming new roles and fear of the anticipated pregnancy, labor, and delivery. The communication skills and techniques of the caregiver will elicit some expression of these mixed emotions from the expectant female.

Physical changes are also expected as pregnancy progresses. At the first prenatal visit, amenorrhea and the positive pregnancy test results may be the only physical proof that pregnancy has occurred. At this time the expectant female becomes scrupulously conscious of the physical changes in her body. The nurse/caregiver should assess these physical changes and the amount of disruption the unpleasant symptoms of pregnancy are causing. Nausea, vomiting, breast discomfort, and fatigue are but some of the physical changes that the expectant female must deal with during the first trimester.

With the expanding role of the nurse, nurses are assuming more important roles during the antepartum period. A certified nurse-midwife may be the primary caregiver in an uncomplicated pregnancy. A nurse-practitioner shares the caregiving role with a physician, whereas an office nurse may supplement the physician by developing the initial client rapport through counseling and offering psychological support to the expectant female. The initial rapport established sets the stage for prenatal counseling and education. It is also extremely important for the nurse to realize that referral to professional colleagues may be the most appropriate action should problems or crises occur that the nurse feels unable to address. Remember that satisfactory accomplishment of one task precedes movement to the next task.

Fetal Embodiment.   The second developmental task of pregnancy identified by Colman and Colman (1971) is that of *fetal embodiment*. It is during this task period that the pregnant woman begins to incorporate the fetus into her body image. A second aspect of this developmental task is for the pregnant woman to restructure her relationships with her mother, on whom she has been dependent in the past, and with her mate, on whom she will become increasingly dependent.

During the accomplishment of this second developmental task, introspection often serves as an important function, allowing the expectant mother to prepare herself psychologically for the arrival of her infant and for her role as a mother. The expectant mother may spend much time thinking about herself, reviewing her own childhood and the quality of mothering that she received. It is also during this period of her pregnancy that fetal movements can be felt, the fetal heartbeat can be heard, and a shift toward focusing on the fetus occurs. The expectant mother may fantasize about the unseen fetus growing inside her; may try to guess its sex and personal attributes; and may question whether her unborn child is developing normally.

Aspects of the nurse's role during fetal embodiment might include allowing the woman to listen to the fetal heartbeat and to discuss her perceptions of fetal movement. These actions will help to enhance the incorporation of the fetus into her body image. Assessing changes in relationships with significant others is yet another important aspect. Explanations as to why her emotions may be different and reassurance that these changes are a normal yet temporary aspect of pregnancy are needed for both the pregnant woman and members of her support system. The nurse should also promote and encourage open communication lines and mutual support among the support systems available to the pregnant woman. It is also appropriate to discuss physical activity, sleep, diet, proper clothing, and general well-being. Anxiety is usually relatively low during this period; a high degree of anxiety may indicate a need for referral to professional counseling.

Fetal Distinction.   After accepting and incorporating the fetus into her life-style, the pregnant woman must begin to view the fetus as an individual separate from herself and begin to formulate a mothering identity for herself (Colman & Colman, 1971). During this time the expectant mother shows increased interest in the baby. She tries out baby names, starts buying needed baby equipment and clothing, tries to interest the expectant father in feeling fetal movements, and attends childbirth classes. The mother's anxiety decreases now that the danger of miscarriage is past. Sexual activity usually decreases.

The nurse's role during this period involves assessing the woman's knowledge of child care practices. It may be necessary to provide information on feeding, bathing, clothing, and other subjects. By discussing fantasies related to the fetus, the nurse can assess whether the pregnant woman's expectations are realistic. The nurse should make clear that the newborn infant will be a totally dependent individual with needs to be fulfilled by the parents. In order to help the woman and her support systems cope with her dependency during this time, the nurse should explain that this dependency forms part of the "qualitative matrix of mothering," terminology coined by Rubin (1975) as she described how women behave while working on each task of pregnancy.

Role Transition.   The final task of pregnancy as identified by Colman and Colman (1971) is to prepare to give up the fetus and become a new mother. During this last trimester of pregnancy, anxiety increases due to thoughts about and apprehension of the impending labor and delivery. Concerns about the condition of the infant also increase the anxiety level. The final trimester is accompanied by the physical discomforts of sleeplessness, pelvic pains, and Braxton–Hicks contractions. These physical discomforts also tend to increase the pregnant woman's frustration and anxiety.

The expectant mother's psychological readiness for labor and delivery is influenced by her knowledge of the birth process; past experiences with childbirth, either her own previous experiences or those of friends and family members; and her cultural milieu. It is also during this time that the expectant mother makes plans for the home while she is hospitalized. Decisions are usually made regarding the method of infant feeding and the question of circumcision for a male infant. Sexual activity during this period is usually low or discontinued.

Cranley's research on maternal–fetal attachment (1984) demonstrated a significant level of attachment of mothers to their fetuses during the third trimester of gestation. Figure 2–1 demonstrates a schematic representation of relationships among variables used in Cranley's study.

Positive correlations were demonstrated with support of health care professionals and family and friends as support systems. Higher levels of perceived stress were related to decreased maternal–fetal attachment.

The nurse's role involves exploring expectations of labor and delivery, assessing the woman's base, her level of preparation, and support systems available. An important all-prevailing guideline should be for the nurse to assess exactly what the expectant female's concerns are before attempting to give guidance. The woman's own preoccupations or concerns may indeed unconsciously impede other educational attempts made by the nurse at this time. Reviewing the expectant female's knowledge of available community resources is also an appropriate action at this time. Overall, the psychosocial aspect of the nurse's role during pregnancy involves many varied assessments. Among some of the assessments identified are: (1) the pregnant woman's adjustment to childbearing, (2) support offered by family members and her cultural milieu, (3) encouragement of open communication lines, and (4) the expectant family's need for information and support.

Regardless of the theorist followed, the general consensus seems to be that the nine months of pregnancy are not *just* for the development of the fetus.

The Expectant Father

Each member of the expectant family must adjust to pregnancy and its associated implications. The integrity of the family unit will depend on resolution of conflicts and acceptance of changes within the family structure. Like expectant mothers, each expectant father has his own unique emotional, and sometimes psychological, reactions to his mate's pregnancy, as he, too, is experiencing a transition of roles. Assessment of the expectant father's perceptions, needs, and concerns is important in planning nursing care. Lacoursiere (1972) studied men who had developed psychological problems after the birth of the first child and concluded that recapitulation and new resolution of earlier developmental conflicts must be adequately resolved by the expectant father or successful adaptation to pregnancy, birth, and parenting will be in jeopardy. Like the expectant mother, it is presumed that the expectant father

Family and Friends Support	+.25		MATERNAL PERCEPTION OF NEWBORNS OUTPUT BEHAVIORS
Health Care Support	+.74	MATERNAL–FETAL ATTACHMENT	
Perceived Stress	−.41	+4.6	

Figure 2–1. Schematic representation of relationships among variables in Cranley's Study (Cranley, 1984, p. 118).

also has developmental tasks to be accomplished. Four developmental tasks of the expectant father have been identified:

1. Acceptance of the pregnancy and attachment to the fetus (Barnhill et al., 1979)
2. Evaluation of practical issues such as financial responsibility (Brazelton, 1976)
3. Resolution of dependency issues (Brazelton, 1976)
4. Accepting and resolving his relationship with his own father (Colman & Colman, 1971)

Like the expectant mother, the expectant father must *accept the pregnancy and form some sort of attachment to the fetus*. Colman and Colman (1971) suggest that touching the pregnant woman's abdomen, attending childbirth education classes, or involvement in purchasing the layette evidence ways that the expectant father becomes involved in accepting the pregnancy and attachment to the fetus.

Concern with practical issues such as financial responsibilities encompasses a second task of expectant fathers. Our society often places this responsibility on both parties as the number of working women increases. With the birth of a baby, expenses are expected to rise, and the curtailment of the pregnant woman's employment before or after birth leads to increasing anxiety on the part of the father. Nurses should not overlook the possibility that the added expenses of medical fees and the cost of feeding, clothing, and housing a child may precipitate problems within the family. Discussion of finances early in the pregnancy may encourage realistic problem solving to meet the anticipated added costs. Providing estimates of costs may also be advantageous.

A third developmental task for the expectant father is *resolution of dependency issues*. The pregnant woman's preoccupation with her own psychological and physical changes often inadvertently lead to her paying less attention to her child's father. Valentine (1982) speculated that some balance of readjustment must be found that meets the dependency needs of the expectant father as he, in turn, meets the dependency needs of the pregnant woman and expected child. The nurse should explore the expectant father's feelings about the pregnancy and explain to him that the emotional changes affecting the woman are normal and temporary.

Hand in hand with the aforementioned task is that of the man's *resolution of his relationship with his own father*. Memories of what it was like to be fathered are his first source about fathering. Becoming a father means giving up being a son, to some extent, and having to face the fathering responsibilities that had always been there for him to criticize within his father (Colman & Colman, 1971). Identifying aspects of his parenting that will be kept or discarded is an important part of resolving his relationship with his own father. It is not uncommon for the expectant father to appear introspective during this time as he spends time thinking of his life, beliefs, relationships, and childhood.

Harding-Weaver and Cranley (1983) developed a paternal–fetal assessment scale to help nurses in assessing a father's behaviors during various stages in the development of the fathering role. Table 2–2 provides sample questions lifted from the Paternal–Fetal Assessment Scale.

TABLE 2–2. SAMPLE QUESTIONS FROM THE HARDING-WEAVER AND CRANLEY PATERNAL–FETAL ASSESSMENT SCALE

DIFFSLF	I'm really looking forward to seeing what the baby looks like. I enjoy watching my wife's tummy jiggle as the baby kicks inside.
INTERCT	I talk to my unborn baby. I refer to my baby by a nickname.
ATTRIBUT	I wonder if the baby can hear inside of my wife. I wonder if the baby thinks and feels things inside of my wife.
GIVINGSLF	I feel all the trouble of being pregnant is worth it. I encourage my partner to eat meat and vegetables to be sure my baby gets a good diet.
ROLTAK	I picture myself feeding the baby. I imagine myself taking care of the baby.
MRITALS	Lately I find that I want to be closer to my wife. I feel I should do more to protect and take care of my wife now that she is pregnant.
BEHAVOR	I have talked to my partner's doctor during her pregnancy. I have taken on extra work around the house (washing dishes, making beds, vacuuming, etc.).
PHYSCAL	I've been suffering from an upset stomach in the last few months. I've had more difficulty sleeping during the last seven months.
HLQ	During this pregnancy, how would you rate your health? _____ Excellent _____ Very Good _____ Average _____ Fair _____ Poor Comment_____

DIFFSLF = differentiation of self from fetus; INTERCT = interaction with the fetus; ATTRIBUT = attributing characteristics to the fetus; GIVINGSLF = giving of self; ROLTAK = roletaking; BEHAVOR = involvement of husband during pregnancy; =MRITALS = feelings and attitudes concerning the marital relationship; PHYSCAL = physical symptoms related to pregnancy; HLQ = physical health
From Harding-Weaver, R.H. & Cranley, M.S. (1983). An exploration of paternal–fetal attachment behavior. *Nursing Research* 32(2);69.

Siblings

While the two most obvious people affected by pregnancy have been discussed, it is of utmost importance to recognize the needs of siblings during pregnancy. In part, the age and emotional maturity of a child will determine the effect that the new baby will have on that child's behavior toward the new family member. The nurse can help parents recognize the sibling's need for educational and emotional support during pregnancy. Changes in sibling behavior might reflect siblings' response to changes in their mother's appearance or changes in her behavior. Perhaps the physical discomforts of pregnancy are altering maternal behaviors, and in turn the siblings form reactions to these changes. Responses may vary from hostility and aggression to confusion or overaffectionate displays once the new baby arrives. Room or space adjustments should be made prior to the time when mother has to go to the hospital. Incorporating siblings into the pregnancy may be accomplished by allowing siblings to feel the baby moving inside the uterus or helping to prepare a special place or room for the baby. After the birth, siblings need to feel they are a part of the family. Some hospitals now allow sibling visitation to help facilitate the introduction of a new family member.

INTEGRATION OF DEVELOPMENTAL TASKS OF EACH FAMILY MEMBER INTO TASKS OF THE EXPECTANT FAMILY

It is the nurse's responsibility to identify the needs, concerns, and functioning of each member of the expectant family and to plan and implement nursing actions to meet these needs. To accomplish this requires integration of developmental tasks of the mother, father, and other family members into tasks appropriate for the family as a unit. Duvall (1962) described the phase within the family life cycle, with the second of these as the *expectant phase*. According to Duvall, the developmental tasks of the expectant family included the following:

1. Reorganizing house arrangements to provide for the expected baby
2. Developing new patterns for getting and spending income
3. Re-evaluating procedures for determining who does what and where authority rests
4. Adapting patterns of sexual relationships to pregnancy
5. Expanding the communication system of present and anticipated emotional constellations
6. Reorienting relationships with relatives
7. Adapting relationships with friends, associates, and community activities to the realities of pregnancy
8. Acquiring knowledge about, and planning for, the specifics of pregnancy, childbirth, and parenthood
9. Testing and maintaining a workable philosophy of life

Each of these developmental tasks involves role preparation on the part of the entire family unit.

POTENTIAL STRESSORS

To facilitate a healthy and happy outcome for the family unit, the nurse must assess the environment for threats to the course of pregnancy and fetal development. Potential stressors addressed here include maternal age; nutritional status; the effects of smoking, alcohol, and drugs on the fetus; and socioeconomic factors.

Maternal Age

Women at either end of the age scale are at risk during childbearing. The birth rate among girls under 15 years of age is increasing. A number of factors tend to complicate an adolescent pregnancy. The adolescent who becomes pregnant is still struggling with Erikson's (1963) developmental task of establishing her own identity while simultaneously facing the additional crisis of generativity. Her immature physical development may further complicate the outcome of the pregnancy. Research by Carey et al. (1981) indicates that the very young adolescent (less than 14 years) is at risk for premature births, low-birth-weight infants, pregnancy-induced hypertension, cephalopelvic disproportion, and iron-deficiency anemia. A most important aspect in influencing the outcome of such adolescent pregnancies is consistent individualized prenatal care.

On the opposite end of the age spectrum are the women above age 30 who elect to give birth. With ever-changing economic conditions, more and more women are choosing careers that require increasing years of formal education and greater job responsibility. These two factors are leading to an increase in the number of births to women over age 30. These women, who have intentionally delayed childbearing, need to discuss the consequences of starting a family at this point in their lives. After being accustomed to a life with time for egocentrism and freedom to focus on a career and a one- or two-person household, it is sometimes difficult to shift the focus to a baby who is totally dependent on its parents for survival. The realities of infant care may indeed be a difficult challenge. Nursing care should include time for listening and counseling and knowledge of when the need for referral is appropriate.

Also among women aged 30 and above are those multiparous women who elect to continue their childbearing years or who conceive during the menopausal period. These women may experience a feeeling of displacement because they feel that pregnancy alienates them from their peer group. Also, the woman experiencing pregnancy as a result of conceiving during the menopausal period may be at risk for hypertension, toxemia, and hemorrhage. Anxiety is usually high due to their perception of pregnancy at this age as "abnormal" and not as the natural happy, welcomed phenomenon it is for younger women. Again, nurses need to allow time for ventilation of these feelings and provide supportive counseling when appropriate. Referrals should be made when the nurse feels unable to provide complete care.

Nutritional Status

Both the long-term nutritional status of the mother prior to pregnancy and her nutritional intake during pregnancy will influence the intrauterine weight gain of the fetus and its subsequent weight and nutritional status. Nutrition counseling is of utmost importance. The American College of Obstetricians and Gynecologists issued the following Policy Statement on Nutrition and Pregnancy:

> A woman's nutritional status before, during, and after pregnancy contributes to a significant degree to the well-being of both herself and her infant. Therefore, what a woman consumes before she conceives and while she carries the fetus is of vital importance to the health of succeeding generations.*

When offering nutrition counseling, the nurse should incorporate significant others, as they are aware of and may influence the pregnant woman's eating habits. By

*From the Committee on Nutrition (1974). Nutrition in maternal health care. Chicago: The   American College of Obstetricians and Gynecologists.

reinforcing the positive aspects of the client's dietary regime, better compliance may be encouraged. Also, by following maternal weight gain according to physician preference, the nurse may reinforce or educate the woman concerning needed changes in her eating habits. There is a discrepancy among physicians regarding maternal weight gain, but it is generally agreed that weight should show little gain during the first trimester, a rapid increase during the second, and some slowing in the rate of increase during the final trimester. See Table 2–3 for dietary requirements for nonpregnant, pregnant, and lactating women.

Other Maternal Risk Factors

Adequate assessment is necessary to identify maternal risk factors. These include problems with previous pregnancies and pre-existing medical problems (i.e., anemia, diabetes, etc.). A social and emotional history may reveal available support systems, the woman's perception of the pregnancy, and her coping mechanisms. A review of the pregnant woman's health status and habits may reveal potential threats

TABLE 2–3. DIETARY REQUIREMENTS FOR NONPREGNANT, PREGNANT, AND LACTATING WOMEN

Food	Nonpregnant	Pregnant	Lactating
Milk (skimmed buttermilk), cheese, ice cream (food made with milk can supply part of requirement)	2 cups	3–4 cups	4–5 cups
Meat (lean meat, fish, poultry, cheese, occasional dried beans or peas)	1 serving (3–4 oz)	2 servings (6–8 oz); include liver frequently	2½ servings (8 oz)
Eggs	1	1–2	1–2
Vegetable[a] (dark green or deep yellow)	1 serving	1 serving	1–2 servings
Vitamin C–rich food[a] Good source: citrus fruit, berries, cantaloupe; Fair source: tomatoes, cabbage, greens, potatoes in skin	1 good source of 2 fair sources	1 good source and 1 fair source or 2 good sources	1 good source and 1 fair source or 2 good sources
Other vegetables, fruits, juices	2 servings	4–6 servings	4–6 servings
Bread[b] and cereals (enriched or whole grain)	6 servings	10 servings	10 servings
Butter or fortified margarine	Moderate amount	Moderate amount	Moderate amount

[a]Use some raw daily.
[b]One slice of bread equals 1 serving.
From Williams, S.R. (1985). *Nutrition and diet therapy,* (5th ed.). St. Louis: Mosby.

to the pregnancy. For example, ingestion of drugs and alcohol may lead to congenital anomalies and/or growth disturbances and therefore pose a threat to fetal well-being. The need to determine the type of drug, the dosage, frequency, and route of administration, and the timing of the exposure to the agent is imperative. Heavy smoking during pregnancy may lead to a reduction in the length of gestation and infants who are small for gestational age (inadequate growth for gestational age). The effects of smoking on the fetus are directly proportional to the number of cigarettes smoked. Understanding of the physical danger of the abused substance will influence its perception by the abuser. Fetal alcohol syndrome (FAS) is a focus of current research. Infants suffering from FAS can demonstrate irreversible growth and mental deficiencies as well as structural or general musculoskeletal anomalies (McCarthy, 1983).

Socioeconomic factors must be taken into account also. The nurse will acknowledge the client's cultural views and values to increase credibility of future teaching efforts. In our fee-for-service health care system, the socioeconomic status of our clients must also be considered. The financial resources available influence the general nutrition of the family unit as well as the quality and the quantity of health care they seek.

COPING MECHANISMS

The survival of a society depends on the reproduction of its members. Reproduction itself can satisfy a multitude of needs. For the expectant female, having a child can be viewed in one of several ways: confirmation of her feminine identity, fulfillment of unachieved career goals, conformity to societal or familial pressures to bear children, or the opportunity to see one's own characteristics passed on to a child. Motivations to reproduce may also be flavored by the relationship with one's partner. The uniqueness of pregnancy and the curiosities aroused by the changes accompanying pregnancy afford a closeness to one's mate that may not be experienced during other times of life.

Nurses need to be aware of the family's present stage of development and its stage-critical tasks. An understanding of the family's health beliefs will afford the nurse the opportunity to offer support and encouragement as they move through this stage of the life cycle.

Society affords relatively little preparation for examining the reality of the tasks accompanying pregnancy and the anticipation of parenthood. Perhaps babysitting and the purchase of the layette are a couple of preparatory-type behaviors, yet neither of these offer the reality of the changes accompanying pregnancy and parenthood. Functional or adaptive coping mechanisms have been identified by Pearlin and Schooler (1978) as those tactics that modify the stressful situation in an effort to alter or eliminate the stressor. Included among these tactics are self-reliance and seeking help from others.

A problem that exists during pregnancy as well as during parenting is the absence of objective standards by which success or failure can be measured during childbearing and childrearing. One would like to surmise that pregnancy results in happiness and anticipation of bringing new life into the world; however, it may be viewed as a highly threatening experience to some. For example, pregnancy may be the result of a pleasure-motivated sexual act with no conscious desire to become pregnant. The way the expectant parents cope with the situation will depend on their cognitive and perceptual evaluations of the event. Pearlin and Schooler posited that no single coping tactic, regardless of its effectiveness, can possibly be effective for the wide range of life strains commonly experienced.

Some of the concerns that challenge coping mechanisms of expectant parents are doubting their competence for parenting; examining their relationship with their mate; reviewing their own childhood and the parenting they received; exploring the possibilities for the unborn child; and anticipating the possible effects this child can have on their lives. By examining these concerns, the couple may reveal positive motivations for the pregnancy as well as deterrents. How the family unit copes will depend largely on their cognitive and perceptual evaluation of the pregnancy.

NURSING ASSESSMENT

In order to provide the best possible care to the expectant female, it is imperative for the nurse to incorporate the family into the plan of care. Utilization of a family developmental framework affords a basis for assessment and planning interventions.

A thorough assessment of the expectant female will provide information about the woman's present condition as well as potential health hazards. The best way to ensure a healthy outcome for both mother and baby is ongoing prenatal care. Ideally, prenatal care should begin soon after the first missed menstrual period. Ongoing prenatal care that begins early in the pregnancy affords the nurse with opportunities to function in a multifaceted capacity. The family-centered nurse should be able to undertake effective health teaching to the expectant family. As a health educator in the prenatal period, the nurse should focus on health promotion and maintenance and can assist in helping the family develop skills to cope with the pregnancy as well as their present health problems or needs. The anticipation of a new baby and the desire to have a healthy newborn may work as a positive enhancement for correcting health problems affecting the expectant mother.

Anticipatory guidance may be an important aspect of the health teaching involved in prenatal care. The nurse should discuss probable events, physical changes, feelings, and situations with the expectant family. Such a discussion offers the opportunity for clarification of ideas, reduction of anxiety, and ways to adjust one's present role to accommodate the changes surrounding the addition of a new baby. Anticipation of, as well as preparation for, the coming event will make it less traumatic for the family. Childbirth classes and sibling education classes offer information that can help in reducing the anxiety accompanying the birth and integration of a baby into the family structure.

History Taking

Antepartal care has traditionally been defined as the care given an expectant female during her pregnancy. As has been reiterated throughout this chapter, the nurse must address the total family unit when dealing with the issue of pregnancy and antepartal care. Initial, and of utmost importance, is the necessity of an accurate and thorough assessment. To begin the assessment, one of the first necessities is obtaining a history from the expectant female. The information necessary for a thorough history may be divided into the following four areas:

1. Menstrual history
2. Obstetric history
3. Medical history
4. Psychosocial history

The *menstrual history* should include the age at the onset of menses (menarche); regularity of menstrual flow; interval between menstrual flows; duration of the menstrual flow; complications associated with menstrual flow (i.e., dysmenorrhea); and the date of the first day of the last menstrual flow.

Some of the necessary components of the *obstetric history* include information on both past pregnancies and the present pregnancy. Information to obtain about past pregnancies includes the course of the pregnancy, labor, delivery, and postpartum period. The date of delivery, the sex, birth weight, and gestational age of the infant, and the present health of the child are also useful information. Determining whether the present pregnancy was planned or unplanned provides clues as to areas where emotional support may be needed. The nurse may also discover information about contraceptive practices of the couple. Assessment of the signs and symptoms the expectant female has experienced that led her to believe that she is pregnant may provide an opportunity for the nurse to give information concerning the signs and symptoms normally experienced with pregnancy.

A *medical history* is also important, as a multitude of diseases pose a threat to pregnancy and the developing fetus. Diseases of a hereditary nature such as diabetes mellitus or cystic fibrosis may have a direct bearing on fetal development and outcome. Kidney disease, heart disease, sexually transmitted disease, thyroid disorders, hypertension, and tuberculosis form a partial list of diseases posing potential difficulty during pregnancy (Carpenter, 1984). A complete drug sensitivity and allergy history should be taken, as well as a list of past surgical procedures the client has experienced. Organized formats for taking the medical history are utilized in most institutions, and the nurse should adhere to institutional policy when collecting the medical history.

Finally, a *psychosocial history* should be elicited from the client. Included in this area are a diet history, educational history of both client and spouse/mate, available support persons, and personal habits. All of the preceding information may not be revealed in one visit; however, as the nurse continues to follow the client's pregnancy, more information may be revealed. Data collected should be classified and identified and may come from a multitude of sources. Data may be obtained from client interviews, objective findings, subjective appraisals, or from other health team members. The assessment phase provides the ideal opportunity for establishing trust between the client and the nurse.

In addition to assessment, the nurse must provide education and help to establish and maintain supportive relationships for the expectant family. Early contact is extremely important due to the vulnerability of the fetus during the first trimester. Helping the family and significant others to understand or at least be aware of the woman's biopsychosocial changes sets the stage for supportive relationships. Anticipatory guidance may be utilized to facilitate the role changes that accompany the birth of a child. Personal growth of the family may either be enhanced or inhibited by the guidance and support the family receives during the antepartal period.

An important aspect to remember is that pregnancy is an additional stress superimposed on the usual life stresses of the family unit. Accompanying pregnancy are changes that will require the use of adaptive mechanisms in order for the childbirth experience to be successfully integrated into the family's total life processes. Although it is easier to focus on the problems and concerns of the expectant female, as the physical changes affecting her are most obvious, her well-being also depends on the well-being of her significant others. Pregnancy is a time when health care workers can utilize preventive intervention to influence the adaptive functioning of those affected by the anticipated birth. By reviewing methods used by the expectant family when dealing with problem or crisis situations encountered in the past, the nurse may identify adaptive mechanisms that may be used by the family in coping with changes surrounding the birth experience. The members of the family unit are faced with the challenge of redefining their present roles, assuming new responsibilities, acquiring new skills, and experiencing significant changes in relationships with others. *The primary goal of health care during pregnancy is to ensure a healthy and happy outcome for the family unit experiencing pregnancy and the events surrounding the birth.*

PRENATAL EDUCATION

The process of educating the expectant family should begin during the very first prenatal visit. In today's era of more educated consumers there is a trend toward a combination of the safety afforded by birth in a hospital setting and the supportive presence of the family unit and significant others. The issue of prenatal education itself raises questions. A very basic question posed is: What content needs to be presented, and when during the pregnancy should it be taught?

During the initial prenatal visit, when the woman is seeking validation of her pregnancy, the nurse can help to set the stage for the course of the prenatal education. Information obtained from the initial assessment can provide clues as to the need for education concerning basic anatomy and physiology of the reproductive system and physical changes accompanying pregnancy. The nurse may provide information on the common discomforts of pregnancy and relief measures for these discomforts. The aforementioned information helps to focus on the initial task of pregnancy (pregnancy validation) and may allay some of the fears and anxieties that the expectant family is experiencing. Nutrition counseling is also appropriate during this time because adequate maternal intake is of utmost importance to the developing fetus.

During the second trimester of pregnancy, the family unit will most likely be receptive to information on fetal development and specific things that the family can do to impact their growing fetus' health.

During the final trimester of pregnancy, the imminence of the upcoming labor and delivery dominates the thoughts of most clients. Traditionally, this is the time period when classes on preparation for childbirth are offered. Content generally taught at this time focuses on the actual labor and delivery itself and may include: signs and symptoms of labor, admission procedures, preparing for the hospital or birthing center, stages of labor, physical changes occurring during labor, breathing and relaxation exercises, role of the support person(s), birthing options, and postdelivery course and procedures.

Forerunners in the development of childbirth education include Grantly Dick-Read and Fernand Lamaze. Dick-Read broached the issue of childbirth education because of an opposition to medical intervention in childbirth. He discussed the fear-tension-pain syndrome, and postulated that the fear and anticipation of pain associated with childbirth arouse natural protective tensions in the body that oppose the forces of dilatation, therefore causing pain. To inhibit this reaction pattern, Dick-Read advocated overcoming fear, eliminating anxiety and tension, and replacing them with a mood of calmness and relaxation. He emphasized a series of physical and respiratory relaxation exercises combined with a consistent coach. The physical and respiratory exercises were devised for the purpose of reducing physical and mental tensions, whereas the coach provides support and alleviates loneliness, believed to generate fear (Dick-Read, 1953).

Dr. Fernand Lamaze, a French obstetrician, developed a method of childbirth preparation based on Pavlovian psychology. The Lamaze method of childbirth preparation is based on the theory that conditioned reflexes minimize the amplitude of the signal received in the brain, therefore altering the behavioral response to the signal received. Psychoprophylaxis is the term given to the exercises of the Lamaze method, which provide strong stimuli necessary to take precedence over signals from uterine contractions (Lamaze, 1958).

In actuality, both of these methods of prepared childbirth are very similar. Both advocate education to reduce apprehension and fear and the presence of a supportive coach. Both utilize respiratory exercises to achieve distraction and relaxation exercises to decrease the perception of pain. The methods differ only in the means by which they achieve relaxation. Many areas in the United States have either altered or combined the above approaches to meet the needs of the more educated consumers who desire more control over their birth experience.

Another factor to be considered when discussing prenatal education is the response of siblings to pregnancy. Their response varies with age and dependency needs. Many institutions now permit some form of sibling visitation in the postpartum period, and there has been an increasing interest expressed in the presence of siblings at the birth. If this is to be an actuality, then it is generally agreed that siblings need to be prepared for labor, delivery, and the changes that accompany the addition of a new family member.

SUMMARY

A most important aspect in the care of expectant families is a willingness to allow the expectant family to exercise some control over their birth experience. The birth experience should meet the needs of the consumer in a safe environment, otherwise if nurses and other hospital personnel cannot be flexible in meeting these needs without compromising the outcome, consumers will seek those experiences in settings which *may* not afford the safety of an in-hospital or birthing center delivery.

CARE PLAN FOR THE FAMILY DEFICIENT IN KNOWLEDGE DURING PREGNANCY

Situation

Barbie Baker is a 17-year-old high school senior who has missed 2 menstrual periods and has not discussed the possibility of pregnancy with her family. She is the oldest of three children. Barbie's parents are devout Catholics and considered leaders in their small town. Barbie states her parents have high expectations of their children and rely on Barbie to be a good role model for her younger brother and sister. Barbie had planned to attend the state university and follow in her dad's footsteps by studying architecture. Barbie has recognized and supported her church's position against abortion, yet she states "I had never dreamed that I would be facing pregnancy myself."

Barbie's boyfriend, Matt Miller, is a freshman at the state university and wants to marry Barbie and have the baby. He plans to quit college and find a job to support the three of them.

Barbie is confused about what is the right choice for her. As a nurse at the local hospital's prenatal clinic, you are in a position to provide care to Barbie. Following is a sample care plan addressing some aspects of this problem.

Nursing Diagnosis

1. Knowledge deficit relating to pregnancy

SAMPLE CARE PLAN

Nursing Diagnosis	Goals	Nursing Interventions	Evaluation
Knowledge deficit: Regarding diagnosis of pregnancy.	The client will gain knowledge about pregnancy during scheduled prenatal visit. The client will discuss with the nurse anticipated physiological changes accompanying pregnancy. The client will discuss community resources available to her during the prenatal visit. The client will make an informed choice about health care for this pregnancy.	Establish a therapeutic relationship. Obtain initial data base: Menstrual history Obstetric history Medical history Psychosocial history Physical assessment 24-hour dietary recall Assess client's reaction to pregnancy. Refer client as indicated by assessment data. Provide information about community resources. Assist client in identifying support systems. Provide care in a nonjudgmental manner and allow opportunity for client to express her needs.	Verbalize correct information presented to her regarding the diagnosis of pregnancy. Continue to come for prenatal care. Display behaviors that indicate compliance to the discussed plan of care. Have received support from family and/or significant others.

Adapted from Aukamp, V. (1984). *Nursing careplans for the childbearing family.* Norwalk, CT: Appleton-Century-Crofts.

REVIEW QUESTIONS

1. Discuss the value of the use of the family developmental approach when assessing the expectant family.

2. Discuss the importance of the nurse's ability to assist in role identification and adaptation as the family unit anticipates a new baby.

3. Discuss how the identification of role-taking behavior can be viewed within the family developmental framework.

REFERENCES

Aukamp, V. (1984). *Nursing careplans for the childbearing family*. Norwalk, CT: Appleton-Century-Crofts.

Barhill L., Rubenstein, C., & Rocklin, D. From generation to generation: Father's-to-be-in transition, *The Family Coordination, 28* (2), 229–235.

Brazelton, T. B. (1976). The parent–infant attachment, *Clinical Obstetrics and Gynecology, 29,* 373–386.

Becker, M. H. (1974). *The health-belief model and personal health behavior*. Thorofare, NJ: Charles B. Slack.

Carey, W. B., et al. (1981). Adolescent age and obstetric risk. *Seminars in Perinatology, 1,* 5–9.

Carpenter, M. (1984). Prenatal risk assessment. In J. B. Warshaw and J. C. Hobbins (Ed.), *Principles and practice of perinatal medicine: Maternal—fetal newborn care*. Menlo Park, CA: Addison-Wesley.

Colman, A. D., & Colman, L. L. (1971). *Pregnancy: The psychological experience*. New York: Herder and Herder, 1971.

Committee on Nutrition. (1974). *Nutrition in maternal health care*. Chicago: The American College of Obstetricians and Gynecologists.

Cranley, M. S. (1984). *The impact of perceived stress and social support on maternal—fetal attachment in the third trimester*. Doctoral dissertation, University of Wisconsin, Madison, 1979. *University Microfilms International*, 80-01134. (Xerox University Microfilms)

Dick-Read, G. (1953). *Childbirth without fear*. New York: Harper & Row.

Duvall, E. (1962). *Family development*. Philadelphia: Lippincott.

Duvall, E. (1971). *Family development, 4th Ed*. Philadelphia: Lippincott.

Erikson, E. (1963). *Childhood and Society* (2nd Ed.). New York: W. W. Norton.

Harding-Weaver, R. H., & Cranley, M. S. (1983). An exploration of paternal-fetal attachment behavior. *Nursing Research, 32*(2), 69.

Lacoursiere, R. (1972). Fatherhood and mental illness: A review and new material. *Psychiatric Quarterly, 46,* 109–124.

Lamaze, F. (1958). *Painless childbirth*. London: Burke.

McCauley, C. S. (1976). *Pregnancy after thirty-five*. New York: Sunrise.

McCarthy, P. A. (1983). Fetal alcohol syndrome and other alcohol-related birth defects. *Nurse Practitioner, 8,* 33–37.

Pearlin, L. I., & Schooler, C. (1978). The structure of coping. *Journal of Health and Social Behavior, 19,* 18.

Rubin, R. (1975). Maternal tasks in pregnancy. *Maternal and Child Nursing Journal, 4,* 143–153.

Valentine, D. P. (1982). The experience of pregnancy: A developmental process. *Family Relations, 31,* 243–248.

Williams, S. R. (1981). *Nutrition and diet therapy* (4th ed.). St. Louis: Mosby.

3

The Family During Childbirth

Elizabeth Farren Pond

OBJECTIVES

Upon completion of this chapter, the student will be able to:

1. Utilize the nursing process to assess the physical and psychosocial needs of the family in the childbirth period
2. Describe the relationship between potential stressors and outcome of childbirth
3. Discuss the variations of adaptation to childbirth and the impact on the family
4. Select appropriate nursing interventions that will help a family to adapt optimally to childbirth

CONCEPTS

Development: a step or stage in growth

Adaptation: a change in behavior that results in better adjustment to prevailing life patterns

Attachment: relationship between two persons

Childbirth is the culmination of nine months of planning, dreaming, wishing, and hoping on the part of the expectant couple. It is the climax of many hours of thinking, talking, and preparation for an event that brings many changes to the lives involved, and whose outcome has a lasting effect on the parents, the infant, and the family. What other life event can compare with the miraculous development and eventual birth of a new life, a new being?

Goals of the health care team for the woman and her family during the process of childbirth include the following: (1) Provide the protection and care needed for the best outcome for the woman and fetus, and (2) facilitate optimal adaptation of the woman and significant others and family to the childbirth process.

This chapter on childbirth will describe ways to meet these goals. Satisfying these goals will require use of the nursing process to correctly assess physical and psychosocial needs in order to appropriately identify needs or problems and plan interventions. The plan must then be evaluated to determine if the goals were met and whether changes need to be made.

INDIVIDUAL AND FAMILY TASKS OF THE CHILDBEARING COUPLE

The childbearing family has individual and family tasks that relate to the period of pregnancy and to the time period beginning with the birth of the infant. There have been no specific tasks identified for the childbirth process itself. However, the work of authors such as Duvall (1977) and Clark and Affonso (1979) suggest some tasks.

During the childbirth process, the childbearing woman and her partner will attempt to accomplish the following tasks. Accomplishment of these tasks will facilitate optimal adaptation of the couple to the childbirth process.

1. Maintaining control over the childbirth events, the amount and type of control determined by the needs of the couple
2. Communicating effectively with each other, family members, friends, and health professionals
3. Maintaining a satisfying relationship with each other, family members, friends, and health professionals
4. Reconciling expectations of the childbirth experience and the actual events
5. Integrating the childbirth experience into ongoing life events.

Maintaining Control

Control over the events in childbirth is an issue that is individual for each couple. Some couples may feel the need to have some control over decisions related to fetal monitoring, intravenous fluids, and perineal preparation and enemas. Other couples are willing to give control over such decisions, related to procedures, to health professionals in the situation.

Communicating Effectively/Maintaining Satisfying Relationships

When the woman and her partner are able to communicate their needs in an open, direct manner, and when they can accept the events occurring during the childbirth process (for example, whether the delivery is a spontaneous vaginal delivery or a cesarean section), satisfying relationships are more likely to be maintained.

Reconciling Expectations/Integrating the Childbirth Experience

As the couple accepts the events in the childbirth process, and as they are able to talk about the events in relation to their lives as a whole, they will be able to integrate the process into their lives. An additional task for the childbearing woman is adapting optimally to the physiological stresses in the childbirth process.

Developmental tasks for family members include some of the same ones as those for the couple. It is important to communicate effectively, maintain satisfying relationships, reconcile expectations of the childbirth process and outcome, and integrate the experience into ongoing life events. The last two tasks carry over into the postpartum period.

POTENTIAL STRESSORS

Stressors Affecting Childbirth

Maternal Diseases.   There are many diseases that may have a negative effect on the outcome of a pregnancy. Conditions such as diabetes, heart disease, Rh sensitization, and pregnancy-induced hypertension, to name a few, can have a great impact on the welfare of the mother, fetus, and/or newborn. Special care is provided in childbirth by the health care team for these mothers. Additional physical support in the form of expert monitoring and treatment as well as additional emotional support are needed to protect the maternal–fetal system.

Maternal Infections.   A mother may have an infection at the time of childbirth. Whether the infection is caused by bacteria or a virus, special attention is paid to the possible effect on the mother and the fetus/newborn. The presence of an infection is a stressor for the mother. When the stress of childbirth is added to an already stressed system, the process and outcome of childbirth, as well as the family unit's adaptation to childbirth, may be altered.

The presence of an infection will have varying effects on childbirth. Depending on the type of infection, the mother may need to be isolated during childbirth. Premature labor has been associated with the presence of an infection in the mother (Moore, 1983; Pillitteri, 1981). An infection might determine the type of delivery necessary. For example, an active case of genital herpes virus would indicate the need for a cesarean section. Following the birth, the infant will be carefully evaluated for signs of infection. The mother and infant may need to be isolated. Both are closely monitored by the health care team, and interventions are instituted as needed to help the family achieve an optimal health status.

Stressors Arising from Childbirth

The birth process itself is a stressor for the mother and fetus. Specific stressors can be categorized according to the critical factors in childbirth, or the four Ps: passage, passenger, psyche, and powers. Any one of the factors can be the cause of dystocia, or difficult labor.

Passage.   The childbirth passage consists of the maternal bony pelvis and the maternal soft tissues within the birth canal. The bony pelvis has three important areas for measurement: the inlet, midpelvis, and outlet. Any of the areas may be smaller than normal and cause a *cephalopelvic disproportion*, or a disproportion between the size of the mother's pelvis and the head of the fetus. Cephalopelvic disproportion may also result when the mother has an adequate pelvis but the infant has a large head.

The maternal soft tissues consist of the uterus and cervix, the vagina, and the vulva. Any abnormalities, such as abnormal position of the uterus, incomplete atresia of the cervix, vagina, or vulva, or the presence of pelvic tumors, may impede labor progress (Pritchard & MacDonald, 1980).

The resulting method of delivery when there is a problem with the passage is usually a cesarean section. A cesarean section is a surgical procedure in which the infant is removed from the uterus through an incision in the abdominal wall and uterus.

Passenger.   The passenger includes the fetus and the contents of the uterus: the placenta, umbilical cord, and amniotic fluid.

Additional stress is created when the fetus is in an abnormal position (occiput posterior, transverse) or presentation (breech, shoulder) or when developmental abnormalities, such as hydrocephaly, are present. Stress is also added when the pregnancy is multiple (twins, triplets, or more), and when the fetus develops symptoms of distress related to cord or head compression or uteroplacental insufficiency.

Problems with the placenta occur when the placenta separates prematurely from the uterine wall (abruptio placentae), and when the placenta is improperly implanted in the lower uterine segment (placenta previa). Both of these situations can cause significant blood loss for the mother and interference with the flow of oxygen and nutrients to the fetus. Thus they are grave threats to the welfare of the mother and fetus.

Anatomical anomalies of the placenta can occur, and usually do not pose a threat to the mother and fetus.

The umbilical cord can become a stressor if it prolapses or a loop slips down past the presenting part. Cord compression then results as the presenting part of the fetus presses on the cord. Blood supply to the fetus is decreased, thus causing hypoxia and decelerations of the heartbeat with contractions. Immediate interventions are indicated: relief of pressure on the umbilical cord, and delivery of the infant.

Amniotic fluid, or the fluid surrounding the fetus in the uterus, may become a problem if there is too much (hydramnios) or too little (oligohydramnios). In severe cases, perinatal mortality is increased (Pritchard & MacDonald, 1980). In rare instances, an amniotic fluid embolism may occur when amniotic fluid enters the maternal circulatory system. Maternal and fetal death may result; therefore, immediate intervention is indicated.

Psyche.   Psyche is defined as being "all that constitutes the mind and its processes" (Thomas, 1981). Psyche as a critical factor in labor includes the psychological and emotional attributes of the mother and her family. Cultural and social factors are also part of the psyche of a mother and her family.

Childbirth has a great impact on the psychosocial parameters of the family. Childbirth can enhance a person's self concept depending on (1) the meaning of the event (self-fulfilling or threatening?), (2) expectations and goals (Were they realistic? Were they met?), and (3) feedback to all participants in the childbirth process (positive or negative?) (Clark & Affonso, 1979).

Childbirth can also produce varying amounts of anxiety for each mother and her family. Sources of anxiety include lack of knowledge of the childbirth process and policies and procedures of the hospital or birthing environment, unmet expectations (the timing is not right; the infant appears different from what was imagined), the presence of strangers (health professionals), fear for self and infant, and many others that are individual for the family (Clark & Affonso, 1979).

The physiological process of labor can be greatly influenced by the psyche, or cultural and emotional factors of the mother and her family. The length of labor can be increased and the perceived discomfort heightened by excessive anxiety. A prolonged labor can in turn place additional stress on mother and fetus.

Powers. The powers in childbirth are the forces, or uterine contractions, that propel the fetus through the birth canal. Dysfunctional uterine contractions can create labor patterns that are hypoactive or hyperactive. These patterns can occur at any time up to the delivery of the infant, and may be due to factors related to the passage, passenger, or psyche, as well as the powers. Both hypoactive and hyperactive patterns of labor can be dangerous for the mother and for the fetus.

COPING MECHANISMS

Coping mechanisms are used by the family during childbirth to facilitate adaptation to this unique process. Adaptation is influenced not only by the physical, psychological, emotional, and social factors already discussed, but also by the environment in childbirth. There are various alternatives related to the environment in childbirth, and an emphasis on family-centered care can be had in all settings.

Adaptation to childbirth can be positive or negative and has an influence on parent–infant attachment and the impact of the birth on the family.

Health Beliefs and Behaviors

Alternatives

Hospitals. Hospitals can provide traditional labor and delivery rooms and birthing rooms. When the traditional labor and delivery rooms are used, the mother is moved from the labor room to the delivery room when delivery is imminent. This usually necessitates a trip in the bed down a hall and transfer to the table in the delivery room. After the delivery, the mother is transferred back to her bed and moved to a recovery room.

When a birthing room in a hospital is used, the mother labors, delivers her infant, and recovers in the same room. These rooms are also called labor/delivery rooms or single-unit delivery systems (SUDS). A variety of criteria are used to determine couples suitable for using birthing rooms. For instance, many hospitals have policies that permit only couples who have attended childbirth education classes and who are at low risk to use the birthing rooms.

The Birthplace at St. Mary's Hospital in Minneapolis, Minnesota, was opened in 1984, and has eighteen childbearing rooms, two delivery rooms, and one cesarean section room (Reed & Schmid, 1986). The childbearing rooms are used for labor, delivery, recovery, and postpartum care. These rooms combine the homelike atmosphere of a birthing room and the technical support of a traditional labor room and delivery room. A central nursery provides care for infants when they are not in the mothers' rooms.

Sumner and Phillips (1981), in their book, *Birthing Rooms—Concept and Reality*, discuss the development of family-centered maternity care at Manchester Memorial Hospital in Connecticut. In 1969, Manchester Memorial Hospital opened the first birthing room in the United States. Now the Manchester Memorial Family Birthing Center coordinates professional and lay organizations to provide a comprehensive program of perinatal services. The features of the program include: (1) physical and emotional preparation of the couple, (2) a single environmental unit for the entire childbirth process, (3) support for the couple by a nurse, and (4) individualization of each childbirth experience. Specific aspects of family-centered maternity care included in the Manchester Memorial Family Birthing Center are presented in Table 3–1.

Birthing Centers. Birthing centers may be located within a hospital setting (alternative birthing center) or outside of the hospital. According to McKay and Phillips (1984, p. 65), alternative birthing centers have been developed as a result of the "home birth movement and . . . consumer pressure for more family-centered and humanized childbirth services." Birthing centers are homelike in furnishings and decorations, but have the same supplies and equipment needed for birthing rooms. The use of intravenous fluids, monitoring equipment, and perineal preps and enemas is uncommon in birthing centers. Obstetric nurses and midwives, backed by obstetricians and pediatricians, provide care to the families. As in the case of couples

TABLE 3–1. FEATURES OF FAMILY-CENTERED MATERNITY CARE MANCHESTER MEMORIAL FAMILY BIRTHING CENTER

Prenatal education
Nutritional consultation
Preparation for birth and parenting
Elimination of routines and risk criteria for eligibility
Individualization of care
Father participation
Emphasis on noninvasive, multiple support techniques
Emphasis on support by experienced obstetric nurse
Nontransfer of the mother for delivery
Recognition of beauty and dignity of birth scene
Recognition of importance of meaningful interaction of mother, father, and infant
Nurturing activities of nursing staff

Adapted from Sumner, P.E. & Phillips, C.R. (1981). Birthing Rooms—Concept and Reality. St. Louis: Mosby.

anticipating using birthing rooms, couples anticipating using birthing centers are screened prenatally for risk factors, and only those with a low risk are permitted to use the facility.

Lubic (1983, p. 1054) reports that a Childbearing Center (CbC) in New York was developed to "demonstrate safety and satisfaction of families electing this type of birthing experience." Evidence has supported the achievement of that goal. Cost was also a consideration, and in 1980, the Center showed that maternity care costs at the CbC were one half to one quarter of those in private hospitals in New York.

Home Birth. The home is chosen by a few couples as the preferred environment for childbirth. Reasons for this choice may be the cost of a hospital delivery, the policies of the hospital, personal beliefs regarding childbirth, and the availability of a hospital. A major disadvantage of a home birth is the danger of unexpected complications, such as hemorrhage or umbilical cord prolapse. A major advantage of a home birth is the chance for the couple to deliver their infant in familiar surroundings with friends and family (Moore, 1983). Careful planning is necessary when choosing a home birth, with special consideration for the needs of the mother and fetus.

Birth Attendant. The health care professional delivering the infant is usually a physician. The physician may specialize in obstetrics, family practice, or general practice. Nurse-midwives may also be the birth attendant, or person who delivers the infant. Nurse-midwives are more readily available and recognized in some parts of the country than in other parts. Whatever the situation in a community, the couple should find someone who can best meet their needs.

Preparation of Siblings. Siblings need to be prepared for the process of childbirth (for example, length of stay in the hospital) and the changes that will occur following the birth (new sister or brother, changes in sleeping arrangements). If they are to be present during childbirth, they will need special preparation; that is, they will need to be made aware of the physical and behavioral characteristics of the mother during childbirth. They will also need an adult support person available only to them. Research on the outcome of sibling participation in childbirth is minimal. Anderson (1981, p. 54), reporting on her research study of 25 families whose children attended a home birth, stated that "I feel justified in saying that children who are prepared for birth are not traumatized by being present but, rather, they experience birth as a happy family event."

Family-Centered Maternity Care. The Interprofessional Task Force on Health Care of Women and Children, composed of the American College of Obstetricians and Gynecologists, the American College of Nurse-Midwives, The Nurses Associations of the American College of Obstetricians and Gynecologists, the American Academy of Pediatrics, and the American Nurses' Association, developed a definition of family–centered maternity care in 1978. Their definition is:

Family-centered maternity/newborn care can be defined as the delivery of safe, quality health care while recognizing, focusing on, and adapting to both the physical and psychosocial needs of the client-patient, the family, and the newly born. The emphasis is on the provision of maternity/newborn health care which fosters family units while maintaining physical safety.*

Although physical facilities and written protocols play a part in family-centered maternity care, the major component is attitude. This attitude is supported by the philosophy developed by the Interprofessional Task Force:

That the family is the basic unit of society;
That the family is viewed as a whole unit within which each member is an individual enjoying recognition and entitled to consideration;
That childbearing and childrearing are unique and important functions of the family;
That childbearing is an experience that is appropriate and beneficial for the family to share as a unit;
That childbearing is a developmental opportunity and/or a situational crisis, during which the family members benefit from the supporting solidarity of the family unit.†

All of the various settings discussed earlier can incorporate a philosophy of family-centered maternity care. To this end, health professionals assist "families to cope with the childbearing experience and to achieve their own goals within the concept of a high level of wellness, and within the context of the cultural atmosphere of their choosing" (McKay & Phillips, 1984, p. 236).

Choice and control are key concepts in family-centered maternity care (McKay, 1982). It is important for the family to be aware of childbirth alternatives and to take part in the decision-making process. It is only then that the family exerts control over what is happening. Education in various forms is absolutely necessary in supporting these two concepts related to family-centered maternity care.

There are two policies in particular which, when used during childbirth, support the philosophy of family-centered childbirth (McKay & Phillips, 1984). One is that every woman should have a support person in attendance during her labor and delivery. This support person can meet some of the woman's physical and emotional needs and thus help make the experience a satisfying one. The support person can be any significant other such as the husband, mother, other relative, or friend. The second policy is that, while safe care is provided for the mother and infant, the parents and the infant should be allowed as much time as possible together after the birth to facilitate the attachment process.

---

*From: Interprofessional Task Force on Health Care of Women and Children (1978). Joint position statement of the development of family-centered maternity/newborn care in hospitals. Chicago: Interprofessional Task Force on Health Care of Women and Children.

†McKay & Phillips, 1984, p. 235.

RESPONSES TO STRESSORS

Coping Behaviors in Childbirth

According to Affonso (1979, p. 368), adequate coping behaviors are "those which do not interfere with the labor process but facilitate the woman's movement into another phase." On the other hand, inadequate coping behaviors are those that do interfere with the labor process. These behaviors appear as the result of increased anxiety and may lengthen labor and affect the mother's adaptation to the process.

Examples of adequate coping behaviors (see Table 3–2) are:

1. *Latent phase (0–3 cm) of first stage* (beginning of labor to complete dilatation of the cervix): exhibits independent role and is able to use childbirth techniques; participates actively in assessment procedures, such as collecting urine and describing onset of labor
2. *Active phase (4–7 cm) of first stage:* a decreased responsiveness to the environment, i.e., less talking; a decreased ability to use coping actions; needs reminders from coach as to when to focus, how to breathe
3. *Transitional phase (8–10 cm) and second stage* (complete dilatation of cervix to birth of infant): decreased awareness of the environment; presence of aggressive behavior; tuned in to inner self and effect of labor on her body; may lash out at support persons, saying "Leave me alone"
4. *Third stage* (birth of infant to delivery of placenta) *and fourth stage* (delivery of placenta to stabilization post partum): attempts to see and touch infant, and verbalizes feelings; may cry; is exhausted but eager to share with those close to her (Affonso, 1979).

Examples of inadequate coping behaviors include (see Table 3–2):

1. *Latent phase:* aggression, hostility, and a preoccupation with details such as contractions or procedures; may exhibit signs of fear in facial expressions and tensed muscles over body

TABLE 3–2. EXAMPLES OF COPING BEHAVIORS IN CHILDBIRTH

	Adequate	Inadequate
First Stage Latent phase	Independent Uses techniques	Aggressive Hostile Preoccupation with details
Active phase	Decreased responsiveness and ability to use techniques	Fantasy Regression Denial
Transitional Phase & *Second Stage*	Decreased awareness of environment Aggressive	Panic Withdrawal
Third & Fourth Stage	Attempts to see and touch infant Verbalizes feelings	Denial Failure to accept reality of infant

Adapted from Clark, A.L., & Affonso, D.D. (1979). Childbearing: A Nursing Perspective. Philadelphia: Davis.

2. *Active phase:* fantasy, regression, and denial; may be unwilling to communicate; may become very verbal and may thrash around during contractions
3. *Transitional phase and second stage:* panic and withdrawal; loses control, may scream and yell; not willing to cooperate with ongoing care
4. *Third and fourth stages:* denial and failure to accept the reality of the infant; does not want to touch or hold infant; does not want to talk about the experience (Affonso, 1979).

Parent–Infant Attachment

Attachment is defined by Klaus and Kennell (1982) as a "unique relationship between two people that is specific and endures through time." The major influences on parent–infant attachment, according to Klaus and Kennell, are the parental background and health care practices surrounding childbirth. Parental background includes factors such as cultural beliefs and practices, genetic makeup, care provided by own parents, and experiences with previous pregnancies and the present pregnancy. Health care practices include the policies of the hospital and the behavior of and the care given by physicians, nurses, and other health professionals. These influences, as well as how the parents and infant respond to one another, will produce effective caretaking and attachment or parental disorders ranging from mild anxiety to disturbed parent–child relationships.

Klaus and Kennell (1982) identify events and tasks that are important to the process of attachment:

Prior to pregnancy
    Planning the pregnancy
Antepartum
    Confirming the pregnancy
    Accepting the pregnancy
    Perceiving fetal movement
    Accepting the fetus as an individual
Intrapartum—Labor and birth
Postpartum
    Seeing the baby
    Touching the baby
    Giving care to the baby
    Accepting the infant as a separate individual

Although there is evidence of a sensitive period (the first hour following birth), which is significant in the attachment process, Klaus and Kennell (1982) emphasize that this does not mean that every parent will develop a close tie to the infant within that time. Also, if the parents and infant are not able to interact during this sensitive period, this does not mean that attachment is hindered or does not take place. The sensitive period is a time when the infant and parents are especially alert and sensitive to one another and, if possible, this period should be taken advantage of to facilitate attachment.

There are behaviors exhibited by the parents that indicate adaptive or maladaptive responses to the infant. According to Cropley (1986), adaptive or positive behaviors are those that indicate attachment and meet the needs of the infant and parents. Maladaptive or negative behaviors indicate lack of attachment and unmet needs of the infant and parents. The following are examples of both kinds of behaviors which might be seen during childbirth (Cropley, 1986).

Adaptive Behaviors	Maladaptive Behaviors
1. Attempts to see infant as infant is delivered	1. Makes little or no attempt to see infant
2. Responds to infant by smiling, talking, touching	2. Makes minimal or no response to infant (may frown, decline to hold, not touch).
3. Asks questions about infant	3. Makes no or negative comments about infant
4. Appears satisfied; may cry from joy	4. Appears dissatisfied, verbally and nonverbally expressed

Impact of Childbirth

The birth of a child alters previous relationships and roles within a family. These changing roles and relationships are influenced by the process of childbirth itself. Depending on the expectations of childbirth, the performance therein, the outcome, and the feedback, the family moves toward integrating and assimilating this new being into its network. The mother, father, siblings, and other family members are all affected by the childbirth process.

Mother.   For the mother, the birth helps her differentiate her infant from herself. They still maintain a oneness, however, as the mother holds her infant and mentally considers the infant a part of herself (Furman, 1982). Even as the infant grows and becomes more independent, the mother still has a considerable self-investment in her child.

In a study in 1983 of 294 first-time mothers, Mercer, Hackley, and Bostrom (1983) found that the mother's perception of her birth experience was less affected by medical management (cesarean birth, medications, fetal monitoring, and anesthesia), and most affected by the emotional support of her mate and early interaction with her infant. A further finding was that the perception of birth score was significantly positively correlated with the mother's gratification in the maternal role and with her mothering behaviors. Thus the mother's perception of the childbirth experience did influence her adaptation to motherhood.

Single Mother.   The impact of childbirth on the single mother can vary according to her emotional and behavioral reactions to her position as a single parent (Tankson, 1986). As a result of having a child, a single adult woman may experience loneliness and social isolation due to the stigma placed upon her by her community. A woman who is separated or divorced from her husband may experience rejection and grief. A widowed woman may experience grief and problems with establishing her independence. These and other problems with single parenthood may bring on difficulties such as family crisis, role change, financial strain, parenting problems, stereotype difficulties, and social isolation (Tankson, 1986).

A study of single pregnant women done in 1974 (Kruk, 1981) found as one of its conclusions that the circumstances of family life after the birth of the infant, as well as the support of the family of origin, are the most important variables in terms of outcome. Another conclusion, or suggestion, was that younger women, single or married, are in special need of support.

From the above information, it appears that perceptions of the childbirth experience from the viewpoint of the single mother would find the same influences as for any other mother, that is, the need for emotional support during childbirth, and early interaction with her infant. Additional influences would relate to her family environment, or family support, and resources related to provision of housing, clothing, food, income, health services, etc.

Father.   For the father, the infant is not an integral component of his body, but the infant is mentally and emotionally a part of him (Furman, 1982). Participation in the birth process led to a great feeling of satisfaction of fathers in a study done by Phillips and Anzalone (1982). This study, done over a 5-year period, resulted in the identification of seven categories of positive experiences for the fathers. These were:

1. *Team event:* the father and mother working as a team
2. *Self-pride:* proud of his performance during childbirth, i.e., not fainting
3. *Heightened respect* for mate: surprised at strength of mate
4. *Completeness:* as a man and husband
5. *Oneness:* with his mate, i.e., "we did it"
6. *New insights:* deeper appreciation of life
7. *Engrossment:* high level of involvement, elation, and interest in birth and infant

There is evidence to support the importance of the father's involvement in the childbirth process. The presence of the father can decrease the distress of the mother (Yogman, 1982). Hangsleben (1983) reports that the father's involvement in the childbearing experience may enhance his later involvement in the father role. In one study (Nicholson et al., 1983), active father participation in childbirth influenced the integration of the experience and paternal self-esteem. Another finding was that the most beneficial type of father involvement depends on the characteristics of the couple. In another study, early extended father–infant contact was found to be important in determining father–infant interaction at 5 months (Palkovitz, 1982).

Adolescent Parent.   The impact of childbirth on the adolescent varies depending on age, physical and psychological maturity, marital status, planned or unplanned pregnancy, and availability of emotional and financial support. The experience of the childbirth process would be very different for a 12-year-old unmarried adolescent, who is planning to place her infant for adoption, and an 18-year-old married adolescent who is experiencing a planned pregnancy and has her husband with her for support.

Individual differences related to physical and emotional maturity, available support, and accomplishment of the task of establishing their own identity must be taken into consideration when assessing the impact of childbirth on an adolescent mother and father. An additional critical factor is the availability and accessibility of health care services. The outcome of childbirth may be positive or negative, depending on these interrelated factors.

The impact of childbirth will be different for an adolescent who keeps her baby and for one who allows her baby to be adopted. The adolescent whose baby will be adopted goes through the grief process and must cope with the loss of her baby. Careful consideration must be given for that adolescent mother's need to bond and then disengage with her baby. The nurse can help by facilitating mother–infant interaction, providing emotional support by listening to the mother's concerns, and encouraging the mother to focus on future goals.

Consideration must also be given to the adolescent father. Information about his needs should be assessed, problems identified, and a plan developed to meet his needs. The adolescent father's adaptation to childbirth will vary, as the adolescent mother's does, depending on his age, maturity, and available support. Other factors impacting on his adaptation are his desired and actual involvement in both the decision making about the pregnancy and in the childbirth process and outcome.

Siblings.   The impact of childbirth on siblings depends on the actual events of childbirth, the impact on the parents, and the age and developmental stage of the child. If the childbirth process progressed as expected, and the mother and new baby are well and come home when expected, siblings will have an easier time adapting to the changes, particularly if they were able to see and talk to the mother and the new brother or sister while in the hospital. The age and developmental stage (preschool, school age, adolescent) of the sibling(s) will determine the strategies used by the parents in introducing the new baby to the sibling(s). For instance, a 4-year-old can be told about the experience of his own birth, and this can be compared to the birth experience of the new baby. Also, while providing private time with the 4-year-old, the parent can encourage appropriate participation in the care of the newborn.

Grandparents.   The impact of the birth of a child on grandparents is given little consideration in current literature. However, the birth of a grandchild can have a positive or negative emotional effect on the grandparents. Some grandparents do not welcome the role of grandparent, and so are not supportive of their son or daughter. Most grandparents, however, do anticipate their new roles in positive ways (Jensen & Bobak, 1985). They enjoy remembering the birth of their own children and reminiscing about their infant behaviors, and want to participate in the birth of their grandchild as much as possible. They may look upon the birth as a guarantee of the continuity of their family.

Impact of Cesarean Birth

The impact of a cesarean birth on a family can vary. In a study done by Affonso and Stichler (1981) of 105 women who were interviewed 2 to 4 days after a cesarean section, 92% said that they experienced feelings of anxiety, fearfulness, worry, and concern about the baby, themselves, and the surgery. Half of the women experienced feelings of frustration, anger, disappointment, and sometimes depression. One third of the women expressed feelings of being happy and/or relieved. Most of the women perceived the cesarean birth environment as being stressful and threatening, and the recovery setting as being one of distortions related to orientation to time, person, place, and events.

In a report of a study done by Affonso and Domino (1981) of fathers whose infants were delivered by cesarean section, it was found that fathers also experience emotional responses. The responses fell into three categories: (1) relief and happiness—54%, (2) worry and concern—90%, and (3) other feelings, usually negative, such as frustration and anger—24%, and disappointment and sadness—22%.

A cesarean birth can also affect the attachment or acquaintance process. Affonso (1981) has identified the following variables that affect the acquaintance process when the birth is cesarean:

1. Circumstances indicating the need for a cesarean section (elective or emergency)
2. Circumstances around the event (information received, support of "significant other")
3. Opportunities to collect data (interaction during and immediately following birth)
4. Factors affecting senses and perceptions (anesthesia, pain)
5. Anxiety about infant (health)
6. Initial reactions to infant (sex, appearance)
7. Infant state of behavior (alert, drowsy)
8. Perceptions of parenting abilities
9. Feelings toward self

Impact of Perinatal Loss and Death

Perinatal loss and death can involve abortion, the death of a fetus, stillbirth, the death of a newborn, or the birth of a malformed or premature infant. In each instance, the mother and father experience extreme disappointment, a sense of failure, and grief. All their hopes and dreams collapse, and the fulfillment of their new roles as parents (or parents of a perfect child) is gone.

As the mother and father progress through their grief, they will experience shock, denial, sadness, despair, guilt, and, finally, resolution and reorganization. The length of time involved in resolving grief may vary from 6 to 24 months (Borg & Lasker, 1981).

The impact of the specific events in childbirth (length of labor, complications, medications, determination of perinatal death or malformation of infant) will be influenced by the support of the health care team received by the mother and family, and by the opportunities for the parents and infant to be together.

NURSING ASSESSMENT

Physical Assessment

Initial Assessment.   The data base should include a present and past obstetrical history and a medical history. The prenatal record and an interview with the woman can supply this information. Data to be collected on admission to a labor and delivery unit include the following items (NAACOG, 1981):

1. Onset, frequency, duration, and character of uterine contractions
2. History of ruptured membranes (time, color, consistency, odor, and amount of amniotic fluid)
3. Presence or history of vaginal bleeding or discharge
4. History of fever or recent infection
5. Physical examination, including: abdominal palpation to determine fetal size, presentation, and position, and vaginal examination for dilatation and effacement of cervix, station, presenting part of fetus, and state of membranes
6. Vital signs and fetal heart rate
7. Time and type of last meal and
8. Review of body systems, to include reflexes

Risk Assessment.   Many health care facilities use a system for assigning a risk score to clients in the perinatal period. Problems that may occur are assigned a number relating to the degree of risk that a pregnancy has for a less than optimal outcome. A total score is then obtained. A low score would indicate that it is unlikely that the mother, fetus, or newborn will have problems. A high score in any period would indicate that there may be subsequent risk to the mother, fetus, and/or newborn.

Fetal Assessment.   Categories of fetal assessment include fetal heart rate, fetal blood sampling, amniocentesis, ultrasound, x-ray pelvimetry, amniotic fluid, fetal body movement, and electronic fetal tests.

Fetal Heart Rate.   The fetal heart rate (FHR) continues to be the most commonly used technique for evaluating fetal status and is a highly reliable indicator. The fetal heart rate may be obtained by using an intermittent or continuous method. Intermittent methods include the use of a fetoscope or Doptone/Doppler, and involve listening to the fetal heart through the wall of the uterus at various intervals of time.

Continuous monitoring involves the use of electronic instruments that can evaluate the fetal heart rate either directly or indirectly over an extended period of time. The indirect method involves attaching an ultrasound transducer, phono transducer, or fetal ECG electrodes to the mother's abdomen at the point where the FHR is heard. A tocotransducer is attached to the mother's abdomen at the top of the fundus, or top part of the uterus, to indicate the occurrence of contractions. Both of these are attached by using elastic belts on the abdomen. They are then attached to the fetal monitor machine, which records and gives a tracing of fetal heart and uterine activity.

The direct method of electronic fetal monitoring involves the use of a fetal ECG electrode, which is attached to the presenting part of the fetus and assesses the fetal heart rate. Uterine activity is assessed through the use of a polyethylene, fluid-filled catheter, which is inserted into the uterus through the cervix. This catheter permits measurement of pressure within the uterus and thus is a way of evaluating contractions.

There are advantages and disadvantages of both the direct and indirect methods of electronic fetal monitoring. However, this method of continuous monitoring of the fetal heart rate is the most accurate in terms of evaluating fetal condition during labor.

Fetal Blood Sampling. Fetal blood can be evaluated during labor if there are indications of fetal compromise or distress. The blood is obtained from a small skin nick in the presenting part of the fetus, and the pH is analyzed to determine if the fetus is acidotic. A maternal blood pH may be evaluated at the same time and compared to the fetal pH.

Amniocentesis. An amniocentesis may be done during labor if it is deemed necessary to have information about the condition or maturity of the fetus. If a pregnant woman is known to be high risk, an amniocentesis might already have been done in the prenatal period.

Amniocentesis is the aspiration of amniotic fluid (fluid that surrounds the fetus in the uterus) through the abdominal wall. The obtained fluid can then be evaluated in several ways. During early pregnancy, amniotic fluid can be assessed for genetic components for the purpose of ascertaining anomalies. During the third trimester or during the intrapartal period, amniotic fluid can be assessed for components that indicate fetal maturity: phospholipids, creatinine, and bilirubin.

The phospholipid lecithin has as a major component surfactant, a substance that permits air spaces in the lungs to remain open after they have been expanded (Gorvine, Hawkins, Fazeka, & Mott, 1982). Measurement of lecithin and comparison of its level with the level of sphingomyelin, another phospholipid, gives an indication of fetal lung maturity. A lecithin/sphingomyelin ratio of 2 : 1 indicates that the fetal lungs are sufficiently mature and that the infant will not develop respiratory distress syndrome.

Creatinine levels in amniotic fluid rise with fetal kidney maturity and increased muscle mass of the fetus. A value of 2 mg/100 ml indicates maturity.

Bilirubin levels in amniotic fluid decrease as the fetal liver and the placenta mature. Bilirubin levels are also an indicator of Rh sensitization.

Ultrasound (Sonogram). Ultrasound involves the use of high-frequency sound waves that reflect off surfaces of varying densities. These reflections are displayed on a screen for viewing and can be photographed. Ultrasound is used during the intrapartum period to evaluate fetal and placental position before an amniocentesis, and to evaluate fetal size by obtaining a measurement of the fetal head. The biparietal diameter obtained is compared to a chart that shows its correlations with fetal weight, thus giving an estimate of fetal size.

X-ray Pelvimetry. The use of x-ray in labor is indicated only if there is a possibility that the mother has a contracted pelvis. Dangers of radiation to the fetus include mutations and an increased risk of malignancy after birth; however, the value of the information obtained from the x-ray may outweigh the dangers of radiation.

X-ray pelvimetry provides exact measurement of two important diameters: the transverse diameter of the inlet, and the interischial spinous diameter. These measurements give an indication of the size and shape of the pelvis. Other factors considered along with these measurements are the size of the fetal head, the force of the uterine contractions, the moldability of the fetal head, and the position and presentation of the fetus (Pritchard & MacDonald, 1980).

Amniotic Fluid. Once the fetal membranes have ruptured, the amniotic fluid can provide some indications of fetal status. Amniotic fluid is usually a pale straw color. A greenish-brown color indicates the presence of meconium. The presence of meconium in amniotic fluid when the fetus is in a vertex or head presentation indicates fetal compromise. Meconium is the first feces of the newborn; it is dark in color and has a tarry consistency. It is believed that fetal anoxia may result in relaxation of the anal sphincter or increased peristalsis, thus producing a release of meconium. Meconium-stained amniotic fluid may be present when the fetus is in a breech presentation, and is usually not a sign of fetal compromise. Yellow-stained amniotic fluid may indicate fetal hypoxia or fetal hemolytic disease, and port wine-colored amniotic fluid may indicate premature separation of the placenta (Jensen & Bobak, 1985).

Fetal Body Movement. Consistent fetal movements felt by the mother are positive signs of fetal well-being. If there is a question about the frequency of fetal movements, the mother can be instructed to lie down for an hour and count fetal movements. Three or more movements in an hour is normal. A frequency of one or two fetal movements per hour, or a sudden reduction in fetal movements, needs to be immediately evaluated by the health care team.

Electronic Fetal Tests. Two tests that utilize electronic fetal monitoring equipment to evaluate fetal status are the nonstress test (NST), or fetal heart acceleration test, and the contraction stress test (CST), or oxytocin challenge test (OCT). These are usually done in the last trimester of pregnancy.

The NST assesses the response of the fetal heart rate to fetal movement. The contraction stress test assesses the response of the fetal heart rate to uterine contractions. Usually the NST is done first, and if its findings are negative, a contraction stress test is done. These tests are usually repeated weekly until delivery, and give an indication of how the fetus will react to the stress of labor.

For the CST, the woman is placed in a semi-Fowler position, and an external electronic fetal monitor is applied. Recordings of the effect of contractions on the FHR are made. The contractions may be spontaneous, induced by stimulating the woman's nipples or by administering intravenous oxytocin. The desired outcome, or a negative test, is indicated by three good contractions lasting 40 or more seconds within 10 minutes with no late decelerations (Olds et al., 1984). A positive test is indicated by late decelerations in more than half of the contractions. A late deceleration is a periodic decrease in the fetal heart rate that begins late in the contraction and ends after the contraction is over.

For the NST, the woman is placed in a semi-Fowler position, and an external electronic fetal monitor is applied. Recordings of the fetal heart rate and fetal movement are made for 20 to 40 minutes. The desired outcome, or reactive test, is shown by at least two accelerations of 15 beats per minute of the FHR with fetal movements. These accelerations should last 15 seconds or more over a 20-minute period. A nonreactive test indicates that the criteria for the reactive test were not made (Olds et al., 1984).

Maternal Assessment.   Assessment of the mother during childbirth includes collection of subjective and objective data. Subjective data include verbal and nonverbal expressions of feelings, sensations, discomforts, and needs. Observations of facial expressions, muscle tension, body position, and character of respirations, as well as verbalizations, can indicate progression in childbirth.

Objective data include: vital signs (temperature, pulse, respiration, blood pressure); frequency, duration, and intensity of contractions; and the progress of effacement and dilatation of the cervix. Effacement and dilatation of the cervix can be determined by performing a vaginal examination. Other data that can be collected during a vaginal examination are fetal position, station, and presentation.

Psychosocial Assessment

The following four areas of assessment were developed by Clark and Affonso (1979).

Expectations of Childbirth.   It is important to assess what the mother and father expect to happen during the childbirth process. Knowledge of childbirth may range from very little to a great deal, and may be based on experiences of friends and relatives, information gained by reading available literature and discussing questions with health professionals, and/or information received in an instructional setting.

Level of knowledge and understanding of the progression of childbirth needs to be assessed, as well as what the couple expects of the nursing and medical personnel, and what the couple expects of themselves. Influences on these expectations and perceptions include cultural background, past experiences with childbearing, and goals for the couple as perceived by friends, relatives, and health professionals. Culture is an extremely important variable to consider, as it forms the basis of many of our habits and beliefs.

Cultural beliefs and practices determine physical approaches and psychological attitudes toward childbirth. Many non-Western nations use upright (kneeling, sitting, squatting) positions for labor, whereas the supine position is most common in the United States, and the lateral Sim's position is the most common in Britain (Brown, 1981). Touch, or tactile stimulation, has been used in a variety of ways by different cultures (Hedstrom & Newton, 1986). Seen less in Western civilization, touch during childbirth has been used to stimulate contractions and to relieve pain.

Psychological attitudes may vary depending on the value of privacy and the idea of whether childbirth is an achievement or atonement. Some cultures expect the woman to deliver completely alone (Talamancan tribe in South America), and others expect family members and friends to be around to offer comfort and encouragement (Navajo tribe). Some cultures treat childbirth as an achievement and believe that the woman is to be highly praised. Other cultures (Laotians) believe that the woman is unclean and must atone for the birth (Brown, 1981).

Cultural beliefs and practices also involve the father. Couvade is an event that occurs when the father experiences symptoms of pregnancy and sometimes childbirth. The father may experience the couvade syndrome, in which he actually experiences symptoms such as nausea or pain. Or he may experience the couvade ritual, in which he pretends to experience the feelings and sensations.

It is important to assess the cultural beliefs of the childbearing family to increase the knowledge and understanding of health professionals. Inclusion of cultural beliefs with assessment of the various aspects of expectations of childbirth will facilitate the planning of individualized, comprehensive care for the childbearing family.

Meaning of the Labor Experience.   Past experiences, level of knowledge, expectations, and cultural beliefs also influence what the childbirth experience means to the mother and father. This can range from being a life-threatening experience to a self-fulfilling experience. When health professionals are aware of the couple's feelings related to childbirth, they can incorporate these into the plan of care in a way that will facilitate their adaptation to the process. For instance, if the nurse is aware that the mother's aunt died in childbirth and that the mother is terribly afraid that she might die too, the nurse can provide the additional information and support needed in such a situation.

Factors That Increase Stress.   Assessment of factors that might increase stress for the individual couple will provide additional information needed for formulating a plan of care. Here it is important to assess the couple's level of knowledge and attitude toward childbearing, their concerns and fears, and their understanding of what is happening in the environment, whether it be hospital, birthing center, or home. Another area of valuable information is the degree of disruption in their daily activities, that is, are other children taken care of appropriately? Is the husband available, or is he out of town due to his job? Perhaps lack of information, environmental elements such as lights that are too bright or noise that is too loud, or concern about something or someone in the couple's everyday life is intensifying an already stressful situation. If the nurse is aware of this, interventions can be implemented to reduce the stressors and thus improve the outcome of the childbirth experience.

Support System.   Another area of valuable information is that of desired support and available support. Whom does the mother want as a companion? Is that person available? This is an important need that should be addressed. If desired support is not available, how can that need be met? Are other friends or relatives available? Can nursing meet this need for the mother?

Childbirth Education. Assessment of knowledge has been discussed. It is also important to know if the mother and father have attended instructional programs related to childbirth, and if so, exactly what was included in the instruction. There are various educational programs available, such as prenatal classes, childbirth education classes, cesarean section classes, and sibling classes. There are no uniform teaching plans for these; therefore, it is necessary to find out exactly what was taught, who taught it, and when and where the instruction was received. This information provides a basis for determining needs of the couple during childbirth.

Table 3–3 provides a general guide for assessment of the family during childbirth.

ALTERATIONS IN HEALTH

It is not within the scope of this book to address illnesses that may occur during childbirth. Detailed descriptions of illnesses during childbirth, including nursing responsibilities, can be found in current maternity texts. However, some of the illnesses, or alterations in health, that may occur during childbirth will be mentioned here.

Acute Alterations in Health

Acute alterations in health during childbirth include those conditions that usually occur during one childbirth experience only. These might include pregnancy-induced hypertension and some infections, especially infections related to premature rupture of membranes. Other acute conditions include acute anxiety associated with fear of childbirth, preterm or postterm birth, and fetal death during childbirth. Dystocia, or difficult childbirth, may be acute if it is caused by an abnormal position or presentation (breech) of the fetus, fetal developmental abnormalities, multiple pregnancy (twins, triplets), abruptio placentae, placenta previa, or prolapse of the umbilical cord.

Chronic Alterations in Health

Chronic alterations in health during childbirth would include those that occur in subsequent childbirth experiences. Some chronic conditions that might compromise childbirth outcome include diabetes, heart disease, Rh sensitization, herpes, and AIDS. Acute conditions may become chronic if they occur in more than one childbirth experience. Examples of these include recurrent premature labor and recurrent precipitous labor and delivery.

NURSING RESPONSIBILITIES

The general goals of nursing care are as stated in the beginning of this chapter. They are to provide safe and protective care for the mother and fetus and to facilitate the family's adaptation to childbirth. Following the physical and psychosocial assess-

TABLE 3–3. ASSESSING THE FAMILY DURING CHILDBIRTH

	Environmental Data
Provisions for Care	Decisions about environment for childbirth, degree of control, techniques to be performed, presence of support person(s); care of other children in family; availability of adequate resources: equipment, health professionals
	Communication Patterns
Mother	Ability to express feelings, needs, desires in understandable, positive way to caregivers, husband or partner, relatives, friends
Mother and Partner	Ability to express feelings to each other; ability to interpret what each is trying to express, verbally and nonverbally
Among Family Members	Use of constructive methods (confrontation, discussion), nonconstructive methods (blaming, yelling); level of participation
	Problem-Solving Skills
Decision-Making Abilities	How and who makes decisions; role of family members in decision-making process
Use of Health Care System	When instituted, location, accessibility, costs, purposes as perceived by family; preparation for childbirth
Support from Significant Other(s)	Support desired vs. availability, areas of strong support, areas of weak support
Societal Interactions	Use of public agencies (welfare; maternal and infant care project; women, infant, and children program), ease and desirability of interaction with these agencies and programs
	Life-Style
Role of New Family Member	Pregnancy planned or unplanned, course of present pregnancy and other pregnancies and childbirth experiences, how new member will fit into family
Socioeconomic Status (SES)	Estimated yearly income, financial assistance, feelings and plans about SES
Family Roles	Traditional or nontraditional pattern, satisfaction with roles
Work Patterns	Wage earners, type of job(s) held, hours worked, anticipated changes
Recreational Patterns	Amount of free time and how used by family members
Safety	Availability of adequate health care; provision for care of other family members during hospitalization; potential hazards (habits such as smoking, or behaviors such as using seat belts)
	Potential Stressors
Interferences with Individual and Family Tasks	Maternal diseases, infections; difficulties with childbirth process due to maternal, fetal, or other problems
Conflict with Society	Societal (including relatives') acceptance of childbirth environment and outcome
Family Response Patterns	Restructuring or reordering goals, priorities; acceptance of events

ment of the mother, fetus, and family, the nurse formulates nursing diagnoses and plans care. Care is individualized to meet the special needs of each mother and her family, whether the mother is an adult or an adolescent, or whether she is single, married, separated, divorced, or widowed. Nursing care during childbirth can come under the headings of anticipatory guidance, education, care giving, and advocacy.

Preventive Measures

Anticipatory guidance involves actions directed at preventing pregnant clients from becoming involved in situations that will deplete them of emotional and physical energy (Clausen, 1979). A great deal of anticipatory guidance is indicated in the prenatal period, and part of it should relate to the process of childbirth. During childbirth itself, the parents, friends, and other relatives will need guidance regarding policies and physical setup of the facility, and expectations, participation, and progression of labor.

Health Promotion

Educator. Education is an important aspect of nursing care and can enrich the childbirth experience for the family. The mother's and family's level of knowledge of the childbirth process is assessed and appropriate interventions planned and implemented (NAACOG, 1981). The nurse supports the mother and family and encourages their participation in childbirth by providing information at regular intervals related to the progression of labor and other aspects of the childbirth environment about which the mother and family need information. They may need information about fetal monitoring, ways to cope with contractions, positions of comfort, reasons for intravenous fluids and minimal oral intake, characteristics of newborns, and parent–infant attachment.

Advocate. An advocate is one who "pleads or speaks for another" (Allee, 1975). A nurse is an advocate for a childbearing couple when he or she assesses the couple's needs and desires and works with agencies and institutions to see that their needs are met. For instance, a nurse might approach the appropriate people and committees in a hospital so that a couple might be able to utilize family-centered childbirth practices.

Counselor. As a counselor, the nurse assists the mother and her family in obtaining the necessary information upon which to base decisions. The nurse provides a nonjudgmental atmosphere and facilitates the progression through the decision-making process. In childbirth, the nurse may act as counselor in high-risk situations, such as premature labor; in situations where there are choices regarding alternatives for childbirth; and in situations such as the death of a newborn.

Caregiver. The nurse functions as a provider of physical and emotional care. Within this context, the nurse's relationship with the mother and her family is a helping relationship. The nurse, other members of the health care team, and the mother and family help one another to develop a plan of care that effectively meets their needs. This helping relationship is characterized by empathy, understanding, respect, and care (Clark & Affonso, 1979).

While providing physical and emotional support for the mother, the nurse also assists the husband or significant other in feeling confident about his tasks and his participation in the process.

An important part of providing care during childbirth is facilitating parent–child attachment. Two significant interventions based on previously cited research are the encouragement of the presence of a support person and early interaction with the infant.

In the situation of perinatal loss or death, the nurse provides care that allows the parents to grieve, such as letting them cry and express their feelings. The nurse can also provide an opportunity for the parents to hold their infant and take photographs. The nurse can be a sympathetic listener and a compassionate source of information (NAACOG, 1984).

SUMMARY

The goals of the health care team when giving care during the childbirth process are to provide a safe and protective environment for the mother and fetus, and to facilitate the adaptation of the mother, infant, and family. The nurse uses the nursing process to plan care directed at meeting these goals. The assessment component of the nursing process includes data collection related to physical and psychosocial factors.

Potential stressors occurring in childbirth include those that are already present in the mother and affect childbirth, and those that arise from the childbirth process itself.

The family's adaptation to childbirth is determined by variables such as alternative birthing environments and family-centered maternity care. Parent–infant attachment is an important outcome and is influenced by parental backgrounds and health care practices.

The impact of childbirth on family members differs for each person and each situation, but there are some commonalities.

The nurse's role in childbirth includes providing anticipatory guidance, education, and care, and being an advocate and counselor.

CARE PLAN FOR THE FAMILY CONCERNED WITH CHILDBIRTH

Situation

Cathy Martin, a 23-year-old white woman, pregnant for the first time, is admitted to a hospital labor and delivery suite at 7:00 AM. She is 39 weeks pregnant, and is accompanied by her husband, Bill. She states that her contractions began 2 hours ago and are about 10 minutes apart. Her "water broke" 1 hour ago. She has had no bleeding.

According to her prenatal record, Cathy has gained 22 pounds; her last hemoglobin was 12 g, her blood pressure has ranged from 110/70 to 120/80, the FHR has been 120–140, and her history indicates no risk factors.

Cathy's present blood pressure is 124/82, pulse is 90, respirations 24, and FHR 136 (auscultated in the right lower quadrant of her abdomen). A vaginal exam reveals that her cervix is 3 cm dilated, 50% effaced, and that the head is at 0 station. Fetal movement is felt by Cathy and the nurse. Contractions are every 5–7 minutes, 40 seconds long, and of moderate intensity.

Cathy and Bill indicate that this pregnancy was planned, and that they are both excited about having a baby. Cathy is a teacher (unemployed at this time), and Bill is in military service. Bill was transferred to this area 1 month ago. Both of their families live great distances from this area. Due to the recent transfer, Cathy and Bill have not been able to attend childbirth education classes. Cathy expresses a fear of childbirth because of her lack of experience and knowledge. Bill wishes their families were closer so that they would have their support. Both describe positive (normal vaginal delivery of healthy infants) and negative (birth of stillborn) childbirth experiences in their family histories.

Nursing Diagnoses

1. Knowledge deficit related to childbirth process.
2. Social isolation related to lack of close proximity of extended family and being new to community.
3. Anxiety related to fear of unknown: process and outcome of childbirth.

SAMPLE CARE PLAN

Nursing Diagnoses	Goal	Interventions	Evaulation
Anxiety related to fear of unknown: process and outcome of childbirth.	Cathy and Bill will recognize their anxiety and use effective coping mechanisms in managing anxiety.	1. Assess level of anxiety 2. Provide physical and emotional support 3. Decrease sensory stimulation 4. Encourage Cathy and Bill to express their feelings, identify coping mechanisms 5. Provide instruction related to relaxation techniques, the childbirth process, and constructive problem solving	Cathy and Bill discuss their anxieties about not knowing what will happen during labor and delivery, and not knowing for sure that their baby will be normal and healthy. They admit that ultrasounds done during the pregnancy have been normal, and that there have been no signs of any problems. After discussing their anxieties, learning more about the childbirth process, and using imagery as a relaxation technique, Cathy and Bill both say they feel better. Their voices are quieter, and facial expressions relaxed.

SAMPLE CARE PLAN *(continued)*

Nursing Diagnoses	Goal	Interventions	Evaluation
Knowledge deficit related to childbirth process	Cathy and Bill will demonstrate understanding of the childbirth process, including stages, and expected physical, emotional, and behavioral manifestations, and participate actively in the process.	1. Assess contributing factors 2. Assess readiness to learn 3. Develop and implement a plan to meet learning needs related to childbirth environment, techniques and procedures	Following instruction related to the childbirth process, Cathy and Bill ask questions about the stages of labor and particularly, what will happen to their baby following the birth. Bill continues to help Cathy through each contraction.
Social isolation related to lack of close proximity of extended family and being new to community	Cathy and Bill will identify the reasons for their feelings of isolation and identify appropriate coping mechanisms.	1. Identify contributing factors 2. Encourage Cathy and Bill to talk about their feelings 3. Assist Cathy and Bill to identify ways to communicate with extended family 4. Identify strategies to meet people in community	Cathy and Bill readily discuss their feelings of loneliness. They discuss ideas for meeting people (military and religious organizations) and communicating with relatives (phone calls and letters).

Review Questions

1. Discuss two aspects of psychosocial assessment and their relationship to childbirth.
2. List three potential stressors and describe their effect on childbirth.
3. Describe the major differences among the various methods of childbirth.
4. Describe the nurse's role in assisting a couple having their first child in a birthing center.

REFERENCES

Affonso, D. D. (1979). Application of psychosocial concepts. In A. L. Clark & D. D. Affonso (Eds.), *Childbearing: A nursing perspective.* Philadelphia: Davis.
Affonso, D. D. (Ed.) (1981). *Impact of cesarean childbirth.* Philadelphia: Davis.
Affonso, D. D., & Domino, G. (1981). A perspective on fathers: A question of facts and fallacies. In D. D. Affonso (Ed.), *Impact of cesarean childbirth.* Philadelphia: Davis.
Affonso, D. D., & Stichler, J. (1981). Impact on women: Feelings and perceptions. In D. D. Affonso (Ed.), *Impact of cesarean childbirth.*Philadelphia: Davis.

Allee, J. G. (Ed.) (1975). *Webster's dictionary.* Ottenheimer.

Anderson, S. (1981). Birth of siblings: Children's perceptions and interpretations. In S. Anderson & P. Simkin (Eds.), *Birth through children's eyes.* Seattle: Pennypress.

Borg, S., & Lasker, J. (1981). *When pregnancy fails.* Boston: Beacon Press.

Brown, M. S. (1981). Culture and childrearing. In A. L. Clark (Ed.), *Culture and childrearing.* Philadelphia: Davis.

Clark, A. L. (Ed.) (1981). *Culture and childrearing.* Philadelphia: Davis.

Clark, A. L., & Affonso, D. D., with Harris, T. R. (Eds.) (1979). *Childbearing: A nursing perspective.* Philadelphia: Davis.

Clausen, J. P. (1979). Anticipatory guidance of the expectant family. In D. P. Hymovich & M. U. Barnard (Eds.), *Family health care.* New York: McGraw-Hill.

Cropley, C. (1986). Assessment of mothering behaviors. In S. H. Johnson (Ed.), *High-risk parenting: Nursing assessment and strategies for the family at risk.* Philadelphia: Lippincott.

Duvall, E. M. (1977). *Marriage and family development* (5th ed.). New York: Lippincott.

Furman, E. P. (1982). Some thoughts on the father–child relationship. In M. H. Klaus & M. O. Robertson (Eds.), *Birth, interaction and attachment.* Skillman, NJ: Johnson & Johnson Baby Products Co.

Gorvine, B., Hawkins, J. W., Fazeka, N. F., & Mott, S. (1982). *Health care of women: Labor and delivery.* Belmont, CA: Wadsworth Health Sciences Division.

Hangsleben, K. L. (1983). Transition to fatherhood—An exploratory study. *Journal of Obstetric, Gynecologic, and Neonatal Nursing, 12,* 265–270.

Hedstrom, L. W., & Newton, N. (1986). Touch in labor: A comparison of cultures and eras. *Birth, 13,* 181–186.

Interprofessional Task Force on Health Care of Women and Children (1978). *Joint position statement of the development of family-centered maternity/newborn care in hospitals.* Chicago: Interprofessional Task Force on Health Care of Women and Children.

Jensen, M. D., & Bobak, I. M. (1985). *Maternity and gynecologic care.* St. Louis: Mosby.

Klaus, M. H., & Kennell, J. H. (1982). *Parent–infant bonding* (2nd ed.). St. Louis: Mosby.

Kruk, S. (1981). Pregnancy and the single woman. In S. Wolkind & E. Zajicek (Eds.), *Pregnancy: A psychological and social study.* New York: Grune & Stratton.

Lubic, R. W. (1983). Childbirthing centers: Delivering more for less. *American Journal of Nursing, 83,* 1053–1056.

McKay, S. (1982). *Humanizing maternity services through family-centered care.* Minneapolis, Minnesota: International Childbirth Education Association.

McKay, S., & Phillips, C. R. (1984). *Family-centered maternity care.* Rockville, Maryland: Aspen Systems Corporation.

Mercer, R. T., Hackley, K. C., & Bostrom, A. G. (1983). Relationship of Psychosocial and Perinatal Variables to Perception of Childbirth. *Nursing Research, 32,* 202–207.

Moore, M. L. (1983). *Realities in childbearing* (2nd ed.). Philadelphia: Saunders.

NAACOG (1984). Perinatal loss and grief: Part I. *NAACOG Newsletter, 11,* 1.

Nicholson, J., Gist, N. F., Klein, R. R., & Standley, K. F. (1983). Outcomes of father involvement in pregnancy and birth. *Birth, 10,* 5–9.

The Nurses Association of The American College of Obstetricians and Gynecologists (1981). *Standards for obstetric, gynecologic, and neonatal nursing* (2nd ed.). Washington, D.C.: NAACOG.

Olds, S. B., London, M. L., & Ladewig, P. A. (1984). *Maternal-newborn nursing–A family centered approach* (2nd ed.). Menlo Park, California: Addison-Wesley.

Palkovitz, R. (1982). Fathers' birth attendance, early extended contact, and father-infant interaction at five months postpartum. *Birth, 9,* 173–177.

Phillips, C. R., & Anzalone, J. T. (Eds.) (1982). *Fathering.* St. Louis: Mosby.

Pillitteri, A. (1981). *Maternal-newborn nursing.* Boston: Little, Brown.

Pritchard, J. A., & MacDonald, P. C. (1980). *William's Obstetrics.* New York: Appleton-Century-Crofts.

Reed, G., & Schmid, M. (1986). Nursing implementation of single-room maternity care. *Journal of Obstetric, Gynecologic, and Neonatal Nursing, 15,* 386–389.

Sumner, P. E., & Phillips, C. R. (1981). *Birthing rooms—Concept and reality.* St. Louis: Mosby.

Tankson, E. A. (1986). The single parent. In S. H. Johnson (Ed.), *High-risk parenting: Nursing assessment and strategies for the family at risk.* Philadelphia: Lippincott.

Thomas, C. L. (Ed.) (1981). *Taber's cyclopedic medical dictionary.* Philadelphia: Davis.

Yogman, M. W. (1982). Observations on the father–infant relationship. In S. H. Cath, A. R. Gurwitt, & J. M. Ross (Eds.), *Father and child—Developmental and clinical perspectives.* Boston: Little, Brown.

4

The Family with a Neonate
First Month of Life

Martha J. Bradshaw

OBJECTIVES

Upon completion of this chapter, the student will be able to:

1. Identify family tasks during the neonatal period
2. Evaluate the impact of the neonate on the family in terms of role adaptation
3. Determine parental responses and expectations to the arrival of the neonate
4. Identify the developmental tasks of the neonate
5. Predict the influence of task accomplishment during the neonatal period on the success of task accomplishment during infancy
6. Recognize potential stressors and appropriate coping mechanisms commonly occurring during the neonatal period
7. Examine threats to the health of the neonate and their effects on individual and family development
8. Describe varied nursing interventions seen during the neonatal period

CONCEPTS

Adjustment to extrauterine life: series of physiologic adaptive processes that enable the neonate to function independently of the mother

Attachment: strong enduring relationship between the neonate and another person

Engrossment: period of intensive interaction between the father and the neonate

Reciprocity: mutually interactive relationship between the neonate and another person

The neonatal period is from birth until the child is 28 days or 4 weeks old (Moore, 1983). During this time the family unit begins to experience growth and changes. Physical size of the unit expands to include this new member, or sometimes members. This is the most obvious change that takes place in a family, because it is an immediate transition. The long-anticipated event has finally occurred, and the new parents and family members experience a myriad of feelings. The cohesion of the family solidifies. The birth of a baby many times creates a family out of what has been a couple or an individual person. Development as a *family* begins, and the family unit begins certain developmental tasks. These tasks have two origins: (1) physical maturity and (2) cultural pressures and privileges (Duvall, 1977). The individual developmental tasks of adults must begin to parallel family developmental tasks that are crucial for functioning in a positive, loving, supportive atmosphere. In cases in which the birth of this baby is the addition of the second, third, or fourth child, the family reinstitutes the various roles and functions that took place with the first child, but with appropriate alterations according to the size of the family and ages of the members.

FAMILY TASKS

The developmental tasks experienced by families as the neonate is added are:

1. Resolving the birthing experience
2. Meeting physical and emotional needs of the neonate
3. Assigning roles
4. Incorporating the neonate into the family
5. Reallocating resources

Certain elements of each task are dealt with by specific family members. As will be seen in this and subsequent chapters, some family tasks are in conflict with certain individual developmental tasks.

Resolving the Birthing Experience

The family members, especially the parent(s), experience varied physical and psychological readjustments after delivery of a baby. The period of childbirth can be looked upon as one of crisis, from which one must recover. Childbirth is also a major occurrence in life that cannot be undone or disregarded. However the family members consider the birthing experience, it is a situation that requires resolution and return to regular patterns of daily living. This recovery period consists of phases that are felt in differing degrees by each member.

The mother recognizes a priority of physical recovery. She initially feels fatigue, hunger, thirst, and perhaps some pain. She then acknowledges the need to care for her body in order to promote involution (return of reproductive organs to their nonpregnant state) and healing. The involutional period lasts approximately 2–3 weeks, and her postpartal recovery is considered complete at about 4–6 weeks.

Reva Rubin (1960) has identified phases or change behaviors characteristic of postpartal mothers. These behaviors are:

Taking-in (first 3 days): fatigue, need to discuss delivery, self-oriented, dependent upon others for care
Taking hold (3–10 days): more active, oriented to present, initiates activities and mothering

They reflect the focus of energy and attention of the part of the mother as she recovers from birth. Evidence now exists that mothers are spending shorter amounts of time in the taking-in phase (Martell & Mitchell, 1984). Much of this is due to the encouragement by nurses of early ambulation and self-care.

The father will also need to recover from the stress, anxiety, and fatigue of the labor and delivery period. Whether he coached and supported the mother during the labor or worried and paced elsewhere while waiting, he also experienced a strenuous period, from which he needs to feel rested and refreshed. Then both parents begin to rejoice over the birth of their baby.

The initial postpartum period consists of an emotional high, from which the new parents must come down. They experience exhilaration, joy, and countless other feelings. They take inordinate pleasure in retelling the birthing experience to anyone who will listen. As with any other critical event in one's life, reliving the birthing experience enables the individuals to deal with all facets of it, and begin to accept the fact that the period is truly over. Also, many couples wish to share their pride in completing a natural birthing experience, or want others to know what their thoughts and feelings were when they first saw their baby. This emotional high may take a few weeks to resolve, and most parents continue to remember the more outstanding instances associated with each child's birth.

The new parent(s) must next accept the reality of the situation, mainly that the baby, which has long been expected, has truly been delivered, and is on the outside for all to see. The parent often gazes in wonderment at the neonate, in order to come to this realization that the baby is indeed *here*. At the same time, the adults must begin to deal with the fact that they are *parents*, and that this calls for certain duties and responsibilities. It is also necessary to begin to relate to or identify with the neonate, to develop the close bond and affectional ties between parent and child.

One of the earliest forms of identification with the baby, which has great significance, is naming the baby. Rubin (1984) points out that naming the baby is a form of claiming the baby, affirming his or her existence and belonging in the family. Most parents give naming a great deal of thought because of its lifelong significance for the baby. This is also one of the first instances in which the parents collaborate on something concerning their new child. Naming can have a great impact on the extended family because of names selected or discarded based upon their association with other family members. Giving the newborn a family name probably heightens the baby's place in the extended family.

As the parents identify with the baby, they also try to learn their baby's early rhythms, personality, and cues. Unfortunately, because the neonate changes in appearance so quickly, sometimes from one day to the next, some parents become confused about their baby's appearance, and wonder when they can be sure they will know what their baby really looks like. After the baby has been settled into the household and the parents become more familiar with him or her, their identification increases. Role acceptance and identification with the baby is at its peak during the first month of life, and seems fairly complete or leveled off by 2–3 months (Rubin, 1984).

Meeting Physical and Emotional Needs of the Neonate

Physical needs are of top priority as individual tasks for the neonate for two outstanding reasons. First, the neonate previously existed in a totally dependent state as a fetus. The baby is accustomed to automatically having all physiological needs met and has never experienced discomfort or deprivation. Second, the metabolic rate of the neonate is quite high, which means he or she will require physiological needs to be met often. Consequently, physical care seems to be the predominant family undertaking during the neonatal period. Sometimes the approaches to meeting these needs can be a source of disagreement or friction among family members. Proper room environment can be a conflict area. Most babies are born in hospitals or clinic settings with environmentally controlled temperature and humidity. Leaving the hospital gives the baby a first exposure to any climate difference. At home, the parent may feel that the baby should have a warm room so that he or she will not catch cold. Consequently, the room temperature may be kept at 85°F, which may be too warm for the rest of the family. In many cases, the baby is born in an air-conditioned hospital, but lives in an unairconditioned or unheated home. In either instance, the major caretaker should attempt to start the baby in environmental conditions as similar to those at the time of birth as possible, then gradually work the baby into a temperature setting that is comfortable for the entire family. This can be done by gradual thermostat adjustments or the use of fans or space heaters.

Family involvement with nutrition for the neonate can be equally shared, or can be quite limited. Much of this will depend upon whether the baby is being breast- or bottle-fed. The type of feeding pattern chosen is often done after great deliberation, mind-changing, and advice-seeking. Breast-feeding goes through phases of popularity in America, with the general population seeing a swing from one to the other method about every 10 to 15 years. These cycles have an interesting historical pattern, based upon research findings on the many properties of breast-milk and on industrial development of a variety of infant formulas. The decision to breast- or formula-feed is often influenced by previous experience or experiences of close friends or family members. Most parents, especially the mother, compare the advantages and disadvantages of each method when trying to determine which to use. While numerous advantages and disadvantages of each type of feeding can be cited, some of the more outstanding advantages of breast- and formula-feeding are cited in Table 4-1. These advantages have a direct influence on the mother and baby, with secondary effects on the other family members. Breast-feeding gives the mother a

TABLE 4–1. ADVANTAGES OF BREAST- AND BOTTLE (FORMULA)-FEEDING

Breast	Bottle
More nutritive value	Less physical demand on mother
Provides immunological properties	More acceptable in public
Sterile	Convenient when mother away
Immediately available	No concerns over maternal diet
Inexpensive	No transmission of drugs
Decreases chances of overfeeding	Psychological or physiological preparation not
Decreases transfer of allergens	needed
More digestible	
Increases maternal contact	
Provides natural nipple shape	

From Ritchey, S. J., and Taper, L. J. (1983) Maternal and child nutrition. New York: Harper & Row.

special time with the baby, but tends to exclude the rest of the family. Small children may be particularly resentful of this, and may try to interfere or interrupt the feeding. This disruption may interfere with the mother's let-down reflex, inhibiting milk flow.

Daily hygiene is practiced by care of the baby following bowel and bladder functions and by bathing. Diapering is one of the first things that comes to mind when one thinks of a baby. Perhaps this is because diapering is done more often than any other aspect of baby care, with feeding being in second place. Also, diapering can become an unpleasant task in many ways. While urine is normally sterile, the fact that it is a body waste makes the handling of wet diapers esthetically unpleasant. For this reason, many new parents or unexperienced family members may have some difficulty with this aspect of care. The stools of the newborn, which may occur more than once a day, are usually soft and not as odorous as those of the infant. Because the odor in stools is from intestinal flora and ingested food, the baby who is breast-fed is more likely to have stools with very little odor.

Bathing the baby can be a most pleasant task and is a time for optimal interaction between the newborn and a family member. Parents are encouraged not to bathe their newborn until the remaining umbilical cord falls off and the stump is healed (after about the 10th day of life). The baby is then slowly introduced into a warm water bath and constantly held with full support of the head and neck. For this reason, it is best that the baby be bathed by an adult, who is more cognizant of the need to support the baby and help him or her feel secure.

All family members can ensure proper hygiene and stop the spread of disease to the newborn by practicing handwashing, especially after diapering. Encouraging each member to avoid breathing directly in the baby's face and controlling what the baby puts into his or her mouth will give further protection.

The family members contribute to the meeting of the neonate's emotional needs while they are simultaneously meeting needs of their own. As shall be seen in the section on individual tasks of the neonate, the forming of the parent–child relationship is one of mutual satisfaction. Initially, the neonate relates to the mother because of her warmth and the physical security of cuddling. The neonate also studies the mother closely as a learning pattern, because hers is often the earliest and most frequent face the baby sees. The mother interprets this as her baby's desire to become acquainted. The father also spends intimate, involved time getting to know his baby. This period of acquaintance is termed *engrossment*. The father becomes acquainted with his baby through visual and tactile awareness—touching and looking at his child. Like mothers, fathers exhibit specific patterns of behavior: the early encounters with the neonate find the father looking for distinct features in his child, especially ones that link the child with himself. This deep physical interaction gives the father a sense of elation and heightened self-esteem. If engrossed, the father will be much more concerned and involved with his child (like the attached mother). This caring paternalism lasts beyond the neonatal period. The father who has had early contact with his child is more likely to sustain contact as the child grows (Greenberg & Morris, 1974).

Throughout the neonatal period, the parents will continue to provide the warm, loving interaction that the baby instinctively craves. In return, the attention the baby gives to the parents will heighten their sense of fulfillment in the new parenting role.

Assigning Roles

Family expansion with the addition of a newborn requires role identification and modification. The family members must re-establish previous roles and launch new ones. Questions that were previously unanswered or were nominally addressed become a target for major discussion and adjustment: Where will the baby sleep? Will that work? Who will feed the baby during the night? Are you going to nurse the baby in the bed with me? Do we take turns with diaper changes? Can you change your work hours?

Adult family members, especially the parent(s), find that besides continuing their personal growth as individuals, their life has taken on the new dimension of parenthood. Hrbosky (1977) feels that the ability to work through this transition to parenthood is largely influenced by the relationship the parents have as a couple. Because the parental dyad is the genesis of the expanding family, its stability is central to the stability of that family. In the case of new parents who are not living together (unwed teenagers, as an example), affectional and supportive bonds are not as strong, and they may not view themselves as a couple. Consequently, they would have more difficulty accepting parental roles thrust upon them.

In established couples, the potential for conflict between individual and parental roles is evident in Table 4–2. This table displays just a few of the roles that exist for parents. An adult who is experiencing difficulty in one of the roles that accompany marriage, such as provider or sexual partner, will experience even further difficulties when a new set of roles is presented. Some roles, such as nurturer, are not exclusively parenting roles but are also seen in spousal interactions. For the single parent, the

TABLE 4–2. ROLES OF THE ADULT FAMILY MEMBER

Provider	Nurturer	Homemaker
Sexual partner	Disciplinarian	Social organizer
Companion	Caretaker	Security figure
Authoritarian	Competitor for spousal affection	

conflicts are of a different perspective. Some of the roles, such as competitor for affection or consistent sexual partner, may never be fulfilled and/or may not be appropriate for that particular family. The single parent finds that, instead of working through role assignment, he or she has the frustrating task of accomplishing the roles alone.

The new parent(s) must not only assign roles for themselves, but for other family members as well. This is usually expected and accepted by the family members, and is viewed as the parents' prerogative. The parent will need to assign, either verbally or behaviorally, the roles the siblings will take. Siblings may experience little change in their lives, or they may add the role of part-time caretaker for the baby. The new grandparents may discover that they are also caretakers, or they may be treated as visitors.

If roles are assumed, rather than assigned, this can cause even greater conflict and confusion. Direct communication is most important in promoting clear delineation of various roles. It is also helpful for the major caretakers to anticipate specific roles that will need to be adopted as the baby changes. This will be easier on everyone than if they learn as they go, making each developmental stage a crisis.

Incorporating the Neonate into the Family

Incorporating the neonate into the family is important for two reasons. First, it will alleviate resentment that develops because the baby is new, and therefore intriguing. This resentment is particularly strong in nuclear family members—siblings and the parent who is competing for affection. Resentment may be mild, and even expected at first, when the newborn is in the spotlight. But if the baby continues to hold this place of importance, the resentment mounts, and can result in inappropriate behavior, anger, and guilt. Second, the contributions the neonate makes to the overall family are symbolic, rather than real (Rubin, 1984). The neonate represents the physical love between the man and woman, and also is an example of the desire of the parents to perpetuate the family line, especially reproducing one's own self. The baby's seemingly purposeless existence (in the eyes of young siblings) can cause his or her needs or demands to seem intrusive and disrupting. Consequently, it is even more important for the parents to begin the incorporation of the newborn as soon as possible, specifically to make everyone feel like *equal* family members.

The mediator of the family, who is frequently the major caretaker, should make the neonate a part of the family. This can be done in a variety of ways, aimed at adapting the baby to the situation, not vice versa. One example is not tiptoeing around the house when the baby is asleep, but conducting usual activities. If all family members are involved in some aspect of baby care, or an attempt is made to give each member a special amount of attention, the baby will not seem so special.

Reallocation of Resources

As families expand with new members, they are confronted with the fact that their income does not usually increase proportionately. With a new baby, there are the usual necessities such as food and clothing, plus additional needs such as baby furniture, toys, and medical expenses. The low-income or strictly budgeted household may not be able to purchase these additional needs, as they may be having a great deal of difficulty with the necessities. Sometimes financial rearrangement is planned before the baby is born, with minor adjustments for specific needs. In some families, the financial area is not considered until the baby is born and the actual needs addressed.

Determining expenditures is usually done by the member or members who have been the wage earners for the family. Some families are organized so that the wage earner also pays the bills and handles finances. In other families, one member earns the money but designates another member to handle the budget. No longer is the father strictly the only or major wage earner in a family. Consequently, financial planning may be a joint decision by all those bringing money into the household. A single parent, living alone, generally has full responsibility, both as provider and in decision making. Families receiving financial assistance find that they may have no say in what monies they receive, and must learn to work within that system to increase their benefits as necessary.

INDIVIDUAL TASKS

The neonatal period is characterized primarily by physical changes. Stabilization of body systems and achievement of independent physiological functioning are priority accomplishments for the newborn. However, development and growth in the neonate are not exclusively physical. The neonate takes in information, integrates it, and establishes a foundation that aids in more complex task accomplishment as an infant and toddler.

Physical Development

The period immediately after delivery is a time of great transition for the neonate. There is a drastic change from a dark, thermally controlled water bath, with maternal sounds and movements, to a colder, drier, noisier, bright environment. The neonate begins to use his or her body and functions independently in the physiological sense.

In the transition to extrauterine life, the first 24 hours after delivery are termed the *period of reactivity*. The neonate progresses through a predictable pattern of adjustment and is observed closely during this time.

The initial reactivity time takes place within the first 15 to 30 minutes after birth and is characterized by generalized systemic activity. Immediate responses upon delivery are cry, exchange of respirations, general motor activity, and blinking as the eyes begin to accommodate. The heart rate increases, the baby makes some facial movements such as grimacing or sucking, becomes alert, and begins purposeful movements, such as exploring. The establishment of respirations is thought to be related to one or several contributing factors: (1) reflex—an action whose mechanism remains unclear, but is thought to be the result of stimulation of airway receptors in the bronchial tree; (2) chemical—as a response to exposure to carbon dioxide; (3)

thermal—the cold environment causes the baby to gasp, thus beginning pulmonary function; and (4) tactile or pressure sensation—the squeezing on the thorax during delivery, plus the new sensation of being handled by people. The initial respiratory rate is irregular and rapid, at about 40–50/min. The neonate may void some very dilute urine, and it is quite common for the neonate to pass the first stool, called *meconium*, as a response to the cephalic pressure from delivery. Meconium is a dark greenish-black substance, of sticky, tarry consistency. It is the waste by-product of fetal life, and consists of mucus, vernix, bile, fats, and cellular by-products.

Maintaining warmth is of top priority for the neonate. As mentioned, the neonate leaves an environment of about 98 or 99°F to enter one of about 70°F. Because newborns have little subcutaneous fat, there is little heat insulation. Newborns do not shiver in response to cold as adults do, because their peripheral neuromuscular responses are not well established.

The cardiovascular system assists in maintaining a proper body temperature. As the baby experiences chilling, vasoconstriction of the extremities occurs, thus shunting blood to vital organs. It is for this reason, along with immature peripheral responses, that the neonate almost always has bluish or pale hands and feet. The newborn further produces body heat by increasing body activity or conserves heat by reassuming the fetal position. These are early signs that the newborn is experiencing chilling or cold stress. If proper warmth has been provided, the skin temperature will stabilize within the first 12 hours of life at 97.6°F.

After the initial postdelivery reactivity, the neonate will be quiet for about 1 to 1½ hours. The heart and respiratory rates will slow, no meconium or urine will be passed, and the baby will sleep, with few responses to stimuli. In the next 2–6 hours, the neonate will experience a second period of reactivity, with an increase in respirations and a varying heart rate. The neonate will once again pass meconium and will present some oral mucus. The neonate is alert to stimuli, and some early reflex actions, such as gagging, are exhibited. It is at this time that the neonate displays some of the effects of extrauterine life and the physiological results of maternal separation. The baby is subject to hypoglycemia, apnea, and a drop in body temperature. There will also be some transient tachypnea, which may be present for several days.

As the cardiovascular system becomes established, kidney function improves. The newborn voids often, but in very dilute amounts. This is because the loop of Henle is short, and the kidney is unable to concentrate urine (Moore, 1983).

Liver immaturity is evident during the early neonatal period. Bilirubin, a by-product of the breakdown of red blood cells, must be converted by the liver to a water-soluble form to be excreted by the kidneys. The liver cannot fully complete this process in the first days of life. Consequently, the bilirubin is not in an excretable form, and it continues to circulate until it is deposited into the subcutaneous tissues, causing jaundice.

Production of clotting factors in the liver is also impaired. The neonatal level of Vitamin K, a necessary component for this process, falls below normal 2–3 days after birth. Typically, Vitamin K is synthesized from ingested nutrients by intestinal bacteria. Until intestinal flora have become established, the steps in the process are delayed.

Endocrine gland activity in the neonate is subject to hormonal influence from the mother. Breast engorgement of both male and female babies is not uncommon, and some newborns have a thin, watery discharge from the nipples called *witch's milk*. Some female newborns experience vaginal spotting. Only small amounts of antidiuretic hormone (ADH) are excreted, which also contributes to the frequent manufacture of dilute urine.

While most term neonates experience this period of reactivity in a similar manner, the first 2 to 3 days after birth are a time for close scrutiny by the caregivers, in order to assess the typical progression or a variation from normal.

Certain physical parameters are normal exclusively during the neonatal period. The neonate often exhibits certain skin findings, which are assessed and noted

TABLE 4–3. COMMON NEONATAL FINDINGS

Finding	Description	Remarks
Skin		
Lanugo	Soft, downy hair; covers body of fetus	Seen on shoulders, arms, back. May be absent in term baby.
Vernix caseosa	White, cream cheese-like substance; water, sebum, oil composition	Protects skin from amniotic fluid in utero; lubricates for passage through birth canal
Milia	White sebaceous cysts found on nose and chin	Disappear in few weeks
Mongolian spots	Dark, bluish-black marking; seen on sacrum and buttocks	Usually seen in black babies; disappears in weeks or few months
Erythema toxicum	Macular rash, usually on trunk	Nonsignificant, disappears in few days
Cyanosis	Bluish or pale tinge common in hands and feet	Extremely normal phenomenon for first 24–48 hours
Hemangiomas:		
Nevus flammeus (Port wine stain)	Macular, purple or deep red marking, anywhere on body	Does not fade; may be treated with laser therapy
Capillary (Stork's beak mark)	Pink patch between eyebrows or at base of neck	Fades until gone by end of first year
Strawberry	Deep red, papular area	Enlarges some until end of first year, then shrinks
Impetigo	Papular rash, crusts	Bacterial infection
Jaundice	Yellow tinge to skin, sclera	From deposited bilirubin or liver irregularity; will fade
Head		
Fontaneles	Anterior is diamond-shaped, posterior is triangular	Anterior closes at 12–18 months; posterior closes at end of second month
Molding	Temporary shaping to allow head to pass through vaginal canal	Normal shape returns after 2–3 days
Caput succedaneum	Edema of scalp at presenting part of head	Edema absorbed and disappeared by third day
Cephalhematoma	Collection of blood between bone and periosteum due to pressure during birth	Requires weeks to reabsorb

Adapted From: Moore, M. L. (1983) Realities in Childbearing, 2nd Ed. Philadelphia: W. B. Saunders

during the routine physical exam. Table 4–3 identifies these more common findings. The neurological status of the neonate is also evaluated by assessing the presence of specific reflexes. These reflexes are indices of the newborn's neuromuscular integrity and also reflect the newborn's habituation with the environment. The tonic neck reflex, for example, dominates the baby's waking time and is a precursor to symmetrical behavior (Gesell, 1955). Prolonged persistence of some of these reflexes could indicate cerebral palsy, and an abnormal finding on a neurological exam could indicate major nerve injury. Table 4–4 describes the more common reflexes and indicates that while some of the findings are exclusive to the neonate, many neurological reflexes that are well developed at birth persist throughout lifetime.

Having progressed through the transitory stage following birth, the newborn

TABLE 4–4. NEONATAL REFLEXES

Reflex	Manner of Elicitation	Age When Disappears	Comments
Moro	A hand clap or slap on the mattress. Consistent absence	from 1 to 3–4 months	Consistent absence suggests brain damage.
Tonic neck	When the baby is supine and the head is turned to one side, the arm and leg extend while the opposite arm and leg are flex in a "fencing" position.	During the first 6 months	If persistent asymmetry and a full response are easily obtained, a cerebral lesion is suggested
Stepping	When held erect and body supported under the arms with soles flat on table top and trunk inclined forward, baby takes regular, alternating steps	6 weeks	Failure to step on several occasions suggests neurological abnormality; stepping with only one foot indicates a unilateral problem
Palmar grasp	Pressing the examiner's finger into the baby's metacarpophalangeal groove causes the baby to grasp the finger	4–6 months	Unequal grasp could indicate unilateral problem
Planter grasp	Pressure on the plantar surface of the foot causes flexion of the toes	8–15 months	
Rooting	Stroking the upper or lower lip or the side of the cheek causes the baby to turn his/her mouth and face toward the stimulus and open his/her mouth.	3–4 months when baby awake; 7–8 months when baby asleep	May be difficult to elicit immediately after feeding
Sucking	Stroking the lips produces sucking	12 months; diminishes at 3–4 months	May be difficult to elicit in recently fed baby; weak or absent in baby with brain damage

Adapted from Moore, M. L. (1981). Newborn, Family, and Nurse, 2nd Ed. Philadelphia: W. B. Saunders.

moves rapidly through physical changes and visible growth. Growth occurs in the areas of height, weight, and volume. Immediately after birth, the neonate loses about 5–10% of the original birth weight, and growth reaches a temporary plateau. This is in response to the adaptation to a different environment—one of the baby's early encounters with stress. After about 2 weeks, there is a noticeable weight gain, and growth continues. Accompanying the increase in size is an increase or refinement of the body systems. For example, the sweat and sebaceous glands begin to function at about 1 month.

One of the outstanding physical/structural changes occurring during the neonatal period takes place within the cardiovascular system. Fetal circulatory structures transport oxygen during intrauterine life. After birth, the neonate's respiratory system takes over oxygen exchange, and the structures are no longer needed. Usually blood pressure changes cause these temporary structures to close, and they are eventually obliterated.

While the central nervous system is immature, both anatomically and physiologically, it is capable of sustaining extrauterine life. Some of the more common and obvious examples of this immaturity are an unstable temperature (due to a young hypothalamus) and uncoordinated gross motor movements. All of the special senses but sight are developed at birth. Because of this, a mother will instinctively hold her baby close in a face-to-face (en face) position to provide better visualization for both.

Of all the senses, touch may be the most significant, because it is linked to affectional responses. Visual perception is best at about 8–12 inches from the eyes. Newborns can hear at birth (if the auditory canals are free of mucus and fluid) and attend to sounds or voices by stopping their activity and turning the head toward the sound. Neonates seem to attend to a higher pitch by becoming more active and alert; a lower pitch is more soothing. Neonates have the ability to taste and prefer sweet over a more bland taste. They are able to smell, and there are indications that the neonate can distinguish his or her own mother by smell (Moore, 1983).

While some instabilities may still be noted, extrauterine transition is considered complete by about 4 weeks (Gesell, 1955).

Nutrition and Elimination Patterns

The breast-fed neonate will probably need to nurse about every 2 or 3 hours until the stomach capacity increases. Because formula is of different composition and slower to be digested, the bottle-fed neonate will probably act hungry about every 4 hours. The usual guideline for bottle preparation and feeding is 2 or 3 ounces of formula (20 kcal/ounce) every 6 hours. This will provide 120 calories/kg of body weight every 24 hours (Whaley & Wong, 1983).

There is a wide variety in stooling patterns among neonates. Some babies stool after every feeding or up to 12 times each day, while some babies stool once a day or every other day. Stooling is more frequent and of softer consistency in the breast-fed baby. Many babies will strain when stooling, but this is not to be considered constipation. A constipated stool is one which is hard and ball-like, rather than soft and loosely formed.

Rest and Activity Patterns

The neonate sleeps approximately 16–20 hr/d in cycles of about 4 hours each time, with gradually longer periods of wakefulness.

During periods of wakefulness, the baby makes use of the senses—especially sight, touch, and hearing. The neonate can stay entertained by watching and listening to something moving, like a mobile in the crib. Many caretakers find that the baby is content to be in a room with a lot of activity and sounds, such as the kitchen. Newborns are also quite happy to finger a textured object, such as a stuffed toy or a piece of towel, and do not have to have constant interaction with people.

The neonate assumes certain levels of consciousness in relation to the sleep/wake cycle. These states are: sleep (deep sleep, light sleep) and awake (drowsy, quiet alert, active alert, crying) (Brazelton, 1973). While babies vary in the amount of time spent in each state, the regulating, organizing, and modulating of these states is a critical developmental task and is a predictor of central nervous system sophistication (Parker & Brazelton, 1981).

Establishing Self-Concept

During progress through the transitory phase following birth, the neonate remains somewhat egocentric, desiring only to gratify himself or herself. In the early months of life the baby's world is limited. This is due to the still developing special senses and also limited to the types of experiences the baby has. All that the baby knows about the environment is what has been experienced. Egocentrism supports this, and the neonate assures himself or herself of initial control of the environment. Gradually, the visual, auditory, and tactile sensations tell the baby that there is something else in the environment. The baby recognizes mother and responds to her. The baby feels a part of the mother as she feeds, cuddles, and talks. But the baby also realizes that she is able to put him or her down and leave. The baby begins to develop the concept of being dependent on, but separate from, the mother. Associated with this, the newborn learns that gratification can come from the self, such as sucking, or from the mother, through feeding or holding. As the baby begins to interact with other members of the family, separate identity is strengthened, especially when the mother is not present. The neonate, discovering crude motor abilities, begins to use them to investigate the environment, thus increasing gratification through increased sucking, manipulation of body parts, or touching things.

The parents consciously or subconsciously contribute to this development of self-concept. Conversing with the baby and providing tactile stimulation helps the neonate to realize the power of the special senses. The mother and father also react to the baby in different ways, which transfers to the baby the notion that he or she, too, should respond to them differently. For example, babies are perceived as more soothable by their mothers than by their fathers (Ventura, 1982). The newborn probably picks up on these cues and exhibits different behavior accordingly.

The development of sexuality does begin in the first year of life, but only to a limited extent during the brief neonatal period. Much of it is related to gender, as shall be seen in the chapter on the infant. Still, certain patterns are laid down during the first weeks of life. Ventura (1982) noted that parents use different coping (parenting) styles with boys than they do with girls. This signifies a transfer of differing expectations about boy and girl babies.

Realizing that he or she is a separate entity causes the newborn to make efforts to relate to the others with whom there is frequent contact. This is the beginning of interpersonal relationships.

Developing Interpersonal Relationships

Initial awareness of others begins with the forming of the mother–infant bond immediately after birth. The mother has an instinctive desire to see, touch, caress, and talk to her baby. The neonate responds to contact with the mother by self-quieting behaviors—cessation of crying, slower movements, fist sucking, or reflexive rooting. As the baby listens to and gazes at the mother, she interprets this behavior positively and continues her maternal responses. This pattern of mother–baby responses has been termed *reciprocity*, and is the earliest, and probably most important, behavior pattern the neonate may exhibit. Magyary (1984) describes the interaction as also being characterized by the eventual development of coordinated responses and a personal communication system between mother and baby—reading and responding to cues. Early attachment between father and baby is influenced by his presence in the delivery room and the amount of caretaking permitted by the mother (Jones, 1981). Thus, familiarity with the baby heightens the relationship.

It should be pointed out that the process of attachment is not only for the neonatal period, but continues over time and is best equated with a more familiar emotional response—love. This lifelong relationship seems to be strongest during the early parts of life, usually with the mother. Bowlby (1982) views attachment as the "attaining or maintaining proximity to some . . . other individual who is conceived as better able to cope with the world" (p. 668). Because the mother is the person who spends the most time with the newborn, she is best able to read cues from the baby to determine the baby's needs. To the baby, she is a buffer between the self and this strange new environment. As she provides for the baby and keeps him or her comfortable and secure, the baby is best able to maintain a sense of equilibrium and interact positively with the environment rather than being threatened by it.

Because the neonate and mother or father are never separated for very long during the first few weeks, the interpersonal tie becomes very strong by virtue of quality and quantity time. As the cue-reading becomes more complex, the newborn develops rudimentary communication patterns—crying, fretting, or change in activity. The newborn realizes that these communication patterns are effective because they receive a response from the parent (reinforcement) and thus the baby continues to communicate.

Competency and Achievement

This task concerns the control of and development of one's own abilities to an optimal level for one's stage of life. As it has been mentioned, the newborn learns about the self and the world through the use of the senses and through exploration. A neurological assessment of the neonate reveals greater strength in the extremities (hands and feet) than in the trunk (neck and sacral area). While sensory development moves in the opposite direction, motor development is thought to progress in a caudal-cephalic direction. Piaget feels that the neonate is in a sensorimotor phase of development, utilizing the senses initially until motor capabilities become refined (Maier, 1969).

The degree to which the neonate can accomplish certain tasks depends in part on the gestational age at the time of birth. For instance, babies born prematurely, especially before 36 or 37 weeks, will exhibit less competency and less use of visual and auditory stimuli due to the immature neurological systems (Magyary, 1984). The term neonate will use the neurological state to bring in information about the immediate environment. The tonic neck reflex is assumed by the newborn in responding to the world. Nurses and parents, in observing the assumption of this position, can recognize that the neonate is using this time for habituation—focusing and attuning (Ambron, 1981).

In using the special senses to learn, the neonate seems to make the most use of vision. While capabilities are limited, the newborn can fixate, although generally not longer than 4–10 seconds. Because the neonate is so curious about the new environment, he or she seems to become bored with fixating on one certain object or person and will soon look around. The amount of visual stimulation seems to have positive influence on motor and cognitive growth (Ludington-Hoe, 1983). This is vital information to be passed on to parents, as they begin to know their baby and provide increasing interaction and stimulation.

Learning continues through the neonatal period by use of all of the senses and by repetition of pleasurable experiences. Parents who have been frequently smiling or gesturing at their baby receive a reward when the baby repeats the gesture or smiles back. This gives the parent such pleasure that the parent gives the baby a great amount of positive feedback so the baby will want to repeat the gesture. The newborn has truly *learned* something and through rewards given by the parent(s) will continue to make further learning efforts.

POTENTIAL STRESSORS

The degree of stress experienced by individuals varies and depends upon such factors as coexisting stressors and adaptive abilities. The neonate may have more than one stressor simultaneously and only primitive adaptive abilities. Since a stressor could have greater impact at this time of life, it must be identified early and altered to promote well-being of the baby.

Physical Stressors

Susceptibility to cold stress, due to temperature instability, has already been identified. The newborn does have one unique property that contributes to thermal regulation. This is the existence of brown fat, a collection of large fat cells with a very rich blood supply (hence their dark color), located in the interscapular, axillae, vertebral, and kidney areas. The location of brown fat protects the major body organs from chilling and comprise 2–6% of the total body weight of the neonate (Davis, 1980). When the neonate experiences chilling, the brown fat cells and stored glucose convert to glycogen, producing energy sources to increase metabolism, thus causing a physiological rise in temperature. While brown fat is a protective mechanism, demands placed upon it can create other problems. If the body temperature falls below 96°F (axillary), brown fat is converted to glycogen, then glucose to produce metabolic heat. This chemical activity creates metabolic acidosis if allowed to continue. If this goes unnoticed, the neonate could experience severe acid-base imbalance due to lack of compensation.

Variations in size and maturity predispose the neonate to any one of a number of physical problems. This creates a stressful situation not only for the baby, but also for family members, who become quite anxious over having a sick newborn. Those neonates born smaller than normal birth weight are classified as either preterm or premature (born before the pregnancy completed the 38th to 40th week, shortening the amount of fetal development and growth), or as small for gestational age (pregnancy progressed normal length, baby is smaller than expected). The other end of this continuum presents newborns who are large in birth weight, and are either postmature (time in utero advanced past the 40th week, usually past the 42nd week) or large for gestational age (birth weight above the norm, often related to diabetes in the mother or an inherent tendency). Problems due to size may have some similarities, but there are also individual differences according to the gestational age. Table 4–5 identifies some of the more common problems found in newborns of varying size and maturity.

Besides brown fat, another protective mechanism in the neonate is the presence of temporary immunities, which the baby receives through placental transfer in utero. Also, a baby who is being breast-fed will receive immunity from certain diseases through the breast-milk. The baby is thus protected from most major childhood diseases (those against which the mother has immunity) until about 6 months of age. The baby does not have immunity against common cold viruses, or such resistance against other pathogens, such as *Staphylococcus* or *Streptococcus*.

TABLE 4–5. PROBLEMS DUE TO SIZE

Premature	Small for Gestational Age (SGA)
Hypoglycemia	Hypoglycemia
Respiratory distress syndrome (RDS)	Hypocalcemia
Necrotizing enterocolitis (NEC)	Anemia
Hyperbilirubinemia	Intrauterine growth retardation (IUGR)
Hypocalcemia	

Postmature	Large for Gestational Age (LGA)
Malnutrition	Birth trauma
Hypoglycemia	Hypoglycemia/Hyperinsulinism
Decreased skin integrity	

Social/Emotional Stressors

Once the neonate adjusts to the stress of extrauterine life, he or she faces more complex stressors. As awareness of the environment increases, the neonate understands that the world around him or her is important and interesting, and there is an instinctive desire to be part of it. In striving to do so, the newborn may encounter interferences with, or poor quality of, interaction, thus creating a new form of stress.

Deprivation of quality interaction may be secondary to a physical stressor. The neonate who is ill or unstable and requires special supervision and care may not be able to be held, cuddled, and talked to by the parents. This causes frustration in the parents: the newborn they have waited so long to see and hold is kept from them for a little while longer. Consequently, when the parents are able to touch their baby in the special care nursery, or are finally able to take the baby home, they initially may have some very hesitant behaviors. It may take some time for the parents to accept the fact that their baby will live and is finally healthy. The baby may be sensitive to these hesitant behaviors and feel insecure. Reciprocal interaction may be missing, and the parents may think themselves incapable of parenting this particular baby (Ventura, 1982). Usually these unsure feelings are resolved by the end of the neonatal period, but they contribute to a difficult period initially, and may lay the foundation for difficulties in the parent–infant relationship.

Conflict with Family Tasks

Occasions can occur in which the birth of the baby, while a joyous happening, can also bring about disruption in family functioning to contribute to family or individual problems.

The mother may be having difficulty recovering from the birthing, either physically or psychologically. She may have delayed uterine involution, difficulty establishing breast milk, or an infection. She realizes that this is all due to her having had a baby, yet knows that her newborn is not really at fault. She may feel guilty for thinking in such a fashion. The new mother may also question her adequacy about her role as a mother and be filled with self-doubt. Either of these two instances can lead to mild postpartum depression, or the postpartum blues. The mother feels that she is not recovering at her desired rate and is anxious. These feelings are most often seen between the 3rd and 10th days postpartum, at the time the mother is newly at home alone, with her baby and her own feelings. Many mothers are aware that the blues may strike them during this time, yet feel powerless to control them. The best solution is loving support from significant others, and a little personal time to cry, rest, or sort out feelings.

The early temperament patterns displayed by the neonate may cause some conflicts with one or more family members. A family eagerly anticipating a warm, cuddly baby that would enjoy being held and passed around may find that they have a slow-to-warm-up or difficult baby who prefers only one or two people. This can cause a lot of dismay and disappointment. Newborn and family members need to adapt to one another, which takes time and understanding. Personality differences, which cannot be totally changed, can be shaped and responded to in a positive manner and need not bring about confusion and negative feelings.

The arrival of the newborn into the home may cause disruption in the integrity of the family beyond the initial reception period. The mother and baby (or father and baby) may have formed such a strong dyad that they act as a wedge, or separate entity, coming between the rest of the family members. The parent seems to send out messages that his or her relationship with this baby is the only one that matters and everyone else is out on their own. This slows the incorporation of the baby into the family unit, impairing smooth functioning. Consequently, family members become resentful of the baby's presence and the parent's attitude toward it, which caused this disruption.

In some families, the newborn is successfully incorporated as a regular family member, but another member may have difficulty adjusting to a new role or roles brought on by this new member. For example, small chores originally handled by the mother may be relegated to the oldest sibling while mother recovers from the delivery and cares for the baby. The sibling may not appreciate an added responsibility that takes away from personal time. Some roles are temporary ones, lasting only the first week or two, or until mother gets back on her feet. Others are more permanent, because they reflect the addition of a member, and may require more adjustment or increased communication among family members in order to clearly define responsibilities and expectations.

COPING MECHANISMS

Approaches to coping are unique to each family system as they foster individual development and promote family stability. Families will embrace and practice specific health beliefs because these are considered to be positive approaches to nurturing—things the family can do to cope with the new member, thus promoting growth and development. While the neonatal period is brief, family members use this time to confirm that their baby is healthy and stable and can be fully incorporated into the family. They can then guide their baby into infancy.

Health Beliefs and Behaviors

Many parents actively use professional health services, generally from the standpoint of illness treatment or prevention. The link with the professional services begins with prenatal care or at the time of delivery. Many new mothers are encouraged at the time of discharge to call the hospital nursery if they have any questions about baby. The pediatrician examines the newborn in the hospital and discusses subsequent health care with the parent(s).

Hygiene is closely guarded in the first few months of the baby's life because the baby is viewed as fresh and vulnerable. Most new parents are not fully aware of the neonate's low level of immunities, but they do know they should protect the baby from germs. As the newborn arrives home, the first hygienic practice is usually care of the umbilical cord stump. The mother is taught to keep the stump dry and clean it daily with alcohol until the cord falls off. Before the navel is well healed, the baby is sponge bathed and then can be tub bathed. This is not only a time for cleansing, but also turns into a time for play and for photographs. The neonate learns the sensation of water on the skin and equates bath time with warm and relaxing pleasure. Perhaps the baby also equates this bath with the amniotic bath during the fetal stage.

Family members also strive to protect the baby from ingesting harmful pathogens. The breast-feeding mother will wash off her nipples before feeding, or the formula-fed baby will be given a sterilized nipple, bottle, and formula. Some overly concerned mothers will sterilize pacifiers, especially if they have been dropped, and will wash the baby's crib and toys. New mothers, however, will soon realize that the baby is exploring and putting a fist or strange object into the mouth, and will give up the time-consuming practice of protecting their baby so strictly.

Close supervision of feeding the newborn is another approach to health. The family is especially cautious during the neonatal period, making sure that their baby has enough milk with no stomach upset or allergy. Feeding is the most common way that families can promote growth of their baby.

As the family watches their newborn grow and change, they make adaptations accordingly in order to meet baby needs. The major caretaker will gradually increase the baby's amount of formula, or the nursing mother may increase the nursing time. Because the neonate is in the cute and cuddly stage, he or she receives a great deal of attention. This aids in refining development tasks of interpersonal relationships and cognition. Family members learn their baby's cues and strive to meet demands. This is one of the best ways they can promote their baby's health.

RESPONSES TO STRESSORS

Adaptive

The major source of stress for the neonate is adjustment to extrauterine life. Achievement of this task and adaptation to independent functioning are critical for life itself before the individual can move on to other tasks (and their accompanying stressors). Consequently, the physiological adaptations through which the newborn progresses are viewed as positive and welcome changes and are the initial regulatory responses to the environment.

Adaptive responses on the part of the parent(s) depend largely on the stressor experienced by the neonate. For instance, the mother of a sick neonate may strive to bring love and comfort to her baby by talking and stroking, even while the baby is bedfast and under life-support systems. Mothers also make it very clear that their baby has been named and will respond well to communications from the professional staff about the baby's status. Positive adaptation to early crises are crucial for strong, loving relationships as the baby grows.

Maladaptive

These responses in the neonate include inability to progress successfully through extrauterine adjustment. Poor respiratory or circulatory exchange, hypothermia, or neurological deficits lead to physiological instability or death. When dealing with interpersonal relationships, the newborn who has a poor attachment relationship with one loving, responsible person may show some physical responses that are early patterns for failure to thrive. The baby may lose interest in the surroundings and feed poorly. A baby who is displaying these patterns as early as the neonatal period requires close scrutiny and observation of interactions with parent(s).

The parent who is having difficulty adapting to the newborn's stressful period may exhibit a range of behaviors. The mother and/or father may avoid going into the special care nursery, out of either fear of the technology or reluctance to see their baby so ill. A neonate who is having difficulty adjusting to extrauterine life may cause a mother to experience postpartum depression rooted in guilt and anxiety. Parents of sick neonates need as much assessment and intervention as their babies do in order to help the entire family overcome this stressful period.

NURSING ASSESSMENT

Table 4–6 provides guidelines for a nursing assessment of a family with a neonate. It is important for nurses to include environmental and social factors, as well as physical parameters, when gathering information about the family.

ALTERATIONS IN HEALTH

The susceptibility of the neonate to illness is largely due to immature body systems or the result of a congenital anomaly. Some babies are more prone to illness because of genetic composition or prenatal factors influencing health. Most acute conditions are responses to extrauterine life following birth or responses by the immune system to the environment.

Acute Conditions

Cold Stress.   The presence of brown fat is the neonate's major defense against organ damage from postdelivery chilling. As has been previously mentioned, the body begins to produce chemical heat (a process called *thermogenesis*) when the newborn is exposed to cool temperatures. This process can also produce metabolic acidosis in the neonate, especially if cold stress is not treated immediately after delivery (Bobak & Jensen, 1984). In the immediate postdelivery period, it is extremely important for the nurse to keep the neonate's metabolic demands at a minimum.

Dehydration.   The term neonate has a very high intracellular fluid ratio. Because of the newborn's high metabolic rate and the inability of the kidneys to concentrate

TABLE 4–6. ASSESSING THE FAMILY WITH A NEONATE

	Environmental Data
Provisions for care	Quality of parent–baby interaction, amount of time spent in actual interaction, method of feeding selected, sleeping arrangements for mother and newborn, measures to meet newborn's daily needs
Alternate caretakers	Relationship to parent, frequency of interaction with newborn, ability to care for newborn
	Communication Patterns
Neonate	Basic temperament, ability to express needs
Between mother and neonate	Mother's interpretation of neonate's sounds or gestures, type of communication (words, baby talk, cooing)
	Communication Patterns
Among family members	Types of communication, amount of communication with mother
	Problem-Solving Skills
Decision-making abilities	Mother's ability to resume decision making, roles of other family members in decision making/implementing
Use of the health care system	Uses for the neonate, accessibility, affordability
Support from significant others	Viewed as positive or negative by mother, areas of strongest support (as viewed by mother, as viewed by nurse)
Societal interactions	Current use of public agencies, anticipated needs
	Life-Style
Role of neonate in family	Pregnancy planned or unplanned, course of prenatal and intrapartum periods, mother's appraisal of neonate (feeding, sleeping, temperament)
Socioeconomic status (SES)	Estimated yearly income, financial assistance, direction of SES mobility, wage earner's feelings about status, anticipated changes
Family roles	Traditional or nontraditional pattern, distribution, level of satisfaction with roles, anticipated changes
Work patterns	Wage earners in family, amount of work hours per day/week, anticipated job change
Recreational patterns	Changes due to neonate, amount of planned activities each week/month, amount of time spent in leisure individually and as a group
Safety	Visible hazards within the neonate's environment, use of safety features (car seats, nonflammable clothing, etc.), adult's knowledge of accident prevention and first aid
	Potential Stressors
Neonate	Physical stressors, adaptability to extrauterine life, quality of interaction with parent
Conflicts with family tasks	Postpartal recovery of mother, acceptance of parenting role by mother and father
Family response patterns	Health beliefs and behaviors, adaptive and maladaptive responses to stressors

urine, maintaining proper fluid balance is necessary to avoid dehydration. Early signs of dehydration include sunken fontaneles and poor skin turgor.

Infections.   Neonates are especially susceptible to infections because of the immature immune system. An infectious disease process early in life seems to occur more commonly in preterm than term neonates and is responsible for 10% of all neonatal deaths (Reeder, 1983). Neonatal infections can be acquired transplacentally, through the vagina during delivery, or from a nonsterile environment postnatally. Also, there is less antibody transfer in preterm babies than in term babies. Preterm neonates have an increased incidence of resuscitation and respiratory support which lead to pulmonary problems, other invasive procedures which also increase the possibility of pathogen introduction, and a tendency for skin breakdown (Moore, 1982). Vomiting, decreased feeding, and unstable body temperature are the first signs of an infection. An infection in an otherwise healthy baby responds well to medical management, but when compounded with other problems can lead to sepsis and death.

Jaundice.   Neonatal jaundice or hyperbilirubinemia is characterized by yellowing of the skin and sclera of the eyes. This coloring is due to an excessive amount of circulating bilirubin, which is deposited in the subcutaneous layers of the body. The Committee on Practice of the Nurses' Association of the American College of Obstetricians and Gynecologists (NAACOG) has classified neonatal jaundice in one of three categories:

> Physiologic: appears 2–3 days after birth with moderate bilirubin blood level, subsides 5–7 days after birth. Usually benign and considered fairly common among neonates
> Breast milk: bilirubin level rises about the fourth day of life, elevated level may last for weeks. While relationship of hyperbilirubinemia and neonatal jaundice seems evident, the cause is unclear (Maisels, 1981). This form of jaundice affects only 1–2% of breastfed babies.
> Pathologic: condition in which jaundice appears within the first twenty-four hours of life, with a rapid rise in serum bilirubin level or bilirubin level is over established "safe" value. Also classified as pathologic if jaundice and elevated bilirubin level persists over one week. Associated with asphyxia, prematurity, or acidosis. Requires more intensive intervention. Pathologic jaundice is seen in hemolytic disease of the newborn, a condition occurring in the presence of Rh or ABO incompatibility between the mother and her fetus. Pathologic jaundice which is not reversed can lead to kernicterus, a depositing of bilirubin in the brain. This can lead to seizures, impaired neurologic functioning, and mental retardation.*

Trauma.   The neonate can experience trauma at the time of delivery as a result of large size in relation to the mother's pelvis and birth canal, due to mismanagement by an inept deliverer, or even from a precipitate delivery. The most common examples of birth trauma are concussion, fracture, dislocation, and nerve plexus.

---

*Adapted from NAACOG Committee on Practice (1986). *Phototherapy and nursing care of the newborn* (NAACOG Practice Report No. 15). Washington, D.C.: NAACOG.

Postdelivery substance withdrawal. The neonate who had adapted to the substance intake from an addicted mother no longer has this circulating substance, so experiences withdrawal symptoms. The abused substance is often a narcotic or non-narcotic analgesic/depressant, so the neonate experiences manifestations usually within the central nervous system (CNS): irregular behavior, inconsolability, disturbed sleep patterns, tremors, incomplete neurological reflexes, and the high-pitched cry characteristic of CNS irritability. Most of these manifestations become obvious within 24–48 hours after delivery.

Along with these CNS symptoms, the mother who had high drug or alcohol intake will most likely have a baby that is small for gestational age, usually due to the mother's uncertainty about her due date and from inadequate prenatal nutrition. The baby born with fetal alcohol syndrome will display growth abnormalities, especially in the maxillofacial area, and have diminished sucking and feeding reflexes.

Hypoglycemia. The condition is particularly common among small-for-gestational-age neonates. The postnatal low blood sugar level is a result of separation from the glucose supply received from the mother. Hypoglycemia usually occurs within the first 12 hours of life, before the baby has received regular feedings. Early signs of hypoglycemia include tremors, shrill cry, change in respiratory pattern, lethargy, and hypotonia. Because the brain relies solely on glucose for cellular nutrition, it is imperative to maintain optimal blood sugar levels.

Infant of a Diabetic Mother. The hypoglycemia experienced by a neonate born to a diabetic mother is the result of glucose and insulin imbalance. In utero, the fetus was accustomed to high circulating levels of maternal glucose and produced insulin accordingly. After delivery, the neonate experiences a dramatic drop in glucose, resulting in hypoglycemia/hyperinsulinism. These conditions require close evaluation and management by the nurse, particularly because of the brain's need for glucose.

Chronic Conditions

Because the neonatal period is so brief, chronic conditions are problems that extend into infancy, such as illness or congenital anomalies.

Congenital Anomaly. The presence of a physical/structural anomaly can cause both an alteration in the health of the neonate and the quality of interaction between the baby and loved ones. Some congenital anomalies are serious, life-threatening concerns, requiring immediate surgical intervention. Diaphragmatic hernia is an example of this: the herniation of the abdominal organs into the thoracic cavity interferes with lung expansion. This loss of full respiratory exchange can bring about severe hypoxia, so surgical intervention is necessary within the first few hours of life.

Some congenital anomalies are surgically corrected after the neonate is a little older and therefore more stable. Until that time, the neonate will need specific nursing care to protect him or her from complications induced by the anomaly. Some examples of this are protection from infection with an omphalocele (herniation of the abdominal organs through the umbilicus) or spina bifida (herniation of the lower segment of the spinal canal into a pouch at the sacral area). The neonate with a cardiac anomaly will need specific interventions to promote oxygenation and circulation.

There are also anomalies considered cosmetic in nature; cleft lip and palate and orthopedic anomalies are examples of these. These may require a series of surgical corrections during the infancy period. The parent(s) can be taught specific measures, such as positioning and feeding techniques, to use in caring for the baby. While these anomalies may be considered the least serious, because they are not life-threatening, some parents react more emotionally to their newborn's less than perfect appearance.

NURSING RESPONSIBILITIES

The family's introduction to nurses and nursing may be at the time of delivery of the first child. Because of this, it is most important for the nurse to establish a good rapport with the family, provide the highest-quality care, and advocate for the family in the health care system. If the family can be comfortable with the system and the health care team, plus receiving optimal care, they will most likely be motivated to continue to seek health care for the growing family.

Health Promotion

A variety of approaches can be taken in the area of health promotion. These approaches should be directed to a goal of developing a family that can independently carry out measures to ensure health, solve problems, and know when to seek assistance within the health care system.

One of the approaches the nurse can take is through providing exemplary care, or *role modeling*. Individuals are often most watchful of nurses because nurses represent certain standards and values. Through role modeling, nurses can demonstrate, educate, and motivate families to obtain optimal health. Some examples of role modeling are: (1) handwashing after diapering; (2) calling baby by name; (3) speaking directly to the baby, slowly and distinctly; (4) cuddling and other forms of affection. In some cases, there can be a fine line between role modeling and taking over in a situation. The nurse who constantly shows or tells new parents how to hold their baby or dictates a structured feeding schedule can create resentment in the parent(s) and precipitate a loss of self-esteem about newly formed parenting skills. While it may be difficult, the nurse may have to relinquish hold and let the parents feel their own way.

In collaborating with parents about baby care, the nurse may discover many opportunities for parent and family education. In assessing early behavioral patterns in the neonate and parent–infant interaction, the nurse may use these findings to enhance the relationship between parent and child. The Brazelton Neonatal Behavioral Assessment Scale (BNBAS) (Brazelton, 1973) measures the neonate's response to stimuli and determines how the neonate deals with the environment. Because this assessment is predictive of infant temperament, the nurse can educate parents about this, so they can begin to direct their parenting skills accordingly. The BNBAS also evaluates infant states (as mentioned in the section on personality development), so the parents can know when to expect optimal interaction (Parker & Brazelton, 1981).

The neonatal period is also an optimal time to promote nutritional health of the neonate. The time of discharge or within the neonatal period is an appropriate time to institute needed assistance through the WIC (Women, Infants, and Children) program. This federal subsidization provides financial aid for food for the mother (if breast-feeding) or formula for the baby. Nutritional health is promoted because the WIC program includes assessment and education of eating patterns and dietary intake for all family members. Nutritional health of the neonate is assessed by parameters such as weight gain, sleep and activity patterns, feeding behaviors, elimination patterns, and neurological activity.

When teaching parents something that directly involves the infant, it is helpful to have the baby present. In this way the nurse can observe the interaction, identify more cues of the infant's behaviors, or have an effective demonstration session. Some new parents are taught baby care skills—how to parent—in structured classes. This is most beneficial because it provides needed information and advice in an organized, meaningful way. Parenting is one facet of life for which adults receive little ongoing, formal preparation prior to the actual experience. Participation in classes strengthens self-esteem. Many new parents are helped by the fact that there is a room full of other adults who feel equally unsure about parenting.

Many nurses enjoy teaching classes of this nature and are challenged by this experience. It is crucial for the nurse to practice sound principles of teaching. The nurse will need to be supportive of observed nurturing behaviors and may need to make allowances for cultural beliefs and values. These approaches to education lay the groundwork for continued family involvement in health care.

Preventive Measures

All aspects of nursing care for the family with a neonate should be based upon the nurse's knowledge of the individual and family developmental tasks of this period. Once the nurse has dealt with priority aspects of care and health promotion, attention can then be turned to anticipatory guidance and education to prevent health problems and interruption with critical developmental tasks.

Preventive measures often evolve from aspects of care while the baby and mother are still in the hospital or birthing center. Observations of the neonate's status or parent–infant interaction, which have resulted in specific interventions, may need further education or guidance to prevent complications. An example of this might be a new mother who is not fully informed on feeding techniques and does not hold her baby properly during feeding or burp the baby as needed. This can result in regurgitation, indigestion, or aspiration. Therefore, the mother (and father) may need more in-depth instruction in feeding techniques to avoid difficulties at home. In addition, the nurse should assess parent–baby behaviors during feeding, to evaluate the quality of parent–infant attachment. Situations in which the baby has difficulty feeding or the mother does not hold the baby closely or talk to him or her could indicate disruptive parenting rather than improper feeding techniques.

The nurse can educate the new parents about environmental safety for their baby. For instance, if a crib is being used, the rails of the crib should be no more than 3–4 inches apart. A bumper pad or padding should be placed between the mattress and the sides of the bed. These measures will help prevent the newborn from lodging his or her head between parts of the bed and strangling.

Because the immunological response to infection is not as efficient as that of an older child, the baby needs protection from infection. Handwashing and other hygienic practices begun in the hospital need to be continued. Parents should avoid exposing their baby to crowds or individuals with known illnesses. Contact between the neonate and anyone with any open lesion should also be avoided (Moore, 1983).

Health Maintenance

The nursing role in the preservation and restoration of health is primarily that of caregiver. The nurse must consistently use the nursing process—assessment, planning, intervention, and evaluation (Yura & Walsh, 1983)—and be current and competent in the provision of care.

One of the first opportunities for assessment of the neonate is in the delivery room. The nurse can use the Apgar scoring system (Table 4–7) (Apgar et al., 1958) to evaluate the neonate's immediate reactions to extrauterine life. While all of the signs are scored with equal weight, proper evaluation of the heart and respiratory systems is crucial, since instability of these systems can be life-threatening. The baby is given Apgar scores at 1 minute and 5 minutes after birth. Most neonates have scores of 8 or 9 at 5 minutes. A score of 6 would mean guarded condition, while 4 or less most likely indicates that resuscitation measures are needed. By using this system to assess the baby's status, the health care team can plan care for the neonate upon admission to the nursery. Besides being a predictor of postdelivery progress, Apgar scores have been a most useful measure in research. The scores have been used as a parameter to evaluate a safe time period for administration of a narcotic analgesic in relation to the

TABLE 4–7. APGAR SCORING SYSTEM

Sign	0	1	2
Heart rate	Absent	Below 100/min	Above 100/min
Respirations	Absent	Slow irregular	Cry; regular rate
Muscle tone	Flaccid	Some flexion of extremities	Active movements
Reflex irritability	None	Grimace	Cry
Color	Body cyanotic or pale	Body pink, extremities cyanotic	Body completely pink

Score is totaled at 1 minute and 5 minutes after delivery.

From Apgar et al. (1958). Evaluation of the newborn infant—second report. JAMA, 168, 1985–1988.

impending birth (Shnider & Moya, 1964). The potentially depressive effects of medications have been demonstrated, through this scoring method, in the neonate's reflexive and respiratory abilities. Similar studies have been conducted evaluating the effects of paracervical and pudendal blocks (King & Sherline, 1981) and epidural anesthesia (Lundberg & Souci, 1983).

After the neonate achieves immediate postdelivery stability, the nurse is then responsible for careful, thorough scrutiny of the baby as he or she progresses in the transition to extrauterine life. This appraisal is incorporated into part of the plan of care for the normal neonate and includes the physical and neurological assessment.

In addition to the physical and neurological assessment, the nurse needs to evaluate gestational age of the neonate. This evaluation measures physical indices of development, such as presence of lanugo or descent of the testes. Evaluation of neuromuscular maturity is done through certain movements and observations of the neonate. Upon completion of assessment, neonates are classified as SGA (small for gestational age), AGA (appropriate for gestational age), or LGA (large for gestational age). This classification enables the nurse to plan appropriate care for the neonate, based upon this baby's specific needs. Other priorities for care of the normal neonate include maintenance of temperature regulation, provision of nutrition, and promotion of safety and hygiene.

In the event of neonatal illness, the role of the nurse as caregiver becomes more intensified. The situation becomes more serious and complex for neonate and family alike.

SUMMARY

In this chapter, the neonate has been introduced as an addition to the family. Strategies for promoting physical and psychosocial well-being of the newborn include attachment with a significant other, selection of feeding method, and the provision of various forms of stimulation.

Early problem identification and intervention and positive support from the health care system are essential for establishing the family with the neonate. Guidance and encouragement from the nurse will prove to be most beneficial as the family begins to incorporate this newest, smallest member.

CARE PLAN FOR THE NEONATE

Situation

Baby K is 38 hours old. She weighed 2800 grams (6 pounds 3 ounces) at birth and had Apgar scores of 8 and 9. Baby K has quiet alert periods in the late morning and late afternoon. She drinks approximately 2 ounces of formula at each feeding and has good elimination patterns. When she cries, she can be consoled by changing her position in her bassinett.

G. K., the mother, is a 20-year old primipara. She has had no prior experience with newborns. Her mother (the grandmother) is present during the waking hours. While the hospital encourages 24-hour rooming-in of babies, the mother only wants her baby from midmorning to about 7:00 PM, when the grandmother leaves. Because Baby K is being bottle fed, the grandmother often does this. G. K. is unwilling to participate in caretaking activities—diapering, feeding, holding—but lets the grandmother do all activities. When G. K. holds the baby, which is usually between feedings, she holds the baby loosely on her lap and talks to her mother or watches TV. G. K. refers to her baby as "squirt," rather than by any chosen name.

Nursing Diagnoses

1. Alteration in parenting related to impaired maternal infant attachment

SAMPLE CARE PLAN

Nursing Diagnosis	Goal	Interventions	Evaluation
Alteration in parenting related to impaired maternal–infant attachment.	G. K. will become more involved in caretaking and interactive behaviors. Baby K will show healthy responses to maternal care.	Explore G. K.'s feelings about being a mother and what she perceives to be important mothering activities. Point out Baby K's positive qualities. Gently encourage more interaction with baby. Praise and support existing caretaking activities.	The patient will verbalize feelings concerning motherhood, expectations of self. She will share impressions of baby and how baby compares with pre-conceived ideas. She will become more involved in care. She will begin to display affectional responses.

Review Questions

1. Suggest ways to promote parent–infant interaction in the following situations: (a) preterm neonate in the neonatal intensive care unit; (b) neonate delivered by cesarean birth, mother experiencing postoperative complications; (c) adolescent parents of normal term neonate.

2. Discuss current societal trends that have influenced the family with a neonate.

3. Prioritize the roles and responsibilities of the nurse when caring for a newly delivered neonate.

REFERENCES

Ambron, S. R. (1981). *Child development* (3rd ed.). New York: Holt, Rinehart & Winston.

Apgar, V., Holaday, D. A., James, L. S., Weisbrot, I. M., & Berrien, C. (1958). Evaluation of the newborn infant—second report. *JAMA, 168,* 1985–1988.

Bobak, I. M., & Jensen, M. D. (1984). *Essentials of maternity nursing.* St. Louis: Mosby.

Bowlby, J. (1982). Attachment and loss: retrospect and prospect. *American Journal of Orthopsychiatry, 52,* 664–678.

Brazelton, T. B. (1973). Neonatal behavioral assessment scale. In *Clinics in Developmental Medicine,* No. 50. Philadelphia: Lippincott.

Davis, V. (1980). The structure and function of brown adipose tissue in the neonate. *Journal of Obstetric, Gynecologic, and Neonatal Nursing, 91,* 368–372.

Duvall, E. (1977). *Family Development* (5th ed.). Philadelphia: Lippincott.

Gesell, A. (1955). *The first five years of life.* New York: Harper & Row.

Greenberg, M., & Morris, N. (1974). Engrossment: The newborn's impact upon the father. *American Journal of Orthopsychiatry, 44,* 520–531.

Hrbosky, D. M. (1977, September). Transition to parenthood: A balancing of needs. In Smoyak, S. A. (Ed.), Symposium on Parenting, *Nursing Clinics of North America.* Philadelphia: Saunders.

Jones, C. (1981). Father to infant attachment: effects of early contact and characteristics of the infant. *Research in Nursing and Health, 4*(1), 193–201.

King, J. C., & Sherline, D. M. (1981). Paracervical and pudendal block. *Clinical Obstetrics and Gynecology, 24,* 587–595.

Ludington-Hoe, S. M. (1983). What can newborns really see? *American Journal of Nursing, 83,* 1286–1289.

Lundberg, G. D., & Souci, L. (Eds.) (1983). Abstract: Studies on neurobehavioral response (Scanlon Test) in newborns after epidural anesthesia with various anesthetic agents for cesarean section. *JAMA, 250,* 2133.

Magyary, D. (1984). Early social interactions: Pre-term infant dyads. *Issues in Comprehensive Pediatric Nursing, 7,* 233–254.

Maier, H. (1969). *Three theories of child development.* New York: Harper & Row.

Martell, L. K., & Mitchell, S. K. (1984). Rubin's "puerperal change" reconsidered. *Journal of Obstetric and Gynecologic Nursing, 13,* 145–149.

Moore, M. L. (1981). *Newborn, family, and nurse* (2nd ed.). Philadelphia: Saunders.

Moore, M. L. (1983). *Realities in childbearing* (2nd ed.). Philadelphia: Saunders.

NAACOG Committee on Practice (1986). *Phototherapy and nursing care of the newborn* (NAACOG Practice Report No. 15). Washington, D. C.: NAACOG.

Neeson, J. D. & May, K. A. (1986). *Comprehensive maternity nursing.* Philadelphia: Lippincott.

Parker, S., & Brazelton, T. B. (1981). Newborn behavior assessment: Research, prediction, and clinical uses. *Children Today, 10* (4), 2–5.

Reeder, S., Mastroianni, L., & Martin, L. (1983). *Maternity nursing* (15th ed.). Philadelphia: Lippincott.

Ritchey, S. J., & Taper, L. J. (1983). *Maternal and child nutrition.* New York: Harper & Row.

Rubin, R. (1984). *Maternal identity and the maternal experience.* New York: Springer.

Rubin, R. (1960). Puerperal change. *Nursing Outlook, 9,* 743–755.

Scipien, G. M., Barnard, M. U., Chard, M. A., Howe, J., & Phillips, P. J. (1986). *Comprehensive pediatric nursing* (3rd ed.). New York: McGraw-Hill.

Shnider, S. M., & Moya, F. (1964). Effects of meperidine on the newborn infant. *American Journal of Obstetrics and Gynecology, 89*, 1009–1015.

Ventura, J. (1982). Parent coping behaviors, parent functioning, and infant temperament characteristics. *Nursing Research, 31*, 269–273.

Whaley, L. F., & Wong, D. L. (1983). *Nursing care of infants and children* (2nd ed.). St. Louis: Mosby.

Yura, H., Walsh, M. B. (1983). *The nursing process* (4th ed.). Norwalk, CT: Appleton-Century-Crofts.

5

The Family with an Infant
1 Month Through 1 Year

Martha J. Bradshaw

OBJECTIVES

Upon completion of this chapter, the student will be able to:

1. Identify family developmental tasks during the infancy period
2. Identify developmental tasks of the infant
3. Identify potential stressors to the development of the infant
4. Describe optimal family patterns and responses during the infancy period
5. Differentiate between adaptive and maladaptive responses to stressors by the infant
6. Recognize interferences to health that are common during infancy
7. Identify nursing approaches that will assist an individual/couple with parenting an infant
8. Identify the roles of the nurse during health promotion for the infant and family

CONCEPTS

Egocentrism: focusing on oneself; belief that self is center of all things

Sexuality: component of personality that deals with gender-related behaviors; perception of self as a sexual person

Temperament: inherent pattern of reaction(s) to a specific situation

Cognition: knowing, learning, and/or understanding

Trust: reliance on, and belief in others

Personality: compilation of personal behaviors, characteristics, responses, and moods

Infancy, which starts at 6 weeks after birth, does not begin as abruptly as the neonatal period does. The family with an infant moves into this period subtly and gradually, just as they will progress into subsequent periods. Some families may have a specific event or milestone that indicates to them that their baby is an infant and no longer a newborn. To some families, arrival at home is the beginning of infancy. To others, it will be the 1-month birthday. The most commonly accepted landmark separating a neonate from an infant is the 6-week physical checkup. At that time, the family is considered released from specific health care and is launched into its own pattern of daily living. Responsibility for future health care is now almost entirely up to the parent(s). The period of infancy lasts until the child is 1 year of age.

The family with an infant may have family developmental tasks that overlap from the neonatal to infancy periods. Much of this is based upon the type and importance of the task and the rate and degree to which the family can resolve it. Resolving the birthing experience and incorporating the neonate into the family may take longer in some families than others. This may be particularly true if the birthing experience was difficult or if the neonate's arrival was of exceptional significance—for instance, after several years of infertility.

FAMILY TASKS

Emotional, psychological, or attitudinal family tasks are long-range and ongoing and do not have to be resolved before entering the infancy period. Along with these ongoing tasks are family developmental tasks unique to the infancy period. The tasks for a family with an infant are to:

1. Promote physical and emotional development
2. Adapt life-style to the changing infant
3. Incorporate new family structure into society
4. Maintain interpersonal relationships
5. Establish goals, priorities, and values

These tasks reflect the dependency needs of the infant and also the importance of continuous family functioning. The degree of family functioning is influenced by success with previous tasks, especially the incorporation of the neonate into the family. Therefore, a goal for the family with the infant would be *to maintain healthy family patterns while resolving new stages of development*.

Promoting Physical and Emotional Development

The family members will express varying degrees of interest in caring for the baby. One member may like to give baby a bottle; another may enjoy dressing the baby for an outing. All family members share the more pleasurable aspects of care while the adults perform the basic, especially the disagreeable, parts of baby care. In some families, task assignment occurs by default, a system that is usually an inadequate approach (Hrbosky, 1977).

Preservation of body temperature through clothing and outer covering is often of foremost concern and sometimes a source of conflict and frustration for the mother and father. New parents and doting grandparents have varying opinions about the amount and type of clothing the baby should wear, and these opinions may be a source of argument among them. Selection of clothing and covering for the baby is based upon climate and environment, and directly reflects the parents' caretaking abilities.

The degree of family participation in feeding the infant will be based upon whether the baby is being breast- or bottle-fed. In fact, some mothers elect to bottle-feed their babies solely because they can have help at feeding time. Mothers who intend to return to employment outside the home, or who will be away from the baby for several hours at a time, often choose bottle-feeding.

Because of the gradual rise in the number of breast-feeding mothers in the United States, coupled with the high number of working women, breast-feeding in the workplace has become a common dilemma. The mother who is committed to nursing her baby finds that she must make arrangements, often inconvenient, to be with her baby every two or three hours. This may take her away from her work, and she may lose wages. In rare instances, the mother brings her baby with her to work until the baby is several months old and then elects to stop breast-feeding. Generally, the breast-feeding mother solves this dilemma by providing the temporary caretaker with expressed milk and then expressing milk from her breasts during work hours. The ideal situation is the place of employment that provides on-site infant care. The mother can then take time off to go feed her baby as necessary and work out suitable time arrangements with the employer.

For the baby who is being bottle-fed, family members can be taught how to properly prepare the bottles and formula and how to hold the baby best for feeding and burping. Because feeding the baby is such a common and frequent task, family members will usually be willing to participate. This is also helpful for the baby because it enables him or her to become familiar with more members of the family. Feeding provides time for baby and the older family member to become acquainted and spend private time together.

As with breast-feeding, introduction of solid food into the infant's diet has also taken a cyclic pattern. For years, solids were not introduced until the infant was almost a year old; then they gradually became introduced at earlier ages. This introduction is based upon whether the baby is being breast- or formula-fed. As he or she becomes older, the bottle-fed infant will not always receive nutrients necessary for growth and will therefore need the added nutrition of solid foods. Most mothers may consult their pediatrician or nurse-practitioner, but usually choose to introduce specific foods on their own timetable. The family becomes much more actively involved at this point, as they may want to experiment with feeding the baby a new food, or the mother asks someone to feed the baby in order to free her to do other things. Sometimes family members can hinder the baby's general nutritional intake by providing candy, ice cream, chips, and soda, instead of more wholesome foods such as fruit, crackers, and juice. Unless supported, the mother may surrender and follow the others, rather than wage a never-ending battle over snacks.

Diapering and perianal hygiene is an ongoing activity carried over from the neonatal period. As the infant grows older, he or she will have fewer wet diapers as the kidneys begin to concentrate the urine. When the infant begins to eat solid foods, the stool will become more formed and heavier. A baby who is formula-fed or is eating some solid foods will have stools with a somewhat offensive odor, due to the bacteria content. Consequently, some family members may be resistant to changing a diaper that contains a fresh stool.

Many families have tried to make the diapering chore a little more pleasant by using disposable diapers. The plastic outer lining keeps clothing, laps, and hands dry, and the diaper can simply be rolled up and thrown away. However, consistent use of disposable diapers is limited to higher-income families, especially in urban populations, because of the expense and ready availability of the diapers. The same is true for a diaper service, which relieves the housekeeper (usually the same person as the caretaker) from frequent laundering. In both cases, the cost of continuing this form of diapering until the infant is toilet trained limits its use to a small segment of the American population.

Bathing the baby is a task that is carried over from the neonatal period, but changes as the baby grows and changes. As mentioned in the chapter on the neonate, bath time can be a very pleasant experience. Siblings may be allowed to take part in this aspect of care after the baby is able to sit up, especially without support. This allows the sibling to see that their little brother or sister can be fun to play with and also helps the baby to become familiar with and trust the sibling. Many parents bathe the infant and older children together, both to save time and promote playtime.

During playtime, family members, either consciously or unconsciously, are promoting neurological and muscular development, as well as contributing to the infant's personality development. Family members and friends pick up the baby, tussle him or her around, and show toys to the baby. The parents may use playtime as an opportunity to evaluate their baby's development. Various means are used to determine head and neck control, arm and leg strength, and the ability to sit up, raise himself or herself up, or roll over. Motor and verbal skills may appear gradually or suddenly, and the parent will always be looking for the baby's new skills. Family members take great pride in discovering that their baby can achieve a milestone such as walking before the neighbor's baby who is 7 weeks older. The infant responds to all this interaction in a reciprocal way, smiling, cooing, imitating, and participating.

Bowel and bladder training are other examples of motor development. Generally, it is useless to start this process seriously before the infant is over a year old, because awareness of bladder and bowel sensations does not begin until the infant is between 9 and 12 months old (Pillitteri, 1981). If parents believed their child was trained during this period, it is probably because they timed the trips to the bathroom and were able to catch the child at the right moment. In such cases, it has been said that it was the parents who were trained.

The family promotes the infant's need for rest by reading cues that indicate sleep is needed. Some infants become irritable and fussy when fatigued; others display physical signs such as shadows around the eyes or pulling at the ears. Efforts on the part of the parents to establish a regular schedule of sleep periods will help the baby meet personal rest needs.

It is most important for the family to overtly and covertly protect the infant from illness or injury. The discussion of physical care pointed out approaches to fostering growth and maintaining health through proper nutrition, hygiene, exercise, and rest. These daily components of life are frequently overlooked as crucial to proper health, but they are the foundation of illness prevention.

Infants need protection from the environment through immunization: illnesses classified as typical childhood diseases have diminished and almost been obliterated due to parental responsibility, accessibility to immunization clinics, and follow-up by health delivery services. Smallpox is an example of this: Because of active, widespread immunization for smallpox through the early 1970s, there are no reported cases of this disease in the United States today.

A schedule of routine physical checkups may vary according to the infant's status and the desires of the health practitioner. Usually, they begin at 6 weeks of age and progress to about every other month until the first year.

Adapting Life-Style to the Changing Infant

This family developmental task is complementary to the task of the neonatal period of incorporating the neonate into the family. The infant needs to become a member of the family, sharing equal status with all other members of the family. The family with an infant should not feel that they should totally rearrange their patterns of daily living and general life-style to accommodate this new member. However, certain modifications in life-style are necessary, usually on a temporary basis, in order to promote the health and optimal development of the infant.

One of the decisions concerning life-style is to determine when, if ever, the previously employed mother should return to work. Kutzner and Toussie-Weingarten (1984) point out that work brings an economic boost, as well as personal fulfillment and gratification. However, the new mother who enjoys these benefits may also experience guilt over a conflict between being in the work force and societal expectations of her as a parent. While fathers are expected to return to work soon after the birth of a baby, society is unclear over the role of the mother in and out of the home.

Some new parents feel they should postpone various activities and stay at home with their baby until he or she is several months old, for the baby's own good. This attitude only makes it more difficult for the infant to adapt to new environments, with resultant guilt in the parents. Also, many parents form a sort of compromise with the baby about schedules. The parent observes the infant's activity state and conducts chores or activities accordingly, doing active or noisy tasks when the infant is active and alert, and doing quiet tasks when the baby is drowsy. Gradually, the new parent realizes that the infant is somewhat oblivious to what is being done for his or her own good. The parent begins to expose the infant to new situations through short trips outside the home, which the infant probably tolerates very well and enjoys. Experienced parents tend to begin this adaptation earlier in the infant's life because they have learned from previous children that their baby reacts positively to new situations.

Adapting the family's life-style needs to be done subtly and gradually so that the focus will not always be on the infant. Subtle life-style changes will aid in the infant's personality development. The baby has a sense of egocentrism (discussed under infant personality) that needs to be resolved. If the baby is held as the center of attention for a prolonged period of time with all family activities revolving around him or her, then the baby will continue to see himself or herself as the center of everything. As the infant becomes older, this pattern becomes more difficult to change without a certain amount of emotional or psychological trauma.

The family needs to "childproof" the physical environment. Infants are totally dependent upon the family to protect them and provide a safe living environment. Parents and older children should be aware of common household perils such as electrical sockets and outlets, poisonous or flammable products, heat-producing appliances, open flames, or carelessly discarded plastic bags. Younger children can be helpful by protecting the crawling baby from open stairs or hazardous work areas.

Away from home, the most important safety measure that a family can enforce for the baby is the use of authorized car seats and seat belts. It has only been in recent years that all 50 states have enacted legislation requiring the use of such child restraints on infants and children under the age of 5 ("State Legislative Activities," 1985, August 23). The importance of this cannot be overstressed, since accidents are the second leading cause of death in infants.

Reallocation of financial resources may also bring about certain life-style adaptations. A new mother who worked before the baby's birth but now stays home may find herself on a budget for the first time. She may be resentful of this or may have difficulty managing her reduced income. An increased number of arguments with the father, who is feeling pressure as the sole wage earner, could result. The mother experiences personal conflict as she tries to cope with her new role of mother, while relinquishing her career and wage-earning capacity. Life-style adaptation as it influences individual members' self-actualization is a common example of a family task that is in conflict with an individual developmental task.

Siblings or other family members living in the home may pick up on this financial strain and feel guilty about this development. Children especially may think that it would be easier for mommy and daddy if there were one less person around, such as themselves. All of the family members may experience some resentment toward the baby, especially in an unplanned pregnancy, as they view it as the source of this predicament.

Families can constructively alleviate their problems by increasing their financial allotments (federally funded programs, military benefits, etc.) and by including the baby as an income tax deduction.

Incorporating the New Family Structure into Society

The family that functions as an open system has interaction with society. The addition of the infant into the family should not limit this interaction, but should increase it. It is at this point that the role of the father becomes more evident. The view is held that the mother is associated with the home, nurturing, and early dependence. Clarke-Stewart (1987) points out that fathers interact more with their infants in play and other social situations, while mothers interact more in caretaking activities. The father is seen more as the link to the outside world (Kiernan & Scoloveno, 1977). This may have evolved from his position as primary wage earner, working outside the home, or from the historical standpoint of the father as the protector of the household by acting as a buffer with society. Over time, fathers have become more interested in their babies and being involved in their care. This has resulted in fathers becoming attached to their babies in the neonatal period rather than later in infancy. Early attachment between father and infant is influenced by his presence at delivery and the amount of caretaking permitted by the mother (Jones, 1981). Mothers are becoming more aware of the valuable relationship and encouraging the father's participation, even as early as the prenatal period.

Some fathers are attuned to the need to get the mother and child out of the home, both for relaxation for the mother and to broaden the infant's experiences. Also, most fathers are anxious to take their offspring out and show them off. It is important that the initial interactions with society be structured in such a way that the experience is a positive one, so that it will be repeated. Therefore, the family will want to go places where their infant is socially acceptable—a place where it will not matter if the baby cries, throws things on the floor, or needs to have a diaper changed. The parents will also be wanting an environment that is appropriate for their child— not one that is smoke-laden, too hot or too cold, noticeably quiet, or expensively decorated. Because of this, couples are temporarily relinquishing their recreational patterns, which may formerly have included bars, water-skiing, and exclusive restaurants. The family develops a change in social patterns and interests and starts to do more family-oriented things.

Introducing the infant to people outside the family and close friends occurs as the family returns to society. For example, as the family attends church, they may choose to leave the baby in the church nursery during the services. While the baby may notice the difference, more anxiety is experienced by the mother. She may feel that the baby has become frightened by the strange environment, is not having personal needs met, or she misses her baby and feels uncomfortable being away from the baby. The experience of leaving the baby with a sitter for the first time can be a major hurdle. Each parent will need some support and encouragement from their significant other in order to work through this first-time separation. This is necessary to permit both parent and child to continue to develop separately from each other.

Maintaining Interpersonal Relationships

This family task is interactive with life-style adaptation and incorporation of the family into society. These tasks are aimed at creating harmonious relationships among family members and between the family and society. This task is also largely the responsibility of the major caretaker, who acts as mediator between the infant and the rest of the family. This caretaker, usually the mother, has assumed this mediator role within the family unit and intercedes during arguments to promote the emotional well-being of each member. Along with maintaining order and morale, the mother strives to spend equal time (in quality, if not quantity) with each person. This becomes more difficult as the family expands, so the role must sometimes be shared with another member. Some mothers, in their conscious efforts to avoid sibling rivalry, may create a jealous father who sees that his children are getting all of the attention. If he points this out to the mother, she becomes angry and frustrated, as she may feel that her efforts have gone unappreciated.

Obviously, open communication between family members is crucial to success with this task. It may also be necessary for the role of mediator to be re-evaluated, but with clear delineation of authority. This will avoid further confusion about who is the decision maker and disciplinarian in the family. Appropriate nursing interventions can guide the family into a solution appropriate to individual family structure and life-style.

Establishing Goals, Priorities, and Values

This task may not be quite as apparent to the family as physical care or reallocation of resources, but it is central to the happiness and success of the family as a continuing unit. New parents will find that their individual goals may undergo alteration, just as individual roles have. They begin to look upon themselves more as a unit, rather than separate entities. The parent will also structure goals for the family as a unit, plus establishing goals for the members. The goals, while unique to each family, will usually include a plan and a desired outcome. They will be achieved at varying times, and some will remain continuous throughout the life of that family unit. Goals may be seen as immediate, short-term, or long-term. Family members may not write such a concrete plan, but they may often verbalize their desired goals for the family. Table 5–1 clarifies the types of goals.

Establishment of priorities may have been minimal or ill-defined prior to the birth of the first child. This is most likely because each parent was prioritizing for himself or herself, and then as a couple. As the baby arrives, the parents need to reassess life-style, plans, and goals, and to agree or compromise on the areas that take precedence. For example, the couple may need to choose between putting money in savings and providing new items for the baby. Decisions will need to be made concerning things the baby needs, without buying to the extent that the budget is strained.

Establishing priorities and working toward goals are more structured and overt

TABLE 5–1. GOALS FOR THE FAMILY WITH AN INFANT

Type of Goal	Goal (Outcome)	Plan	Initiated by
Immediate	Help baby recover from a cold	Encourage rest and fluids. Reduce fever with prescribed medication	Major caretaker
Short-term	Wean baby by first birthday	Substitute bottle with cup often	Any family member
Long-term	Develop values and behaviors accepted by this family	Express approval or disapproval	Parents
		Explain certain values as child grows	

tasks than determining values for the family. Developing a value system is gradual and subtle, and often remains rather abstract. New parents may have approaches toward the development of values, but eventually find that it takes a great deal of discipline to hold on to the approach. A parent may begin with a rigid behavior standard, but gradually relax it. This may be exemplified in caretaking skills. A primipara may begin motherhood by vowing that she will always quickly respond to her baby's cries in a gentle, patient manner, whether it be day or night. However, Mercer (1986) determined that, of a group of primiparas under study, only 28% of those did actually respond in a consistent manner. Other mothers tended to ignore their babies' cries, or pick up the baby and put him or her in bed with them. For some mothers, over time, the desire to meet personal needs is in conflict with meeting the needs of the baby.

On the other hand, the behavior pattern may reverse itself. New parents may agree, before the birth of their first child to be open and accepting of their baby's behavior to allow him or her individual growth. Later they find in themselves a different perspective toward parenting, and become more structured in their discipline to cause the baby to conform to their or society's standards. This does not mean that values are dropped; they need to be altered to become more realistic and obtainable.

INDIVIDUAL TASKS OF THE INFANT

The developmental changes that take place in the infant are proportionately more rapid than during any other period of life. While the physical changes taking place in the neonate (birth to the end of the first month of life) may seen more profound than general growth of the first year, the psychosocial characteristics are much more evident for the infant (beginning of second month to the end of the twelfth month of life). This first year may be considered a "critical period" in a persons's life. Duvall (1977) states that critical periods in human development occur at the times when specific organs or other aspects of an individual's growth are undergoing most rapid change. It is at this time that a person is most vulnerable to environmental factors. This is how many people view an infant—as vulnerable. We experience progressive development, beginning with the physical realm, then moving into the psychological (Mussen, 1979). The individual developmental tasks of the infant reflect this physical, then psychological, progression. The tasks for this period are:

1. Physical development
2. Release of egocentrism
3. Developing a concept of sexuality
4. Expanding interpersonal relationships
5. Establishing communication patterns
6. Developing competency and achievement

Physical development during infancy often receives priority attention at the expense of other tasks. Psychosocial growth and other accomplishments must also be well established during this first year of life in order to contribute to the total development of the individual.

Physical Development

Body growth and weight gain is one of the most outstanding physical characteristics of the infant. It is most typical for this growth to be in spurts, not constant, and delays should be expected (Ritchey & Taper, 1983). These spurts are more noticeable during the second half of the first year of life. The infant will gain about 1½ pounds every month during the first 6 months of life, then will experience sporadic increases. The baby's birth weight will most likely have tripled by the first birthday. Body length will increase one inch per month during the first 6 months, and birth length will have increased by approximately 50% by the first birthday. Bone development seems to be more rapid in black babies than in Caucasian and is also more rapid in females than in males (all races) (Ritchey & Taper, 1983).

The major body systems increase in proportion to the skeletal structure. The heart, lungs, gastrointestinal tract, genitourinary system, lymphatic system, and the brain increase 50% in size by the end of the first year. The least amount of growth is in the genitalia. Identifiable marks or characteristics present on the neonate may gradually disappear. The infant gains more subcutaneous fat, and the skin does not seem so transparent and thin.

The digestive system is fully functioning at 3 months. The ability to concentrate urine increases, but glomerular filtration rate remains low for several months. Timing of stooling is regulated by 6 months (Tackett & Hunsberger, 1981), but actual awareness of the need to defecate or void does not become apparent before about 1 year of age.

Infants are instinctive nose breathers initially. Use of the respiratory system is augmented when the baby learns to breathe through his or her mouth. The body recognizes this only as an alternative, as in the case of congested nasal passages, since mouth breathing does not warm, humidify, or purify the inspirations.

The fetal circulatory structures, which are not needed after birth, should have ceased to function immediately after birth or during the neonatal period. Delayed or improper closure causes cardiopulmonary problems in the child during the infancy or toddler periods. These structures are described in Table 5–2.

The baby gradually establishes motor control with purposeful movements. By 16 weeks, increased cortical function causes better sensorimotor behavior, especially with ocular and manual activity (Gesell, 1955). This allows the infant to have better

TABLE 5–2. FETAL CIRCULATORY STRUCTURES

Structure	Location	Time of Obliteration
Foramen ovale	Between right and left atrium	1 year
Ductus arteriosus	Junction of pulmonary artery and aorta	1 month
Ductus venosus	Liver, at inferior vena cava	2 months
Umbilical arteries	From descending aorta	2–3 months
Umbilical vein	Between placenta and liver	2–3 months

interaction with the environment and to do more exploring. By ten months, motor control extends the infant's environment. Use of this motor control is discussed in greater depth in the section on activity and play.

Nutrition.   The rapid growth of the infant, especially in the vital organs, demands proper nutrients. Protein is particularly needed for central nervous system development, so it should be the major element in the baby's daily intake. Daily protein and calorie requirements vary with the amount of activity. Infants have the instinctive sense, like animals, to eat when they are hungry and not by a timetable. The parent who feeds the infant by a rigid schedule may develop a child obsessed with food and mealtime. Constantly offering the baby a bottle or finger food develops eating habits linked to oral gratification for security or a positive reward. This results in an obese child with a need to always be eating. Because the kidneys are better able to concentrate urine, the need for fluid replacement reduces slightly as the child grows older. Proper fluid intake is still a priority in infant nutrition, but fluids are no longer the sole source of nutrients. Table 5–3 indicates the recommended daily requirements of critical components for infant nutrition.

Introduction of solids is not considered necessary before 2½ or 3 months of age. It is easy for the parent to gradually begin certain foods, as the infant readily accepts new things at this age. The extrusion reflex is fading, and the infant will retain a solid placed in the mouth. It is often recommended that solids not be introduced into the infant's diet much before 5 months of age, due to the limited digestive capability of the stomach (Whaley & Wong, 1983). Because neonatal iron stores are used up by about this same time, this is a good time to begin specific foods that will replenish the iron, such as cereal. Because the infant begins teething at about 6 months, he or she enjoys having something to chew or bit that can be swallowed. Crackers or cookies especially made for the infant are particularly good. Table 5–4 lists suggested ages for introducing new foods.

Sleep/Activity Patterns.   Sleep requirements gradually decrease during the first year of life. By about 3 months of age, the baby eliminates one daytime nap, will take a long morning or afternoon nap, and dozes briefly during the other part of the day. The baby will sleep approximately 12–14 hours during the night, but will generally awaken for a feeding. By 9–12 months of age, most infants will sleep all night, especially if they are weaned, are eating solid foods, and do not have to be fed as often. With the gradually increasing periods of wakefulness, the infant spends more time

TABLE 5–3. CRITICAL COMPONENTS OF INFANT NUTRITION

Component	Age	
(per kilogram of body weight)	*6 months*	*1 year*
Kilocalories	105	900
Protein	2.0 g	2.0 g
Fluids	130–155 ml	120–135 ml

From Ritchey, S., & Taper, L.J. (1983). Maternal and child nutrition. New York: Harper & Row.

TABLE 5–4. AGES FOR INTRODUCING NEW FOODS

Age (in months)	Food
1–3	Fruit juice
4	Strained cereal (rice, oatmeal)
4½–5½	Strained vegetables and fruits
5½–6	Strained meats
7–9	Firm finger foods (crackers, meat sticks)

From Ritchey, S., & Taper, L.J. (1983). Maternal and child nutrition. New York: Harper & Row.

interacting with the environment. The increased neuromuscular development and longer energy span cause the infant to seek ways to stay busy. As will be seen in subsequent chapters on early childhood, play is the child's work and is a source of fulfillment. The infant likes to learn more about the self, and derives great pleasure from discovering his or her own image in a mirror. Infants also enjoy learning special sensations over the entire body, such as the feelings brought by bare contact with a fur rug or the water in a bath. The infant learns through play and is challenged in the areas of fine and gross motor skills by being given a piece of sticky tape, squeeze toys, or an activity box, or being placed in a walker.

Release of Egocentrism

As self-identity is evolving, the infant learns certain restrictions. By being demanding, he or she is able to receive rapid gratification and feel that he or she is the center of a somewhat limited environment. However, the infant gradually becomes aware of the fact that some demands are not always immediately met. The infant does not receive immediate attention and becomes more demanding—out of fear, frustration, egotism, and the desire for gratification. These incentives result in aggressive behaviors.

The parent(s) tries to help the infant become aware of the fact that one cannot always control the environment and that needs cannot always be immediately met. The baby discovers that the most basic needs will indeed be met and that he or she will receive necessary comfort and attention. The baby learns that he or she is treated more favorably—cooing, tender handling—with certain behaviors, and sometimes needs are met more quickly. The infant gradually learns to relinquish certain unsuitable behavior modes for more positive, pleasurable, acceptable ones (Maier, 1969). The baby realizes how enjoyable favorable responses are and strives to repeat those behaviors that will bring them. The infant learns that, while still being the focus of a small, personal world, he or she needs and responds to others. Major caretakers are incorporated into this world, and the infant becomes less egocentric.

The gradual release of egocentrism frees the infant, allowing the infant to let go of the self and take in and learn from the outside world. In the early months of life, the infant knows of object permanence only in relation to the self. If something can be seen, touched, or heard, then it exists. Once removed from the limited world, it ceases to exist. At about 7 months, the infant is more attuned to the surroundings and will search for an item removed from the immediate view. For example, in the early months of life, a small block placed under a cup is quickly forgotten. The 6-month-old infant, however, will search for a block if it is hidden, and take great pleasure in finding it. These discoveries are, of course, aided by the infant's progressing motor development.

Developing a Concept of Sexuality

Sexuality is a component of personality and is extremely influential upon interpersonal relationships. The infant is not aware of a distinction between male and female of any age. Concepts concerning the infant's own gender and appropriate roles are gradually acquired through observation. The infant learns what is sex-appropriate behavior for him or her because it will be reinforced, especially by the parent(s).

Parents have their own ideas on how they want their child to develop, what they want their child to be, even before the baby is born. Despite the increase in sexual equality, the fundamental physical and psychosocial differences continue to be recognized by new parents, and the baby is treated accordingly. The sex of the child influences parental responses to him or her and the direction of training and discipline. Fathers are more likely to handle their daughters more delicately, speak more softly, coo more, and feel more protective toward them (Parke et al., 1979). For male infants, separation from the mother and incorporation into the masculine environment is likely to occur at an earlier age. Fathers and other family members are more likely to roughhouse sooner with a boy, with fewer protestations from the mother than if the rough play involved a female infant. Jones (1981) found that fathers had more positive perceptions of high-irritability boys and low-irritability girls and also verbalized more to the girls. This seems to indicate some of the parental expectations for the new baby, thus influencing future personality development.

Infants are not cognizant of presexual behavior; adults are. The values of the adults having most of the interaction with the infant are transferred to him or her. Increased exploration and manipulation of body parts results in handling of the genitalia, especially in later infancy, as sensations in that area increase (Hymovich, 1980). The parent may not give this much consideration at this young age, interpreting it for what it is: exploring and learning about the body, or associating it with early toilet-training behaviors. Some parents are most embarrassed and distraught by genital handling and slap the child's hand away. As these behaviors persist into the preschool years, the child's increasing sexual identification may be complicated by guilt.

Further value transfer takes place by dressing the baby in gender-appropriate clothes and colors, and frequently placing the baby in the company of family members of the same gender. Gender identification may be particularly difficult for a male infant born to a single mother, especially if he lives in a strongly maternally oriented household.

Expanding Interpersonal Relationships

The chapter on the neonate described the establishment of a close, very special relationship between the baby and one other individual. The bond formed by attachment and reciprocal behaviors enables the baby to learn about others and how to interact with them (Klaus & Kennell, 1983). Because of the neonate's limited self-concept, the strong attachment figure is perceived as present only to gratify the baby. The infant, however, is learning more about the external environment and is developing increasing awareness of others outside of the self and the mother. As the infant gains stronger control over the body and special senses, exploration and interaction increase. The infant begins to respond more and receives responses from a variety of people and situations.

It is at this point that the personality of the infant becomes more apparent. Personality is individuality; it is the compilation of personal behaviors, characteristics, responses, and moods, all making us what we are. As the infant begins to display certain behaviors and moods, family members realize that this baby is more than just a cuddly little body, but also has a real person inside.

Family members, especially the mother, gradually learn the baby's personality based upon his or her temperament. Temperament is a reaction pattern that is an inherent characteristic of all infants. It is not formed by the major caretaker, but may undergo some changes as the infant adapts to the world. Most likely, it is the major caretaker who learns to adapt to the infant, attuning to cues from the child and anticipating a slow or fast reaction to a specific situation. This has been termed a process of *mutual modification*. Temperament is seen as being composed of these qualities (Thomas & Chess, 1977):

1. Level of activity
2. Physiological rhythm
3. Approachability
4. Adaptability
5. Intensity of reaction
6. Distractability
7. Persistence
8. Mood
9. Threshold of responsiveness

Awareness of these aspects of temperament guide the mother in her care for the baby and responses to his or her behavior.

Formation of strong attachment behaviors leads to the establishment of trust. Erikson (1963) has indicated that it is crucial for the infant to learn to trust both self and others, for his or her own internal security and as a foundation of interpersonal relationships. Trust includes the reliance upon others, a certain dependence upon others, and the belief that a person or persons will provide such pleasurable aspects of life as gratification and companionship. As trust is internalized, the infant learns that he or she must also trust himself or herself to communicate properly with others in order to make needs known. The infant trusts his or her own bodily urges, and relies on others for the continuity of care (Erikson, 1963). As needs are met, confidence is established, and the infant can turn attention to other aspects of environment and self, attuning to needs of a higher order, thus increasing inner growth.

Attachment behaviors and the trusting of others occur in differing degrees with different people. In a family, depth of attachment behaviors occur at different levels:

the infant places the family members in a hierarchical pattern according to the amount and quality of care and interaction. One of the most common examples of this would be the infant's preferences for mother, father, older sibling, etc.—in that order, based upon who the infant perceives as best able to "read" him or her and care for needs. In a broader sense, the infant may exhibit some attachment behaviors with a variety of people—those who are known to him (grandparents, babysitter, neighbors, etc.)—but forms the attachment bond with only a select few (Bowlby, 1982). Because of repeated displays of positive, secure loving and caring, the infant knows who can be trusted and is consequently more closely attached to those people. The evolution of trust through security is one of the biggest hurdles for the infant to overcome. It is the foundation for future interactions; it is a requirement for later interpersonal relationships. Failure to establish trust can result in infantile schizophrenia. In the adult, failure to accomplish this task is manifested as withdrawal into depressive and schizoid states (Erikson, 1963). A trusting person is able to interact in a positive, meaningful manner with others and the environment.

Establishing Communication Patterns

As the infant realizes the value of interactions with others, he or she begins to develop a method to communicate in order to express needs or desires. This is done through speech (preverbal and verbal linguistic sounds) and language (vocabulary and word usage according to the native tongue of the immediate environment). The young infant learns that he or she can make a variety of sounds, which he or she likes to hear. While this brings the infant enough pleasure that he or she will continue these nonsensical utterances, the family recognizes this as the early stage of talking and reinforces it through positive gestures and repetition of the infant's sounds. As the family members begin reinforcement, they will need to understand the importance of speaking to the infant distinctly. The infant needs to hear clear, distinguishable speech patterns and words in order to learn proper language and to foster speech development.

The infant develops more refined control of the facial muscles and the tongue at about 2–3 months and can then begin to coo, squeal, and babble. Between 6 and 8 months, the infant can imitate speech sounds, and by 9 months can make all basic sounds. The first word is usually "Ma-ma" or a facsimile. Some fathers are upset when their baby chooses this word, but it easier for the infant to form an "M" with the lips than a "D" with the gums and hard palate. Since the vowel sound in "Ma-ma" and "Da-da" is the same, then "Da-da" is usually the second word spoken, especially if the baby has been receiving a lot of repetitive reinforcement of the formation of the "D" sound.

Between the 9th and 12th months of life, the infant will know his or her own name and begin building a vocabulary by associating sounds with meanings. For example, the word-sound "meow" to him means "kitty." At 1 year of age, the baby will have a vocabulary of about six words, usually nouns and verbs concerned with daily life—cup, bed, eat, play, etc. Beyond the inherent ability in each infant, progress in language and speech is related to the amount and quality of verbal interaction, the further development of the speech structures, and individual curiosity.

Because the young infant has no concept of the *meaning* of words and generally sees them as symbols, it is possible for the infant to develop bilingually. This may be done deliberately by the parent(s), or as a result of parents/caretakers from two cultures. In Mexican-American homes, the mother may speak Spanish with her baby, while the father, who has more contact with the English-speaking community outside the home, may feel it is important to also teach the baby English. The baby may come to accept the fact that one set of words is used with the father and another set with the mother, perceiving this to be part of each parent's personality.

Developing Competency and Achievement

Every individual has an inner need for achievement. Through successful achievement of a task or goal, one gains self-satisfaction and strong personal integrity. Achievement requires a certain amount of competency—the underlying knowledge and skills necessary to complete the goal or task. Competency is accomplished by the taking in of certain information and by the practicing of the specific skill(s). Achievement is then reached when one is able to apply personal competency to the situation.

These concepts of competency and achievement are also true for the infant. While the tasks or goals of the infant may seem, to adults, to be very rudimentary—grasping a toy, learning to speak—they require as much effort, learning, and practice on the part of the infant as is needed for an adult to present a major project.

Jean Piaget theorized that learning in infancy evolved from combined intellectual and affective (emotional) functions (Maier, 1969). Piaget identifies learning and development as results of adaptation to the environment. He views the adaptation as cognitive striving by the person to find equilibrium between himself and his environment. It involves assimilation—use of the environment according to the individual's perceptions—and accommodation—incorporation of the environment as it truly is. The two forces balance each other in an effort to obtain affective, mental, and biological equilibrium.

Piaget postulates that intellectual organization is just beginning by 1 year of age. In preparation for that, the infant begins to imitate, relate to objects, and utilize depth perception. The infant learns through the use of schemata—patterns of cyclic, meaningful behaviors that promote cognition. The infant takes in a certain aspect of the environment and categorizes it according to its meaning. An example of this is that the infant looks at mother's face, recognizes it, and associates it with pleasure and gratification. Through the use of schemata, the infant achieves accommodation and assimilation to gain knowledge of this new world outside of the self. While Piaget established approximately 1 year of age for true intellectual development to occur, the work of Wolff (1969) and Brazelton and associates (Parker & Brazelton, 1981) indicates that forms of learning (such as recognition of the human face or imitation) begin in the neonatal period. In the infant, early learning comes from primitive neurological organization and repetition. As the infant grows older and possesses greater neurological organization, increasing alertness, and an expanding environment, the existing schemata change, and new ones are developed as the baby learns.

At approximately 7 months, the infant can effectively use the palmar grasp to rake an object or perform a hand-to-hand transfer. The baby can spontaneously lift his or her head, turn over, and sit without assistance. The ability to perform these movements allows the infant to take in more of the world and attune to something of interest. By 10 months of age, the infant can purposefully use the pincer grasp, may begin to creep, and will be observed doing a specific movement to attain a goal, such as rolling over, scooting or creeping, then raking in a toy. Erect posture while standing is possible at about this age, and by the first birthday, most infants are able to walk with their hands held.

As parents reflect upon their infant's development by the end of the first year of life, they realize how much their baby truly has accomplished. The infant, through competency and achievement, has been able to broaden the environment and become more independent. The stage is set for more refined learning during the toddler period.

POTENTIAL STRESSORS

The infant is susceptible to stressors from many sources. The immaturity of the infant's body potentiates possible physical illness. The physical, emotional, and psychological dependence of the infant causes him or her to rely on others to have needs met. In circumstances in which caretakers and family members are unable to appropriately meet these needs, the infant becomes a helpless victim.

Physical Stressors

The young infant still has unrefined body systems and low immunity to certain diseases. Consequently, it is easier for an infant to contract certain illnesses, and the course of the illness may be more severe than in an older child. The rapid metabolic rate of the infant contributes to more profound symptoms, such as high fever or rapid dehydration.

For the infant with a congenital anomaly, the physical/physiological effects of the anomaly may become more evident during the first year of life. The infant who is chronically ill or experiences prolonged hospitalization may experience interference with other developmental tasks because of physical incapacity. Opportunities for play, interaction with other family members, and learning may be rather limited during illness.

Many infants are exposed to typical childhood diseases from contact with siblings and other children who have the disease. Unless the infant has passive acquired immunity, he or she may experience a course of the disease. An infant who is chronically ill or has a weak health status may be seriously affected by an illness that is considered common and of no consequence in many other babies.

Adequate nutritional intake and preventive health care, especially immunizations, are the most significant measures that can be taken to prevent physical stress. The infant in an environment in which there is inadequate caretaking and little access to health care is at greatest risk for physical problems.

Social and Emotional Stressors

Potential stressors to social or emotional development come from the infant's striv-
ings to establish relationships with others and as the infant learns and tries to become
a part of this newly discovered world. Because all of the infant's initial dealings with
others are with the mother and father, these are the most important relationships,
and can cause the most anxiety.

In the first few months of life, the infant is balanced between egocentrism and
the early formation of a trusting relationship. Any factor that interferes with this
equilibrium, thus disturbing the parent–infant relationship, causes the infant to
regress and become mistrustful. For example, separation, due to illness in either the
baby or the mother, decreases the mother's perception of competency in dealing with
the baby at a critical time, lowers her self-esteem, and disrupts the attachment
process. These factors in combination lead to poor or inconsistent mothering and
result in the infant being confused about being able to safely depend upon someone
to meet his or her needs. This causes the baby to have difficulty establishing a strong
bond with other caretakers. A conflict between parental perceptions or expectations
and the actual infant behavior will also lead to a disturbed parent–infant relationship. A parent who does not understand the baby, or a baby who is identified as being
difficult, results in a tense emotional environment.

Concerning parental preference, Lamb (1977) determined that in a stress-free
environment, the infant seems to have no parental preference, and will feel comfortable with father or mother. Given a situation in which the infant perceives stress—a
new environment, for example—the infant prefers a parent over a stranger. Also, the
infant will prefer the mother over the father when both are present.

Conflicts with Family Tasks

Difficulties often arise within the family as it works to include the infant and as the
infant gradually learns about the family. The problems can be short-term, in the
presence of an acute situation, or more long-term and in-depth, such as the problem
of poor parent–infant relationship. If the baby is unwanted, he or she could very
likely be rejected by the parent(s) and never made a part of the family. If the
pregnancy is unplanned, the parent(s) may experience resentment. Many family
members may feel rivalry or jealousy directed to the baby, and may express these
feelings either directly to the baby through rough handling or neglect, or may disrupt
the family patterns through regressive behaviors.

Failure to incorporate the infant may be unintentional. The new parents may
prolong the special atmosphere around the baby and keep him or her as the center of
the family, yet not a part of it. This delayed incorporation causes the infant to have
delayed release of his or her egocentrism, sometimes to the point that the infant will
be somewhat self-centered. Efforts to keep the baby at the cute newborn stage may
impair the infant's motor and language development. All of this attention to the baby
results in resentment by other family members, especially siblings.

Failure to progress with family developmental tasks following the birth of the
baby could also be due to improper or unequal role assignment. Perhaps the mother

finds she is expected to do all the caretaking, household activities, and a full-time job, while the father continues in his status quo as if the baby had not been born. Conversely, the mother and father could be competing for the role of major caretaker and neglect their role of spouse. Some families also experience difficulties because they are not able to successfully deal with the financial shift or schedule changes.

Some families experience a situation in which the birth of a baby must take second place, because there is a priority need by another family member. Because family patterns are already well-founded among existing members when the baby is born, those ties are stronger and may receive attention. The priority could be an illness of a family member or activities to help a member achieve a major goal, such as admission into college or a promotion at work. The illness of another child can be particularly devastating, especially in the case of a terminal disease. The ill child may not understand the nature of the sickness, or may think that the parents will be all right if he or she dies because they have a new baby. If the new mother has a complicated intrapartum period, then the family not only has an ill member, but is without the major caretaker. Prolonged illness in a family involves time, money, and physical and emotional energy that should be channeled toward the new baby and involvement with the family. The main effect on the infant is that he or she may not become attached to any one person; the mother and father are at the hospital with their sick child, or daddy was killed and mother injured in an automobile accident. During these stressful periods, the infant may have multiple caretakers, or one major one who knows that this is a temporary position and keeps a certain emotional distance. The baby may also have difficulty establishing rhythmicity patterns due to the family's erratic schedule.

Conflicts in Parenting

Parenting is fraught with obstacles, real or imagined, threatening or perceived as such. As with other components of family development, these conflicts may or may not be experienced by each family. Some of the conflicts may have a greater impact upon the family than others, and each family handles the situations in unique ways that optimize its functioning.

Possibly one of the most common types of discord stems from the parents as a couple. It is crucial for this dyad to be established with assigned roles and common goals before it can expand and take on new ones. Interference with this establishment can occur in a number of ways.

Nontraditional Order. A common yardstick for family and life patterns has been termed *sentimental order*. In American society, the pattern is dating, engagement, marriage, an extended honeymoon period, then a child, then perhaps another child or children. This pattern is both highly romanticized and publicized. The media do much to display this route as the pursuit of the individual American dream, especially for the female. (Of course, this does not take into consideration career goals or other contributions to society by both the male and female.) A couple who "has to get married" because of an unwanted or unplanned pregnancy interrupts this pattern. Each of them may have a sense of loss, grieving for irretrievable experiences. He would have liked to have more time to get to know her better or make some financial plans; she feels deprived of a long engagement, her picture in the newspapers, bridal showers, and other attention. This sense of loss creates anger that is first directed at each other, then later toward the baby as it becomes more of a reality. In the mother, the anger may be manifested as prolonged postpartum blues or a feeling of entrapment. The father may view the baby as an unwanted financial burden and threat to freedom. The couple may begin to bicker over a variety of problems, and try to place blame on each other for their present circumstances. One or both parents may abuse the infant, as he or she seems to be a major source of their unhappiness. While the situation cannot be reversed or reordered, it can be optimized. The couple needs to ventilate their feelings with a professional counselor, and then be shown some individualized alternatives that will help to compensate for their losses.

The Extended Family.   The mention of the words "in-laws" evokes quite a variety of responses from couples. While many people enjoy a most favorable relationship with the second family, unfavorable or disharmonious relationships are the ones most frequently mentioned in conversations, jokes, and marital strife.

Sometimes the problems arise when the dyad has not established themselves as a couple, either because they live in the home of one of the sets of parents or because they are beginning their family through the nontraditional route. Consequently, they become parents before their unity is well founded. In these circumstances, one or both parties still strongly identifies with the family of orientation, tending to side with them over the partner in an argument, not encouraging interaction between spouse and family, or perhaps displaying to their family dissatisfaction with their partner. Any of these behaviors tells both the partner and the family of orientation that the bonds are not strong enough between the pair to allow them to break off and begin their own family.

On the other hand, the establishment of the particular dyad may be the cause of in-law trouble. Perhaps it was a "had to" situation of a sudden marriage, and everyone was faced with disappointment, embarrassment, grief, anger, and many other emotional responses. This often results in a lack of family loyalty. One member of the pair senses, or is certain of, lack of support or any positive feelings from the partner's family. The source of conflict is evident here because the partner has to choose between spouse and parents (Duvall, 1977). At the birth of the baby, the new parents realize they are missing some support they sorely need at this time of change and stress. Sometimes the birth of a baby fills a need for the new grandparents, who consequently develop more positive feelings for their in-laws. The new parent may recognize that it was the baby, not themselves, that brought about this change and a great deal of resentment may occur, being directed toward the baby.

Even in families that have harmonious interaction with the members of the extended family, the arrival of an infant can cause some changes in this interaction. One or both of the parents may find it difficult to assign roles to the new grandparents, aunts, etc. Each parent may be reluctant to assume a responsibility for role assignment that may cause friction. However, if roles remain unassigned, individuals within the extended family may either assume an inappropriate role or withdraw from involvement with the baby. This lack of communication within a family demonstrates how parenting can have difficult beginnings.

Parenting Versus Individual Goals.   Progressive societal views are recognizing, accepting, and encouraging the contributions that the adult female member of the family can make to the professions, business, industry, and the general work force. Many women are finding that not only are they able to contribute in a significant manner, but they are in some instances able to successfully compete with their male counterparts in the job market. Women of childbearing age who recognize that they enjoy working outside of the home and prefer the opportunities and challenges that the work world provides are often reluctant to relinquish that completely in order to stay home specifically to raise children. This becomes a particular problem when they are linked with a partner who is more traditionally minded or holds the view that it is more beneficial for the child that the mother remain at home until the child is a specific age (usually anywhere from 6 months to 1 year, or until school age). This is a major philosophical argument that can only be resolved according to each specific situation, family, and life-style. The parents need to discuss this and work out a practical compromise.

With the increase in career-oriented women, there is also a trend in which women are delaying childbearing until a later age. Through conception control and later marriages, women are opting to establish their business, profession, or job seniority first in order to meet personal self-actualization. For childbearing women, a conflict occurs when they are confronted with career responsibilities and motherhood. This role confrontation may be viewed as a conflict when, to the individual, the roles are seen as being incompatible. Pickens (1982) examined a group of over-30, career-oriented primiparas. By choosing to interrupt their careers in order to have children, these women were faced with this role confrontation. They seemed to positively deal with the conflict by comfortably accepting a personal definition of self, which was sometimes opposed to society's definition of the working mother. Pickens found that these new mothers had a strong sense of identity and were desirous of combining roles. In fact, many of them anticipated giving stimulation and input into their child's development, viewing motherhood as a task similar to a job. Consequently, the mother who anticipates or experiences role conflict should be helped to define her personal role for herself. This role could include goal-setting and task accomplishment that could be applied in any environment. The mother could then determine realistic expectations for herself as she fulfills her maternal and career roles.

Romantic Versus Realistic.   Many new parents may not be experiencing some of the specific problems previously mentioned, but are finding a general disillusionment with what it is like to have a baby and become parents. Advertising media have done a great deal to portray what a desirable home life is like with the baby, and many people are led to believe that this is average. When their baby is not as cuddly and even-tempered as the one on TV, the new parents begin to wonder what other disappointments are in store for them. This form of reality shock occurs more often with first-time parents, but can happen in families with the second or third child. As the family grows, the parents take on more responsibilities, find more friction in the household, and begin to wonder if perhaps they should not have stopped their family expansion a child ago.

Parents experiencing this disillusionment need to understand the realistic aspects of parenting. As their social support system grows to include other new parents, they will all find that certain problems are quite common, to the point of being normal. In some cases, they may even find that their own situation is not as bad as someone else's.

Sibling Rivalry. Couples having their second child may have a much brighter outlook, since they feel they have more experience in childbearing and childraising, and are more able to cope with the needs of the newborn. However, the presence of an older child in the home sparks a type of jealousy and presents a new area of conflict never before encountered. The types of responses made by the child toward the baby often create guilt in the parents. Even if they felt they were providing equal attention to both children, it may never seem quite right. Some parents, so burdened with guilt, wonder if they made a mistake in having this baby, especially if it was to be a companion for the older child. A more detailed discussion of sibling rivalry is found in Chapter 6.

Change in Social Support and Life-Style. Having a child can add stability to some families or bring unwanted restrictions to others. Many couples who have been enjoying various activities individually or as a couple find a curtailment or cessation an unwelcome sacrifice. This could be due to the fact that the couple is unwilling to replace one type of fulfillment for another, or is not ready to take on the responsibilities of parenthood. This may be particularly true of the couple who has not progressed in "sentimental order" and has not had the opportunity to enjoy themselves as a couple. Or, if the childbirth occurred to couples who have been married for several years but have remained childless, certain well-established routines become upset. This is frequently seen in couples who, being childless for many years, eventually adopt a child. Their parenthood may be accepted with mixed feelings: joy over finally adding to their family and reluctance to give up certain freedoms.

As individuals grow and change, their interests and external support systems change with them. A couple who has previously enjoyed the company of couples the same age has a shifting of values and priorities once they have a baby. They become more interested in staying at home in the evening. Or their choice of recreation may become limited because there are some activities, such as water-skiing, where bringing the baby along would be quite inconvenient or impractical. The couple will enjoy the pleasure of their baby, yet long to relax with friends. From the perspective of the other couples, they may not fully understand the deep sense of responsibility the new parents have, or are mystified that their friends can easily give up their old routine of late-night partying. The new parents will find that they will gradually begin to acquire a new set of friends in the form of other young families. Opportunities to acquire these new friends abound—other couples from the childbirth education class, other families using the same babysitter, families at church. As the parents' interests change and focus on their baby, they become more aware of other couples who share commonalities.

COPING MECHANISMS

The family with an infant will continue to utilize the effective coping mechanisms that were established during the neonatal period. The family will gradually develop new ways of coping that are appropriate to the frequently changing needs of the infant.

Health Beliefs and Behaviors

The importance of early health care was introduced in the chapter on the neonate (see Chap. 4). By the time the baby enters the infancy period, the family most likely is familiar with a health care practitioner or agency. Since many parents recognize the infant's vulnerability to illness, they will generally adhere to the schedule of routine checkups and immunizations.

Hygiene.   On a daily basis, families will transfer many personal health beliefs and behaviors to the infant. For instance, parents who bathe every day will probably bathe the infant daily. A full daily bath is not always necessary for an infant; the infant's typical daily activities, with perspiration and exposure to bacteria, are not to the same extent as an adult's. It is not advisable to bathe the infant every day in the winter, since the cold, dry air, in combination with soapy water, will cause excessive dryness of the tender skin. Nurses should recommend to most families to bathe the infant every other day and only wash the face, hands, and genital/anal areas daily.

Feeding and Elimination Patterns.   Maintaining feeding and elimination patterns is equal to hygiene in importance and concern to parents in the early months of infancy. The mother will follow the advice of the health care agency concerning feedings: amounts in a 24-hour period, progression to juices and solids, and the use of vitamins. In most families, the tendency is for the parent to be more strictly in line with the doctor's or nurse's recommendations about dietary intake. With subsequent babies, the mother frequently does what seemed to work best with the first child.

Maintaining proper elimination of bodily wastes is usually not difficult for the infant, as the infant instinctively responds to pressure on the sphincters and voids or defecates at will. Given normal circumstances, family members evaluate adequate hydration through a tally of wet diapers for the day. A normal pattern is kept through the feedings: an occasional juice or water, especially in hot weather.

The infant will gradually set personal rhythms for bodily functions. A baby may not have a bowel movement every day, or may have two on some days. These changes from a daily bowel movement at an expected time may cause the mother some unnecessary concern and calls to the pediatrician or clinic. This pattern should not be thought of as constipation. The baby is probably constipated if there has not been a stool in about 3 days, or if the stools seem quite dry and the baby strains to pass them.

It is not unusual for the young infant to pass whole undigested foods, such as corn, due to the inability of the gastrointestinal system to properly digest highly fibrous foods. The parents may, at first, interpret this as diarrhea or a similar disturbance. Diarrhea is generally identified as the passage of several stools per day or stools that are watery and malodorous. Parents can be consoled about these patterns and told what to do for the baby to relieve any discomfort and re-establish a normal routine. Treatment for diarrhea is aimed at slowing intestinal activity and conserving fluids by giving juice, electrolytes, or liquid Jell-O (Whaley & Wong, 1983). For older infants, adsorbent foods, such as bananas or applesauce, will increase stool consistency.

Comfort.   Promotion of comfort can be difficult and frustrating for parents, because the infant is unable to specifically express needs or desires. Some comfort provisions are learned easily, such as positioning. The major caretaker, either consciously or subconsciously, learns that the baby sleeps best on a certain side, likes to be burped in a certain position, and detests sitting in an infant seat. A proper amount of clothing is often the most difficult to assess. In their efforts to protect the baby from catching a cold, plus desire to dress him or her up, parents and grandparents will apply layers of clothes and covers until the baby becomes fretful. The best rule of thumb is for the parent to dress the baby in a weight and number of clothes comparable to what they themselves are wearing that day, then also have a wrap or cover handy in case of drafts.

Teething.   Eruption of teeth at about 6 months of age often causes a change in the infant's behavior. Because of the irritated, tender gums, the baby is often fretful and likes to gnaw on whatever is handy. Teething takes the blame for many simultaneous problems in the baby—gastrointestinal disturbances, sniffles, and a cranky temperament are the common occurrences. Because teething is a universal process, parents know the family or friends will understand the excuse of "The baby's fussy today—I think she's teething."

Teething is also one of the first developmental milestones in a family. Many parents save the first tooth after it comes out, or even save objects showing tooth prints from gnawing during teething. Delayed teething causes some parents to generalize and become anxious over other delays—especially in the cognitive/behavioral areas and in motor development. Dentition is not related to these other areas, but is an inherent, physiological process. Conversely, early dentition is not related to precociousness.

Besides gnawing during the first year of life, many infants like to suck. Infants who at feeding time have not satisfied their desire to suck will usually suck their thumb or finger(s). Many parents try to restrain this natural desire by striking the hand from the mouth. Some do not feel thumbsucking is socially acceptable, but the general concern is when thumbsucking persists past 4 years of age or when the permanent teeth erupt (Whaley & Wong, 1983). To alleviate this anxiety, the parent may wish to provide a pacifier, which is softer, relinquished earlier than the thumb, and will thus preserve skin integrity of the thumb or finger(s).

Play/Activity. The use of play as a time of interaction and for evaluating motor abilities has been discussed. Parents also provide opportunities for play as a form of entertainment. The infant can be quite content with solitary play, which many parents encourage in order to receive a brief break from parenting.

As the baby grows older, the desire for more activity increases. This is a result of increased awareness of the environment, curiosity, and more refined motor skills. Parental responses to the infant's play needs include new forms of diversion, and skill-appropriate toys, such as blocks and squeeze toys. Play is the time of learning and work for the infant. The parent can structure the playtime in such a manner as to specifically guide the baby through a phase of development. As an example, fine motor skills can be enhanced through stacking blocks. The parent can begin by showing the baby how to stack two blocks, repeating the process until the skill is achieved. The next step would be to stack three blocks, then build a pyramid, and so forth. This playtime provides interaction plus meaningful activity. The process of structured play should be particularly appealing to the career-oriented mother or father, who will enjoy organizing the play period and determining a goal.

Responses to Stressors

Adaptive Responses. Since physical needs are a priority, stressors such as cold, hunger, and fatigue more readily upset the infant. In the first few months of life, the infant has learned that increased sounds and movements attract the attention of the major caretaker, who in turn provides whatever the baby needs to promote comfort. The infant gradually builds a vocabulary associated with needs: "bottle," "toy," and "mother" are prime examples. The mother, as major caretaker, learns her baby's individual sounds and is thus able to meet the needs more accurately.

Exploration is used by the infant to make contact with the outside world, thereby increasing learning and decreasing anxiety over the unknown environment. The infant learns about strangers, the rest of the home in which he or she lives, and what dogs, chairs, and kitchen floors feel like. The infant also learns that caretakers set limits on this exploration, or learns (the hard way) what it feels like to fall downstairs.

As the baby matures, he or she becomes more of a social being and encounters stressors in those areas as well. Once the infant begins to cope with stress, the way he or she deals with it can be predictive of a resolution of future stressors and developmental tasks.

Parents vary in their abilities to recognize or admit to stress. The positive or desirable responses to stressors are based on this recognition and attempts to alleviate or adapt to the stressors associated with parenting an infant. Ventura (1982) observed that parents' perceptions of their own caretaking abilities can have an influence on family integrity and perceived need for support or assistance. Parents who were anxious or depressed felt the need for more social support than those parents with less anxiety. These anxious parents also perceived of their baby as less soothable or as a difficult baby. Parents who viewed their infants more positively (easy baby) were those more likely to use positive coping behaviors that would maintain family integrity.

Some individuals readily seek advice and guidance from others. In many cases, it is a person who is trusted and respected for childrearing abilities: mother, sister, grandmother. Some parents like to seek out "genuine" authorities and read books on aspects of baby care and parenting. On the other hand, some parents choose to provide for the baby on their own and proceed with caretaking through instinct and experimentation. Results may vary, depending upon the parent's problem-solving skills or luck. Still, parents develop a great sense of pride in being able to say, "I raised her without any help."

Use of health services varies according to access to the system, the adults' confidence in their own parenting skills, knowledge about preventive health care, and the health status of the baby. Visits to the pediatrician's office or the public health clinic may range in frequency from annually at about the birth date, to only at immunization time, to persistently with every stuffy nose or rash. New parents need information about appropriate health checkups and reassurance about their care for their baby during time of minor illness.

With parenting being a 24-hours-a-day, 7-days-a-week job, many adults feel a strain from this constant demand. Continuous contact with the infant also can create some stagnation, boredom, and fatigue, especially in the major caretaker. Many parents alleviate the situation by taking a small vacation from the baby. This does not have to be something as elaborate as a flight to Acapulco, but anything that will break the daily routine: arranging for care for the baby, then going out of town for the weekend is very effective. Best resu' .s are achieved when the *parents* leave home, rather than sending the baby, since the parents are more likely to benefit from the change of scenery. This break in routine helps revitalize the parent(s) and contributes to strengthening the marital relationship by temporarily excluding parenting, so the couple can concentrate on themselves.

Maladaptive Responses.   Some individuals exhibit maladaptive behaviors, which are unhealthy responses to their present set of circumstances. In the infant, especially in the earlier months of life, maladaption is characterized by responses on basic levels of functioning, such as difficulty in feeding or disturbed sleep patterns. The baby seems unregulated (hyperexcitable) and unresponsive to others. This will progress to inanimate, impersonal involvement, which is typical of early autistic patterns (Greenspan, 1981).

The most serious distress pattern in the infant is called *failure to thrive*. This is defined as growth failure (below the third percentile on a standard growth chart), for which no organic cause can be found (Barbero, 1982; Johnson, 1986). Usually it is caused by a problem between the infant and the primary caretaker, and while it can be caused by poor parenting skills, it is most often the result of a disturbed emotional relationship. Sometimes it is secondary to familial/marital problems or low self-esteem in the caretaker, resulting in lack of interest in the infant. In either case, this inadequate nurturing results in a "reciprocal process in which both parent and infant fail to thrive" (Johnson, 1986, p. 185). Besides weight loss or curtailed weight gain accompanied by malnourishment, failure-to-thrive infants exhibit developmental slowness and signs of diminished interaction: little communication or smiling, and no interest in the environment. Failure-to-thrive infants often succumb to malnutrition or related diseases or to developmental problems. When identified early enough, a situation of this nature can be corrected before the infant suffers permanent damage or dies.

Parents also exhibit maladaptive parenting behaviors. Conflicts in parenting and difficulties with incorporating a new family member have already been discussed. The negative outcome of one of these conflicts would be directed toward the baby, who is perceived as the source of the problem. Consequently, the parent's behaviors is directed to the infant on a level that the infant may most likely interpret as punishment—unfulfilled physical needs. Some parents elect to punish the baby by withholding feedings or not changing diapers. This may bring some satisfaction to the parent, but the baby has no concept of punishment and will not understand why needs are not being met. The baby then becomes fussy and more irritable, which may anger the parent further, bringing on more punishment.

Another type of neglect is the withholding or lack of positive, affectionate interaction. This can be from punishment, actual lack of interest in the baby, or an unwillingness to form an affectionate bond with the child. These behaviors begin early in the baby's life and are characterized by depersonalizing the infant (calling the baby "it") and a lack of reciprocal interaction. In the later months of infancy, the parent may handle the baby roughly, converse with him or her in an abusive manner (or not at all), and not play or interact positively, generally ignoring the baby.

An even more unhealthy response is physical abuse: deliberately beating, burning, or maiming the baby as a form of punishment. The profile of the parent as an abuser may be found in Chapter 9 on the young adult.

The parent who is unable to develop a positive, healthy relationship and is also unwilling to continue to be a parent may simply abandon the baby. Hospitals, churches, orphanages, old cars, or trash dumps are common sites for discovery of an abandoned baby, many times a neonate. After attempts to locate the parent, the child is usually placed in a foster home. Even though the baby has been abandoned, signifying lack of an emotional bond, this type of situation may have a better outcome than leaving the infant in the original environment.

NURSING ASSESSMENT

The nurse who is establishing a relationship with a family that has an infant member will need to examine physical, behavioral, and environmental aspects of both the infant and the entire family. Table 5–5 gives guidelines for this evaluation.

TABLE 5–5. ASSESSING THE FAMILY WITH AN INFANT

	Environmental Data
Provisions for care	Who is major caretaker, how much time is spent in actual interaction with the baby, availability of food, sleeping arrangements, clothing, comfort measures
Alternate caretaker(s)	Relationship to parent, frequency of care of infant, number of children in that person's care, cost of care
	Communication Patterns
Infant	Level of verbal or preverbal sounds, person to whom infant turns when frightened, fatigued, hungry, etc., temperament of infant
Between caretaker and infant	Level of vocabulary, presence of baby talk, caretaker's interpretation of infant's sounds or gestures
Among family members	Constructive methods (confrontation, discussion), nonconstructive methods (yelling, abusive language, blocking), level of participation by each member
	Problem-Solving Skills
Decision-making abilities	How are major decisions made, does caretaker make any decisions independently from adults in household, roles of family members during decision making/implementing
Use of health care system	When instituted and for whom, location, accessibility, cost, purposes as perceived by family
Support from significant others	Viewed as positive or negative by major caretaker, areas of strongest support, areas of weakest support (as viewed by caretaker, as viewed by nurse)
Societal interactions	Use of public agencies (welfare, crippled children's, etc.), ability of caretaker to deal with or circumvent the system when appropriate, business communicative skills
	Life Style
Role of infant in family	Pregnancy planned or unplanned, course of prenatal and intrapartum periods, position of infant in household, caretaker's appraisal of infant (feeding, sleeping, temperament, etc.), family's evaluation of impact of infant on their life-style
Socioeconomic status (SES)	Estimated yearly income, financial assistance, direction of SES mobility, wage-earner's feelings about status
Family roles	Traditional or nontraditional pattern, distribution, level of satisfaction with roles
Work patterns	Wage earners in family, amount of work hours per day or week, anticipated job change
Recreational patterns	Use of free time, amount of planned activities per month, amount of time spent in recreation/leisure by each family member, amount of group recreation

TABLE 5–5. *(continued)*

Safety	Visible hazards (broken steps, exposed electrical outlets, glass in yard, etc.), use of safety features (car seats, latches on medicine cabinet, etc.), adult's knowledge of accident prevention, first aid, poison control
	Potential Stressors
Conflicts in parenting	Parent(s)' perception of parenting role, own recognition of conflicts, potential for unrecognized problems
Interferences with family tasks	Goals of family members, present health of family members
Conflicts with society	Incorporation of infant and involvement with society, societal acceptance of family and infant
Family response patterns	Restructuring or reordering of goals, determining priorities, identifying realistic, practical approaches to meeting goals, changing family structure or life-style

ALTERATIONS IN HEALTH

Deviations from wellness during infancy can be categorized as acute and chronic. Many of these alterations in health, especially those in the chronic category, were in existence during the neonatal period and are carried over to infancy. Most of the acute conditions are so common, they are considered to be part of being an infant. Often these acute illnesses reflect the infant's changing physiology. Other health alterations are a result of the infant's increased motor control and mobility, leading to accidents or skin problems. Through identification and understanding of the alterations in the health of the infant, the nurse has a strong foundation for the provision of care.

Acute Alterations in Health

Infections.   The most common infection in the infant occurs in the gastrointestinal tract and is characterized by diarrhea. While diarrhea is considered a symptom in older people, it becomes a diagnosis in the baby, especially if it is associated with fever, vomiting, and decreased feeding. Diarrhea can also occur spontaneously at about 6 months of age. This is usually the time of life when the acquired immunity from the mother is lost, making the infant more susceptible to pathogens. Contrary to popular thinking, there does not seem to be any relation between this spontaneous diarrhea and teething, which is also occurring about this time. In the absence of an infectious process, controlling the diarrhea and restoring or maintaining the fluid and electrolyte balance are the major foci for care.

Along with gastroenteritis found in the gastrointestinal system, other infections most prevalent during infancy are associated with these systems:

- *Respiratory:* bronchitis, tracheobronchitis pneumonia
- *Neurological:* meningitis, encephalitis

Anemia. Iron deficiency anemia, as a result of inadequate dietary iron, is the most prevalent nutritional disorder in the United States (Whaley & Wong, 1984). This anemia can be seen in infants starting at 6 months of age. Often it is the result of high milk intake coupled with low solid-food and vitamin-supplement intake. Because milk is high in protein and fat and a poor source of iron, the infant may be gaining weight, but show poor muscle development and a tendency to infections. An acute infection, particularly in the younger or less healthy infant, may cause a destruction of erythrocytes, resulting in hemolytic anemia.

Normochromic, normocytic anemia can be found in infants 3 or 4 months of age who were born prematurely (Pillitteri, 1981). Generally this is due to an immature hematopoetic system that is unable to handle the physiological demands of extrauterine life. Once erythropoesis is stimulated, aided by dietary iron, hemoglobin levels return to normal and the anemia can be corrected.

Allergies. An allergy is the result of a specific antigen/antibody interaction and is characterized by an adverse physical reaction, usually involving the skin, mucous membranes, and vascular endothelium (Ritchey & Taper, 1983). Infants are particularly susceptible to sensitization until about 6 months of age (Moore, 1982). Food allergies are the most common type in early infancy and are caused by foods with a high protein content. The most prevalent foods in the diet of the young infant are milk, wheat, and eggs (Ritchey & Taper, 1983). If an immediate family member has a history of food allergy, the infant should not be given cow's milk or specific high-protein foods until after 6 months of age. Food allergy is most often characterized by eczema, asthma, rhinitis, and decreased appetite (which affects growth and development of the infant). Infants may also exhibit an allergic reaction from animal hair, dust, pollen, cosmetics, or medications—all of which are commonly found in American life-style. An allergy of this nature is also characterized by asthma and rhinitis and especially eczema if the infant is in contact with the allergen.

Skin Problems. Skin problems are a common occurrence during infancy and can come from a variety of sources. Probably the most well-known skin problem is diaper rash. This dermatitis is the result of prolonged and/or repetitive contact with an irritant. Diaper rash is not always from the ammonia in urine and feces, but can be caused by chemicals in detergents or bath soap, and even friction from a too-tight diaper.

Impetigo is a skin disorder with a bacterial cause. Manifested by a macular, then vesicular rash, impetigo can spread easily because of the infant's low immune state. Pruritus is common, and the infant may rub the itching area, thus breaking the vesicles or scabs and delaying healing.

Infants can also have eczema as a dermatologic manifestation of an allergy. This eczema is characterized by erythema, edema, pruritis, and the development of papules. Elimination of this and other skin problems is enhanced by proper hygiene, but is dependent upon identification and elimination of the causative factor. This task is not always easy for the family of the infant and may seem somewhat like solving a mystery.

Trauma. Trauma as a result of accidents is commonly an outcome of the infant's exploration, or due to negligence on the part of the caretaker. Most of the accidents are due to falls, inhalation of a foreign object, aspiration, poisoning, burns, or drowning (Pillitteri, 1981), and are one of the leading causes of death for this age group. Falls or blows due to a motor vehicle accident have declined in number due to legislation on infant car seats ("State Legislative Activities," 1985, August 23).

Sudden Infant Death Syndrome (SIDS). Known to the lay public as "crib death," SIDS is an unforeseen, traumatic infant demise, with the common incidence at 2–3 months of age (Tackett & Hunsberger, 1981). The cause of SIDS is unknown, but may be linked with hypoxia or anoxia in utero. The baby, who appears normal in every way, develops severe pulmonary edema and death by suffocation.

   The loss of a baby through SIDS, perhaps more than any other circumstance, weighs heavily on the parents. Grief and guilt are the most prominent feelings. The parents will always wonder what they could have done differently, why they did not know their baby was in trouble, or if it was a genetic factor that caused the death. The nurse can be most valuable in counseling the parents, helping to diminish unrealistic feelings and allay guilt.

Chronic Alterations in Health

Congenital Anomalies. The physiological characteristics of, and interventions for, birth anomalies are extensive and are not appropriate for this text. The nurse does need to be alert to the life-threatening abnormalities: those of the heart, lungs, and brain. Generally, the baby with a defect in another body system can be stabilized first, then undergo surgical correction later.

Metabolic Disorders. During infancy, most metabolic disorders are related to growth problems or inability to properly utilize nutrients. A pituitary tumor or deficiency, while rarely found in infancy, can be detected at an early stage by the baby's failure to progress along standard growth charts.

   Cystic fibrosis is a condition caused by a dysfunction of the exocrine gland (pancreas). It becomes evident at about 1 month of age, then even more so as the baby increases feedings, because the baby seems to be unable to digest fat, protein, and some sugars. The stools have a thick, greasy consistency. Tenacious mucous secretions pool in the bronchi, causing respiratory infections and decreased lung functioning. Cystic fibrosis is one of the more common chronic diseases of childhood.

   Examples of other disorders in this category are phenylketonuria (PKU), an irregularity of amino acid metabolism, and Tay-Sachs disease, a problem with lipid metabolism. These are autosomal recessive inherited disorders causing mental retardation. Screening for PKU may be done during the neonatal period, with appropriate follow-up, but Tay-Sachs is not usually identified until about 1 year of age.

Malnutrition. This may be considered a chronic disease because the condition has persisted for some time, gradually worsened, and the results may be irreversible. In the United States, malnutrition is seen mainly as a vitamin or mineral deficiency and is not limited to a specific socioeconomic level, race, or ethnic group. In some cases, it occurs in a baby of a mother unknowledgeable about proper vitamin intake, such as one who only provides limited food types (or milk only) and does not use vitamin supplements. Protein deficiencies are common in children of vegetarians, especially those of the strict dietary following. Beriberi, rickets, and pellagra, diseases usually associated with Third World countries, may be seen among poverty-level families.

Failure to Thrive. Failure to thrive (FTT) is a classification for infants whose weight and body length fall below the third percentile for their age (Barbero, 1982; Johnson, 1986). FTT can often be categorized as having organic and inorganic causes. Organic causes are physical/physiological conditions that interfere with nutrient intake and absorption, such as a congenital anomaly or cystic fibrosis. Inorganic causes are psychosocial; lack of growth is the result of inadequate stimulation and affection. Because the FTT infant often has irregular sleep/activity patterns, he or she can be viewed as being difficult because of unpredictable behaviors (Morant, 1979).

    Marasmus is a general malnutrition of calories and protein and may be considered a subdiagnosis in the infant classified as FTT. As mentioned in the section on stressors, the infant with FTT will quite likely be suffering from the most outstanding psychosocial disorder of infancy, an attachment disorder. This inability to establish a close reciprocal relationship with one significant person can result in emotional lability and poor feeding, and is a precursor to autism. In most identified cases, the infant will be hospitalized for nutritive buildup and given a lot of tender, loving care. The nurse can work closely with a social worker and counselor in dealing with the parent(s) about strengthening the parent–infant relationship or finding a foster home.

NURSING RESPONSIBILITIES

The nurse who provides care for the infant and family has a myriad of opportunities and approaches to meet needs. By using the nursing process and by prioritizing needs, the nurse enacts various roles, such as preventor of accident/illness, promotor of health, and caregiver. It is through these approaches that the nurse can be assured that the family has a greater likelihood of achieving and maintaining optimal health.

Preventive Measures

With the thrust of health care directed more and more to self-help and illness prevention, nurses have a key role in guiding the family in maintaining wellness. Through assessment of the family structure, function, and stressors, the nurse can identify areas that need strengthening or potential problems that need resolution.

    It is often necessary for the nurse to spend time counseling, to guide the family and the individual members in problem solving, to provide an outlet for ventilation of feelings, or to bring support and encouragement. Some new parents may be having difficulty with the transition to parenthood. The individual may be grappling with one of the conflicts to parenting and may be unable to smoothly adapt to the new role. Talking with the parents about role changes associated with parenting may uncover even deeper marital problems that are now compounded by the addition of the baby. The nurse may be able to effectively guide the family to a workable solution, thereby avoiding potential stress and conflict.

The nurse should also be able to provide the parent(s) with anticipatory guidance about developmental changes and needs of the baby. With each health visit, the nurse can do spontaneous teaching, so the parent will be prepared for the infant's changes. The nurse may remark, "Your baby will probably be crawling the next time I see him," or "When she is ———— months old, you may start feeding her ————." As the nurse observes the infant in the familiar environment, predictions can be made about upcoming behavioral changes—when the child will be pulling up to the sofa, what cabinets he or she will want to explore, etc. The parent(s) may then want to "childproof" stairs, drawers, or cabinets, and protect precious mementos.

Encouraging regular immunization is probably the most common preventive measure that families can practice. The current schedule for routine immunization for the infant is*:

> DT (diphtheria and tetanus toxoids)   2, 4, 6 months
> TOPV (trivalent oral polio vaccine)   2,4 months

The timing for these coincides with routine checkups, which helps to ensure parental compliance. Parents should be given praise and positive feedback for keeping their child's immunizations current. It is an extremely important area of health protection.

Automobile safety measures are critical to accident prevention. With each family, nurses must determine the presence of an infant restraint to be used while riding in the car. Agran and Winn (1985) report that while restraint usage has decreased the number of fatalities and serious injuries in young children, some injuries do occur because of improper restraint usage. Therefore, the nurse should assess the consistency of restraint use and discuss specific precautionary measures. For instance, parents can be taught to ascertain that they have the proper size of seat and seat belt for their child, and that the child should not be placed near a protruding object, such as a stereo speaker.

Health Promotion

While nurses are meeting the needs of infants and families, they can simultaneously be providing measures to promote health. This health promotion not only safeguards existing behaviors and conditions, but also enables the family with the infant to avoid any complications that may occur due to a concurrent illness of further debilitation.

---

*From: Center for Disease Control, New Recommended Schedule, *Morbidity and Mortality Weekly Reports*, 1986, September 19.

Health promotion can be accomplished through many approaches. Common methods are standard health care practices and structured and unstructured education. Standard health care practices include hygienic measures, nutrition, and time for sleep and play—all areas vital for the growth and development of the infant. At the time that the infant's physical status and the family's health beliefs and behaviors are being assessed, the nurse can also take the opportunity for some unstructured teaching. For example, an 8-month-old infant is receiving a routine physical exam by a nurse-practitioner. As the nurse notices the infant's three teeth, he or she may begin to question the parent(s) about use of a toothbrush. If the child has not yet had these teeth brushed, the nurse can point out that, even though these baby teeth are not permanent, it is important to begin good dental habits early. Brushing the infant's teeth helps him or her to become accustomed to the feel of the brush and toothpaste. Dental care can easily become part of the child's daily routine.

Another unstructured approach to teaching for health promotion is role modeling on the part of the nurse. Because many parents value the knowledge and standards possessed by nurses, they will often strive to emulate them. As a result, the nurse's behaviors may frequently be incorporated into the family's care for the infant. For example, during a period of hospitalization, the nurse can demonstrate desirable practices such as:

- Washing hands after diapering
- Providing a safe environment
- Slow, deliberate spoon feeding
- Instituting developmentally appropriate play

Not only can nurses be central to physical health promotion; they can also be instrumental in enhancing the family integrity and the parent–infant relationship. Giving new parents encouragement about specific parenting behaviors will often give them a much-needed boost to the self-esteem. It is also most important for nurses to assess the reciprocal behaviors that exist between the parent–infant dyad. Identification of a potentially maladaptive situation, with specific interventions, can do much to strengthen the family unit. For example, in working with parents of an older infant, the nurse may ask them to complete a revised Infant Temperament Questionnaire (ITQ) (Carey & McDevitt, 1978). This enables the practitioner to use temperament classifications by Thomas and Chess (1977) to point out the baby's basic personality. By doing so, the parent gains more insight into their child's behavior, and can accept the fact that the child is "difficult," "slow to warm up," or, in a relative sense, an "easy" baby.

The nurse may be able to use interaction time with the parent(s) to teach about nutrition—not just for the baby, but for the entire family. Through assessment of appearance, life style, and dietary habits, the nurse may identify some areas in need of change. Parents who are both overweight, with skin, teeth, or hair in poor condition, may bring in their baby, who is in the upper range of weight on the growth chart. The nurse can infer that this family has a chronic eating problem—high caloric intake, frequent feedings, etc.—and needs education and counseling about meal planning, food intake, and eating control.

Parents of an infant with a chronic disease may be particularly in need of education. They may need instruction in performing special treatments or information on dietary changes for the child with anemia or cystic fibrosis. The parents of a baby with a genetically linked disorder may want more background on this, particularly in guiding family planning.

Acute Caregiver

Nursing activities included in care of the hospitalized infant may involve both symptomatic treatment and therapeutic or alleviative measures. For instance, when caring for the infant hospitalized with anemia, the nurse will need to develop a plan of care that will minimize the baby's oxygen needs. In the case of an infant undergoing surgical correction of a congenital anomaly, the nurse must also provide the necessary preoperative and postoperative care, plus consider the infant's underlying status associated with the condition. As an example, the infant with a cleft lip and palate may be somewhat undernourished because of difficulty with feeding and may therefore require more intensive nutrition therapy.

The nurse who is caring for an infant must have professional and ethical competency and an awareness of the complex problems and needs of the family with a hospitalized infant. For the infant experiencing an acute illness or condition that requires hospitalization, the time in the hospital may only be two or three days. During this time, the nurse provides the needed care for the baby and can also assist the parent(s) in the areas of promotion and prevention. The nurse can take advantage of spontaneous moments for teaching, especially in the areas of nutrition, anticipatory guidance, or accident prevention. For example, for the baby hospitalized with diarrhea, the nurse can explain how diarrhea can sometimes be food-related and what approaches the parent(s) can take to control the diarrhea with foods, rather than medication. Nurses can also point out how easily the infant can become dehydrated and measures that can prevent this, so that in the event the baby has further episodes of diarrhea, it may not be necessary for him or her to be hospitalized.

For the infant with a chronic condition who must be hospitalized for surgery or other therapeutic reasons, it is quite likely that this is one in a series of several hospitalizations. The infant who receives warm, nurturing care can learn to trust the people whom he or she has come to associate with the hospital. As the infant grows into a toddler, fears over hospitalization may be decreased.

The nurse should involve the parents in the care of the infant as much as possible, for several reasons:

- Provides as much parent–infant interaction as possible
- Recognizes the value of the parent, making them a part of the health care team
- Helps decrease anxieties about the baby's condition or the technology associated with care
- Assists the parent in maintaining some control over their child and the course of the hospitalization

To promote this involvement, the nurse can take such measures as:

- Encouraging, but not requiring, 24-hour parental stay
- Including the parent(s) in planning, implementing and evaluating the care
- Allowing hands-on experiences with intensive care babies or for certain procedures
- Keeping parents informed of the child's progress and anticipated changes in care

The nurse should strive to keep communication lines open, allowing parents to ventilate their myriad feelings and verbalize their needs or wishes. For example, the family of an infant who has died will probably be feeling grief, anger, denial, and guilt. It will be necessary for the nurse to discuss death and the loss of a child in a meaningful, therapeutic way.

SUMMARY

This chapter has examined the growth, development, and socialization of the infant as a family member. One is able to better understand the infant and recognize how stressors, including illness, affect this maturation. The role of the infant's parent(s) is most important because of the dependency of the infant. The nurse provides care directly to the baby and gives direction and guidance to the parents as they strive to attain optimal family functioning.

CARE PLAN FOR THE INFANT WITH ALTERATION IN FLUIDS AND NUTRITION

Situation

M. W. is a 3-month-old infant hospitalized for surgical correction of pyloric stenosis. He was hospitalized 2 days prior to surgery for fluid and nutrition therapy, and is now 1 day postoperative. While M. W. still has some vomiting in small amounts, he is able to tolerate small feedings of glucose. He continues to receive IV therapy, and a nasogastric tube is in place. M. W. has 5–6 wet diapers during a 24-hour period. He sleeps 14–18 hours every day, and rarely exhibits any distress that could be interpreted as discomfort. When he is awake, M. W. moves about in his crib, looks around his immediate environment, and gestures toward items within reach. He will be hospitalized at least 2 more days.

Mrs. W. is present continuously, except for 2-hour periods in which she returns home to bathe and change clothes. She frequently asks questions about M.'s status, and hovers around the bedside when the nurses are providing care. She remarks, "I guess my 6-year old is feeling a little neglected. I'm not even sure how he gets to school every day. I hope his father is managing all right." The father visits every evening for approximately 1 hour, leaving the 6-year old with a neighbor.

Nursing Diagnoses

1. Post-op infant, experiencing alteration in fluids and nutrition
2. Alteration in family process (temporary)
3. Mother experiencing anxiety and fatigue

SAMPLE CARE PLAN

Nursing Diagnoses	Goal	Interventions	Evaluation
M. W. in stable condition, displaying normal infant behaviors. Fluids and nutrition a priority	Recovery from surgery and normal growth patterns	Maintain intake, gradually introduce infant formula Assess output by number of wet diapers Keep IV site patent, monitor fluid therapy	Vomiting episodes diminished, intake increased, output increased
Alteration in nutrition and fluid and electrolytes	Fluid, electrolyte, and nutrition needs met		
Mrs. W. appears anxious and fatigued. Hovers over bed when nurse provides care Mrs. W. also preoccupied by worrying about other child at home Alteration in family process (temporary)	Decrease in role conflict experienced by Mrs. W. Positive family functioning with stable relationships	Involve Mrs. W. in M.'s care—feedings, bathing. Ask her to provide various forms of infant stimulation Continue to apprise Mrs. W. of M.'s status Encourage Mrs. W. to spend more time with other child. See if Mr. W. can stay at hospital one night	Mrs. W. became actively involved in M.'s care, seemed less anxious, asked fewer questions Mr. W. stayed at hospital. Mrs. W. seemed much more relaxed next day

Review Questions

As families progress from the childbearing to childrearing stages, the role of the nurse focuses on two major areas: education of the parents about the infant's current health needs, and provision of anticipatory guidance for developmental changes.

1. Discuss how the nurse can explain developmental tasks to parents in terminology that they can understand

2. Give examples of developmental tasks to which parents can be alerted

3. What could be some disadvantages to anticipatory guidance? How can this be avoided by the nurse?

4. Apply strategies of counseling to the following situations:

   a. A woman, over 35 years old, has given birth to her fourth child. The baby has some congenital anomalies and will most likely be retarded.

b. A couple in their late twenties, whose first child died at age 3 months of Sudden Infant Death Syndrome, is unable to decide about having another child.

c. A new father says he was abused as a child, and is afraid he'll abuse his infant.

d. A young couple with their first child continues to compare their newborn daughter with their six-month-old nephew.

REFERENCES

Agran, P. F., & Winn, D. G. (1985). Motor vehicle accident trauma and restraint usage patterns in children less than 4 years of age. *Pediatrics, 76,* 382–386.

Barbero, G. (1982). Failure to thrive. In Klaus, M., Leger, T., & Trause, M. A. (Eds.). *A round table: Maternal attachment and mothering disorders.* Skillman, N. J.: Johnson & Johnson Baby Products.

Bowlby, J. (1982). Attachment and loss: Retrospect and prospect. *American Journal of Orthopsychiatry, 52,* 664–678.

Carey, W. B., & McDevitt, S. C. (1978). Revision of the infant temperament questionnaire. *Pediatrics, 61,* 735–739.

Center for Disease Control, (1986). New recommended schedule for active immunization of normal infants and children (1986, September 19). *Morbidity and Mortality Weekly Report,* 577–579.

Clarke-Stewart, K. A. (1987). And daddy makes three: The father's impact on mother and young child. *Child Development, 49,* 466–478.

Duvall, E. (1977). *Family development* (5th ed.). Philadelphia: Lippincott.

Erikson, E. (1963). *Childhood and society* (2nd ed.). New York: Norton.

Greenspan, S. I. (1981). Adaptive and psychopathologic patterns in infancy and early childhood. *Children Today, 10*(4), 21–26.

Hrbosky, D. M. (1977). Transition to parenthood: A balancing of needs. In Smoyak, S. (Ed.). Symposium on parenting. *Nursing Clinics of North America.* Philadelphia: Saunders.

Hymovich, D. (1980). *Child and family development: Implications for primary health care.* New York: McGraw-Hill.

Johnson, S. (1986). *High-risk parenting* (2nd ed.). Philadelphia: Lippincott.

Jones, C. (1981). Father to infant attachment: Effects of early contact and characteristics of the infant. *Research in Nursing and Health, 4*(1), 193–201.

Kiernan, B., & Scoloveno, M. A. (1977). Fathering. In Smoyak, S. (Ed.). Symposium on parenting. *Nursing Clinics of North America.* Philadelphia: Saunders.

Klaus, M., & Kennell, J. (1983). *Bonding: The beginnings of parent–infant attachment.* St. Louis: Mosby.

Kutzner, S. K., & Toussie-Weingarten, C. (1984). Working parents: The dilemma of child rearing and career. *Topics in Clinical Nursing, 6*(3), 30–37.

Lamb, M. (1977). Father–infant and mother–infant interaction in the first year of life. *Child Development, 48,* 167–181.

Maier, H. (1969). *Three theories of child development.* New York: Harper and Row.

Mercer, R. (1986). *First-time motherhood: Experiences from teens to forties.* New York: Springer-Verlag.

Morant, J. (1983). A baby who is failing to thrive. *Nursing Times, 79*(14), 23.

Moore, M. (1983). *Realities in childbearing* (2nd ed.). Philadelphia: Saunders.

Mussen, P, (1979). *The Psychological Development of the Child* (3rd ed.). Englewood Cliffs: Prentice-Hall.

Parke, R., Power, T., Tinsley, T., & Hymel, S. (1979). The father's ;role in the family system. *Seminars in Perinatology, 3*(1), 25–33.

Parker, S., & Brazelton, T. B. (1981). Newborn behavioral assessment: Research, prediction, and clinical uses. *Children Today, 10*(4), 2–5.

Pickens, D. (1982). The cognitive processes of career-oriented primiparas in identity reformulation. *Maternal-Child Nursing Journal, 11,* 135–164.

Pillitteri, A. (1981) *Child health nursing* (2nd ed.). Boston: Little, Brown.

Ritchey, S., & Taper, L. J. (1983). *Maternal and child nutrition.* New York: Harper & Row.

State legislative activities concerning the use of seat belts—United States. (1985, August 23). *Morbidity and Mortality Weekly Report 34*(33), 505–508, 513.

Tackett, J. J. M., & Hunsberger, M. (1981). *Family centered care of children and adolescents.* Philadelphia: Saunders.

Thomas, A., & Chess, S. (1977). *Temperament and development.* New York: Brunner/Mazel.

Ventura, J. (1982). Parent coping behaviors, parent functioning and infant temperament characteristics. *Nursing Research, 31,* 269–273.

Whaley, L., & Wong, D. (1983). *Nursing care of infants and children* (2nd ed.). St. Louis: Mosby.

Wolff, P. (1969). Observation on newborn infants. *Psychosomatic Medicine, 21,* 110.

6

The Family with a Toddler and Preschooler 2–5 Years

Marion E. Broome

OBJECTIVES

Upon completion of this chapter the student will be able to:

1. Discuss the concept of the reciprocal nature of the relationship between a parent and young child
2. List the developmental tasks of: (1) a toddler, (2) a preschooler, (3) parents of a preschool child(ren)
3. Describe the potential stressors for a family with preschool children
4. List assessment techniques used to determine the health status of toddlers and preschool children
5. Analyze the significance of the reaction of the young child to separation from the parents during a stressful procedure or event
6. Differentiate between adaptive and maladaptive responses to demands of parenting
7. Discuss the development of competence and coping in the young child
8. Discuss selected concepts from various adaptation and developmental theories to develop (1) a family anticipatory guidance plan with a normal toddler during the 2-year-old well-child visit, and (2) a preparation program for a preschool child who will be hospitalized

CONCEPTS

Advocacy: the active participation of the child health nurse in issues and concerns of families with young children. *Case advocacy* refers to actions on the part of the nurse for individual families; in *class advocacy* the nurse acts on behalf of groups of families

Adaptive Potential: the capacity of a young child to cope actively with stressors

Anticipatory Guidance: the provision of information to parents of a young child regarding upcoming developmental milestones and associated concerns

Coping: the verbal and nonverbal behaviors used by a young child to adapt to external or internal demands

Potential Stressors: demands placed on the young child that exceed the child's initial ability to expend energy to meet the demand

---

The family with a toddler and/or preschool child is experiencing a busy, exciting, and demanding time of family life. Parental role changes and the accompanying demands during infancy have abated somewhat. Parents begin to settle in for a quieter, more relaxed time with their child, only to find the next four years to be in many ways more demanding and requiring a great deal of psychic and physical energy. While they are attempting to meet the challenges of parenting a young child, the parents' physical, social, and emotional needs often continue to be neglected. In single-parent and dual-career families these adult needs may be even further compromised.

FAMILY TASKS

The family of a young child has to attain and master several different tasks during each stage of development. One difficulty families have in mastering the necessary developmental tasks is that these tasks may frequently interfere or conflict with the developmental tasks of individuals within the family. An example of this in a family with very young children would arise when the parents have little time to communicate in order to reach a consensus about a pressing financial problem because their 2-year-old and 5-year-old require so much of their attention and time. Developmental tasks of the family of a young child include:

1. Maintenance of physical health needs of members
   a. Nutritional needs
   b. Physical fitness needs
2. Development and maintenance of social relationships inside and outside the family
   a. Marital relations
   b. Parent–child relations
   c. Community relations

Maintenance of Physical Needs

This involves (1) the initiation and maintenance of a special place where the family lives together, usually referred to as a home; and (2) meeting the requirements for physical growth and well-being (air, food, safety).

A major concern of parents of a toddler revolves around the decision about the spacing of subsequent children. Some couples decide to postpone further children indefinitely, while others choose to attempt to conceive again very soon after the birth of the first child. Many considerations enter this decision, including the family's financial status, career goals of both spouses, and their beliefs about the importance and effect of siblings on their child's development. If the couple decides to enter the childbearing phase again at this time, the woman will experience the same physical demands as in the first pregnancy. However, additional stress is evident during this phase of the life cycle as a result of the parents' having to meet the needs of their first child. Many mothers who are pregnant for the second time will report how, while they may feel wonderful, they are experiencing much more fatigue with this pregnancy. Although it is tempting to attribute this fatigue to many things, certainly the energy used to provide and care for the toddler or preschooler in the family is considerable. These mothers need to be encouraged to evaluate their busy schedules, perhaps delete some activities, and plan for others that will enhance their ability to relax.

If a couple chooses to postpone childbearing, either temporarily or indefinitely, the choice of a relatively long-term birth control method will be necessary. Again, this choice depends on the financial status, past experience, physical status, and personal preferences of the couple. Some types of birth control are more effective than others, and certain ones can produce unpleasant side effects (see Chap. 9). The nurse who is working with young families needs to be knowledgeable about all birth control methods—their techniques of use, user-effectiveness rates, cost, and side effects—to effectively assist these couples in making a decision that is right for them.

Nutrition.   The parent of a young child has a very busy and hectic schedule. Over 50% of mothers with preschoolers work, placing additional demands on their time (Hofferth, 1979). Nutritional requirements for the young adult are presented in Chapter 9. The ritualistic three-meal-a-day patterns of young families are changing. More individualism is evidenced in when and what food is served and eaten by the family. Parental and child activity schedules determine whether food is eaten at home. The nurse needs to make a thorough and detailed assessment of families' nutritional intake over several time periods to get an accurate picture of their eating behaviors and whether they are in accordance with recommendations that are made to optimize health and well-being. Table 6–1 presents an assessment guide that can be used to assess the dietary patterns of a family with a preschool child.

Fitness.   Over the past decade, Americans have become much more interested in their health and have engaged in exercise programs at an unprecedented rate. Most healthy, young people find that 30 minutes of exercise three times per week will increase their sense of well-being and decrease appetite and fatigue. The exercise does not necessarily have to be part of a structured program. Having a young child often places the couple in a position of finding it difficult to find time to engage in exercise activities in which the toddler cannot participate. Walking on one's lunch hour or in the evening or use of video or audio exercise tapes are two examples of exercise activities that adults with young children could engage in.

TABLE 6–1. ASSESSMENT OF DIETARY PATTERNS OF YOUNG CHILDREN

| | Food Group | | | | | | | |
| | Milk and Cheese | | Meat and Eggs Poultry and Fish | | Fruit and Vegetable | | Cereal and Bread | |
	Child	Parent	Child	Parent	Child	Parent	Child	Parent
Breakfast								
Lunch								
Dinner								
Recommended Servings per day	4	2	1	2	2	4	2	4
Actual Intake								
Recommendations								

From: Phipps, W., Long, B., & Woods, N. (1983). Medical-surgical nursing: Concepts and clinical practice. St. Louis: Mosby. (Adult requirements)
Slattery, J., Pearson, G., & Torre, G. (1979). Maternal and child nutrition: Assessment and counseling. New York: Appleton-Century-Crofts. (Child requirements)

Development and Maintenance of Social Relationships

The young couple with children find less and less time to devote to their relationships as a couple as their children grow older and they themselves become more involved in community activities such as sports, church, and civic and professional organizations. Most working couples report their social activities are the first to decrease as family-related activities take more and more time. The marital relationship finds itself highly stressed with the first child, with additional pressures reported as more children are added (Steffensmeirer, 1982). Couples report little time for themselves and each other and find they must make a concerted effort to communicate and meet their needs. Some couples with young children make time for a weekend away without their children, although others who do not have extended family or friends to care for the children find this difficult. Even a regularly scheduled lunch date that allows the couple time to talk about things important to them as adults will help to improve communication levels and increase family cohesion.

The emotional needs of young adults require stimulation, affection, and feedback from other adults. The parents of a young child often find themselves feeling trapped in a world of toys and baby talk. It is particularly difficult for the single parent who often has no one to share the responsibility of meeting the demands of a child. A parent may find that the need for rest, time alone, quiet, and exercise conflicts with the needs of the child for rest, activity, and nourishment. It often takes some planning on the part of the parent(s) to see that time and opportunity is provided for adult needs to be met. This sometimes requires asking others to trade off time to sit with the child.

Parent–Child Relationship.   Just as parents differ in their personality and temperament, so do they differ in their childrearing styles. Diana Baumrind (1967) has identified three major types of parental styles that have been used in research of families and measured the relationship between a particular style and child behavior. Baumrind's three categories paralleled those commonly referred to as *authoritarian*, *authoritative*, and *permissive*. These terms are based on the degrees of warmth and control evidenced in the parent–child relationship (see Table 6–2).

In subsequent research with preschool children, Baumrind (1967) as well as White (1978) found that parents who were authoritative had children who were best able to handle stressful situations, who best utilized adults in meeting their needs, and who were able to express themselves in order to obtain what they wanted. Children of permissive parents were often found to be immature and unable to rely on themselves to meet the demands of a situation.

This has many implications for research in health care for the family with a young child. Child temperament has received much attention of late, and yet researchers also need to study how childrearing patterns can affect a child's health behavior and responses to illness and developmental demands.

There are many activities that will promote quiet time together between parent and child. The parent of a toddler finds that the child is able to comprehend much more than he or she can verbalize. Toddlers enjoy being read to by their parents. This reading time also promotes physical contact.

Discipline expectations and affection are transmitted from parent to child through multiple daily interactions. Parents need to encourage the toddler in attempts to be independent and try new activities while placing firm limits and defining acceptable and negative behavior. The toddler will begin to develop a sense of family identity as he or she internalizes parental expectations.

Grandparents often become more involved with the toddler as he or she grows older. This is especially true if a second or third child has been added to the family. The quality of the relationship between the grandparents and the toddler's parents can influence greatly how much interaction occurs between the grandparents and the child. Oftentimes the grandparents can provide extra attention for the toddler.

TABLE 6–2. PARENTAL CHILDREARING STYLES

	Level of Warmth and Control	
	Warmth	*Control*
Authoritarian	Low	High
Authoritative	High	High
Permissive	High	Low

Adapted from: Baumrind D. (1967). Parental control and parental love. Children, 6, 230–234.

Interaction with Community. Social support systems have been found to enhance parenting abilities (Norbeck, 1981). With the increase in mobility of young families, any community involvement they choose will assist them in developing a supportive social system. Friendships and involvement in activities with other couples with young children allows role modeling to occur. Parents share much information on an informal basis in such relationships. Socialization into cultural norms occurs largely as a result of interactions of this type.

Sometimes these interactions with the community occur through play groups (groups of mothers with young children), church membership, day care enrollment, etc. Although each of these vary somewhat, they will all provide the parent and child an opportunity to observe other similar individuals.

INDIVIDUAL TASKS

The child who is 13–16 months of age is commonly referred to as a *toddler*. This label reflects the priority that mobility and motor skills have in the development of the young child. Ambulation normally begins anywhere from 9–15 months and becomes more coordinated as the child grows older. Skill development is progressive and builds on previous skill attainment. For a concise presentation of developmental milestones during the toddler and preschool years, the reader is referred to Table 6–3.

The developmental tasks of the toddler include:

1. Physical development
2. Emotional development
3. Social development

Physical Development

The tremendous growth spurt of infancy begins to slow dramatically during the second year of life and remains steady until adolescence, when the second fast growth period during the life cycle begins. The toddler will slow weight gain to about 4–5 pounds per year (2 kilograms) and will gain 3–4 inches in height. All children grow at different rates, and the nurse will assess each individual child's rate of growth by plotting height and weight on a growth chart. These growth charts allow one to see how the child compares to other children at the same age. Over a period of time, the nurse is then able to effectively diagnose any sudden growth declines, spurts, or inconsistencies. Parents often enjoy seeing where their child is on the growth chart and how he or she compares to other children. Use of the chart will emphasize to the parent the individuality of each child's development. That is, if a child is consistently plotted on the 20th percentile, has adequate intake, small parents, and is developing normally in other areas, the parent can be assured that there is nothing wrong with their child. Another parent whose toddler is in the 90th percentile for weight and 50th percentile for height may better see that he or she weighs too much for the achieved height and is not just a big girl or boy.

TABLE 6–3. GROWTH AND DEVELOPMENT OF THE YOUNG CHILD

	18 months	24 months	36 months	48 months	60 months	72 months
Gross motor skills	Stands alone; walks well; most can walk backward; begins to move up steps	Kicks and throws ball and walks up steps	Most pedal tricycle; begins to jump in place	Can perform broad jump; climbs well	Catches ball; hops on one foot; runs well	Coordinated ambulation achieved
Language skills	10–20-word vocabulary; identifies 2–3 body parts; uses gestures to communicate	200-word vocabulary; talks in 2–3-word phrases; speech intelligible	Uses simple sentences; 900–1000-word vocabulary; names 1 color; tells name; expresses basic needs	Up to 1500-word vocabulary; recites songs from memory; questions why; sentences are 5–6 words long	Up to 2300-word vocabulary; repeats 4–5 digits; continues to question meaning fully; prints name	Up to 2500-word vocabulary; can relate composition of objects and relates stories; recites numbers, poems, etc.
Fine motor adaptive skills	Pinches, grasps; stacks 2 blocks; used pencil to scribble spontaneously	Stacks 4 blocks; uses pencil to draw lines	Copies O; stacks tall tower of blocks	Discriminates between length of objects; copies	Draws stick figures with 3 or more parts and uses pencil to draw name	Draws a square; adds more parts to stick figures; can play simple game like checkers
Social skills	Parallel play; drinks from cup; temper tantrums	Imitates adults in activities; begins cooperative play	Puts on clothing; peer play favored; separates from mother easily	Able to follow directions in group play; forming friendships outside the home	"Buddy" system evident; prefers to be with children; responds to requests	Responds well to other adult supervision; able to concentrate for longer periods

From 12–24 months, the toddler is still often clumsy and falls frequently while walking and running from place to place. The abdomen protrudes, and it appears as if the spine is abnormally curved (toddler lordosis). This curvature will disappear at about 4 years of age when the back muscles strengthen. The toddler's legs and arms grow more rapidly than the trunk, and it often seems that the legs are rotated inward with a bowed appearance.

Brain growth is 75% complete by 3 years of age. The limbic system has matured, and the toddler's sleep-wake cycles are more regulated. The child's rapidly expanding cognitive abilities are a result of this increasing maturation of the brain and the greater number of experiences and stimuli available to the toddler.

Nutritional Requirements. The growing toddler needs about 1200–1300 calories per day, with 23 grams of protein, which will support the rapidly growing muscular tissue (Slattery et al., 1979). Toddlers prefer to eat those foods that they can take with them, more commonly referred to as finger foods, such as cheese, dry cereals, hot dogs, or slices of fruit. Large meals are likely to be refused by the toddler.

Toddlers often use meal times to assert their independence. If parents engage in a struggle and force the child to eat, conflict can result that may have long-reaching effects on future eating habits and parent–child relationships. It is best to offer small frequent feedings to the child during these years and to set limits on the amount of junk foods allowed. These limits will encourage the toddler to eat any available nutritious food offered when hungry. Many parents worry a great deal over what at first appears to be the small amount of food a toddler eats. It is not uncommon for the toddler to go on food binges and refuse favorite foods while eating only vegetables, meat, or some other food. In order to accurately assess the actual amount and type of food the toddler eats, it is usually most helpful to have the parent keep a daily record of everything the child consumes for three different days. This record can then be analyzed for deficiencies in either caloric or nutrient intake and assist the nurse in helping the parent to better manipulate the toddler diet.

Bowel and Bladder Control. The bladder size and capacity to hold urine increases during these early years, and sphincter control is attained after the child is ambulatory. Most children are ready to begin toilet training somewhere between the ages of two and three years of age. Before toilet training is begun, the child must (1) be able to verbally express awareness of the need to urinate or defecate; (2) be able to maintain sphincter control; and (3) walk to the toilet and sit on the commode. Most parents who find toilet training to be an opportunity to allow and encourage independence in their toddler and who wait for signals of readiness report the training period to be of short duration. These same parents will ignore accidents that result from active involvement in play or temporary regression.

Other parents feel pressured by their own schedules or by advice from others to toilet train soon after the child's first birthday. These parents will take the toddler to the bathroom on a scheduled basis (every 2 hours) and encourage him or her to urinate and defecate in the commode. Any unscheduled voidings are highly discouraged. Often the young toddler will, in fact, learn to use the bathroom facilities on schedule. However, the maintenance of toileting behavior depends heavily on parental compliance with the schedule, and any changes in routine will quickly affect the ability of the child to remain toilet trained.

Once a parent decides the child has demonstrated the three aforementioned behaviors, toilet training often is achieved in a short period of time. There are children's books available that the child and parent can read together that will give them an opportunity to discuss how they will approach the activity and exactly what is to be done. Throughout the training period, the parent should praise the child's efforts and ignore any mistakes.

Activity Patterns.   Another major concern most parents verbalize about their toddler is in regard to sleep and activity patterns. A toddler needs 12–14 hours of sleep per night, and most usually still take a nap during the day. It is difficult for the very young child to give up a very busy, stimulating, and exciting activity to go to bed at a predetermined time. Separation fears are also common in the young toddler (12–18 months), which adds to dislike for bedtime. At the same time, parents feel a need for some time alone in the evening. If allowed to escalate, struggles over bedtime can become a power struggle between parent and child. Several developmental authorities recommend that parents develop a ritual that precedes bedtime, such as, reading a story, bathing, and brushing teeth. This not only gradually slows the busy toddler's activity and promotes relaxation but also prepares the toddler for the upcoming event. Some parents use a timer that is set for 15–20 minutes, and the time limit is adhered to. Ritualism will also allow for a special time for the parent and child to be together—something all toddlers enjoy.

Emotional Development

The child aged 1 to 3 is in Erik Erikson's (1963) stage of autonomy versus shame and doubt. The toddler must resolve several conflicts during this maturational crisis period and become more independent in order to feel good about the self and the world. Shortly after the infancy period, most toddlers learn to walk and, with this advanced motor skill, become more able to explore and interact with their world. During this time the young child begins to master not only part of his environment but also additional parts of the body. Burton White (1978) states that this period (9–18 months) is the most critical in the development of a child's sense of competence. He states that the toddler must be provided an environment that is safe *and* stimulating to intellectual and cognitive growth in order to continually test out and learn new skills.

The toddler's emerging verbal abilities are coupled with this increased striving for independence, and oftentimes this produces negative responses to any attempts parents make to guide actions. *No* is one of the first words learned and most frequently used during this period. Ambivalence is another hallmark characteristic of the struggle for autonomy. The toddler continually evidences *push-pull* behavior when trying to develop self-control over impulses while still remaining very dependent on parental love and guidance. Parents, too, sometimes have a difficult time dealing with their own feelings of pride at their child's accomplishment and fear of letting go too soon.

Cognitive Development

The child makes the transition from the sensorimotor period of cognition to representational intelligence from ages 18 to 24 months (Flavell, 1963). The child begins to symbolize events mentally and thus can now learn about the world in ways other than just by physical interaction or manipulation. Whereas the infant actually used a trial-and-error approach, the child is now able to begin to utilize the mind to try out varied solutions to problems. The toddler is also able to imitate people and events after the fact. All of these new skills are reflected in the play of the toddler. Favorite activities include a game of hide-and-seek (reflecting attainment of object permanency) and reading short stories.

After the age of 1½ to 2 years, a process Piaget called *symbolic function* begins and enables the child to represent an event or object by means of a signifier (Flavell, 1963). This attainment allows the child to express a need (although this may remain confusing when the child's personal definition for an object is not universally recognized). This symbolic function ability will develop further during the preoperational period in the preschool years.

Social Development

The most influential factor in the toddler's social development remains the relationship with the parents. Family relationships, particularly those of parent and child, are recognized as the prototypic relationships on which all others will be based throughout an individual's life (Bowlby, 1969). A child's parents are primarily responsible for structuring an environment that is safe, stimulating, and enables the toddler to challenge and refine developmental skills.

Play is the vehicle through which toddlers begin to develop social skills, refine motor skills, and test out emerging abilities. Toddlers do not engage in interactive play. That is, they are not yet sufficiently developed to understand the rules and give and take of group play. The toddler is much more interested in exploring the self and how the environment expands or restricts use of the self.

Parents also serve as the young child's role models in the conception of gender identity. Although there is controversy over exactly when boys and girls realize they are of one sex or the other and different from each other, most developmental experts believe the discovery is an exciting one for children and one they spend a great deal of time thinking about (Powell, 1981). The toddler is generally aware of gender differences and begins to imitate in small ways the parent of the same sex. The purpose of this imitation is an identification process that will intensify in the preschool years and continue throughout childhood and adolescence.

The traditional mother–father roles have been expanded a great deal with the increase in mothers of preschoolers who are employed outside the home. Fifty-three percent of mothers of children under 5 years old work, and the number is expected to increase. Although current research has revealed no clearcut benefits or deterents to children of working mothers, it is obvious that alternative caretaking arrangements provide the young child with increased exposure to other children and adults that add to the child's repertoire of imitative behaviors and socialization levels (Hofferth, 1979).

Sibling relationships are often also a very significant influence for the toddler's development. Some families feel it is better to have their children 1½ to 3 years apart. The presence of a sibling will provide an opportunity for the toddler to evaluate the relationship with the parents and his or her own self-esteem. The younger child (12 months to 2 years) will often become withdrawn and even hostile after the birth of a new baby for a period of time. Parents will need to understand the toddler's reactions, structure ways of spending special time with the older child, and praise efforts at self-control in order to help the child to overcome negative responses toward the new baby.

INDIVIDUAL DEVELOPMENTAL TASKS OF THE PRESCHOOL CHILD

Physical Development

The preschool child, ages 3 to 5 years, is very stable physiologically. During these 3 years, the young child will grow relatively slowly but steadily and gain about 4 pounds and 3 inches per year. Increasingly, the child becomes more adultlike in appearance with most of the body fat, abdominal protrusion, and apparent shortness of the extremities disappearing.

Nutritional Requirements. The preschool child needs 1800–1900 calories per day and 30 grams of protein to sustain growth (Slattery et al., 1979). Foods from all four groups need to be encouraged daily. Foods high in roughage and fiber (vegetables, nuts, grain cereals) are often underrepresented and can precipitate problems with constipation. High activity levels and need for play will often be more important to the preschooler than the need for nourishment. Foods that can be eaten on the go are still very popular during this time. Examples of these foods that are high in nutritive value include peanut butter, raisins, fruits, hot dogs, and cheese.

Activity Patterns.   The preschool child is usually more amenable to bedtime rituals and will respond more readily to rational explanations than the toddler. Preschoolers require 10–12 hours of sleep per night. Most preschoolers will discontinue taking a nap during the day. However, many preschool and daycare programs encourage a rest period during which many children sleep. Most preschoolers are enrolled in some sort of daytime educational activity outside their homes, which requires earlier awakening times and encourages earlier bedtimes. On the other hand, television becomes much more interesting to a child after 3 years of age and will provide a great deal of competition for the more active forms of play. Parents need to limit television time and encourage the child to engage in more active play.

Personality Development

The child from 3 to 6 years of age must develop in such a way as to resolve the maturational crisis labeled initiative versus guilt (Erikson, 1963). The child is now much more independent; language ability has progressed rapidly so that the child is able to express needs and is able to separate from parents for increasing amounts of time. People outside of the home become more influential helping the child to learn about the world. The preschooler has a very active imagination and is incessantly questioning about events and people. A sense of initiative is evidenced in the child's attempts to further explorations, stake out territory, and to be more active in setting goals. More responsibility for toys, body, activities, and friendships can be assumed.

Cognitive Development

Much intellectual growth occurs in the child from age 3 to 6 years. This period was labeled by Piaget the preoperational stage (ages 2–7 years) (Flavell, 1963). During this time the child further develops the ability to use symbols and can now think of past, present, and future events. Early in the preoperational period, the child is unable to think conceptually and will generalize a label for one person, object, or event to several others with similar characteristics. An example of this is calling all large four-legged animals "horse."

After the age of 4½ the child enters the intuitive period of thinking. The child can now provide reasons for behavior, even though these often are egocentric and one-sided. Other characteristics of the preoperational phase are: (1) egocentrism—the inability to see things, people, and the self the way others see them; (2) centration—the focusing of one aspect of a situation to the exclusion of all others (an example of centration is the inability of the preschool child to understand that although an injection is painful, it also conveys physiological benefits); (3) animism—the tendency to believe that inanimate objects are real and possess the ability to think; (4) fantasy—the belief that thoughts and gestures can command things to happen like magic; and (5) fears—fears of both real or imaginary things, frequent during the preschool period. Misinterpretations of events are common, and fears will be unique to each child. Preschoolers are not always capable of verbalizing their fears and may instead evidence them in their play or drawings.

Social Development

The preschool years are a time of widening experiences, particularly with other individuals outside the family. Many preschoolers are enrolled in either day care or nursery school programs where they come into contact with other adults and children. Socialization, especially the learning of accommodation to others, is intensive during this period. The preschool child is more able to share with others, engage in more complex games, and withstand longer periods of separation from the family.

Gender identity solidifies during the preschool years. Girls and boys prefer the company of same-sex peers and, due to ambivalent feelings, become very sex-typed in their ideas about appropriate games, toys, and jobs for girls and boys. Sexual exploration is an extension of this striving to achieve a secure idea of their identity and also results in part from the high level of curiosity preschoolers demonstrate. Parents often become concerned when finding their preschool child engaging in sex play with either themselves or other children. Oftentimes sex play is an attempt to play out roles such as mother, father, and baby. Parents need to realize these activities are normal, and if they find their child engaging in sexual activities to simply divert the child's attention to other activities. A private discussion with the child is also helpful in helping the child to feel comfortable about being curious and yet realize there are more acceptable ways to channel energy and curiosity.

POTENTIAL STRESSORS

Physical Stressors

Toddlers and preschool children are particularly susceptible to trauma and injury of an accidental nature, due to their high level of activity and relative immaturity. In addition, nutritional demands remain high while the child's interest in eating declines, predisposing the child to vitamin and mineral deficiencies.

Socioemotional Stressors

During the toddler and preschool years, the child's sense of competence and self-esteem is being developed. The parent–child relationship is the most critical one during this period, and the parent must provide the child with nurturance, firm guidance, limit setting, and warmth in order for the child to test his or her capabilities. When the parent is experiencing stress or is unable to nurture a child due to emotional deficiencies, the child is at risk. The nurse should assess the parent–child relationship at each visit. Guidelines for the assessment are listed in Table 6–4.

If the parent–child relationship appears strained, the nurse should talk with the

TABLE 6–4. GUIDELINES FOR ASSESSMENT OF PARENT–CHILD RELATIONSHIP

Physical Proximity

Does the child maintain close proximity to parent in high-stress situation; venture out in nonthreatening situation?
Do the parent and child initiate eye contact and touching at various times?
If parent leaves child with stranger (i.e., nurse), does parent prepare child, provide distraction?
How does child respond when parent leaves? Distressed, crying, avoidance?

Communication Patterns

Does the parent talk to child about aspects of environment?
Does child express needs to parent using clear verbalization?
Is parent's nonverbal and verbal behavior regarding child consistent?
If two parents are present, is their verbal perception of the child's behavior consistent?

Discipline Methods

Does the parent set firm limits on the child's behavior?
Does the parent provide rationale when refusing child's request or setting controls on behavior?
Is control balanced with a degree of warmth?
Does parent state child is a "good" or "bad" child in comparison with peers/siblings?
Does child consistently push limits set by parents?
If both parents are present, do they agree on limits and controls?

parents about other events in their family life. Referral to a family counselor may be necessary for families with multiple or severe stressors.

Child abuse is a symptom of extreme stress in a family. Most parents who abuse their children have been abused themselves. As a result, they have not learned appropriate parenting skills. They often have unrealistic expectations of their child. Recent findings have demonstrated that the child may play an important role in child abuse (Millor, 1979). That is, certain children are more susceptible to being abused— those who are unattractive, have a defect, or are strong-willed. Families who are suspected of child abuse need much support and counseling.

The nurse should also assess how much freedom the child has in his or her environment. Some parents are very protective and actually hinder the young child's exploration of the environment. This overprotection could stem from an early threat to the child's well-being or prolonged separation of child and parent that resulted in parental fear of loss of the child. These parents do not feel they can allow the child to explore anything that could possibly injure him or her; thus they hinder the child's testing of body limits and mastery over the environment.

Sibling relationships should also be explored. A new baby is often introduced into the family during these years and initially can produce strain in both the marital dyad and the parent–child relationship. This disruption is usually only temporary. The nurse can assist the family by exploring with them their plans to prepare the older child during pregnancy and how they feel they will deal with the child's feelings and behavior after the baby comes home.

The nurse should recommend to the parents that they talk about the baby during pregnancy and involve the toddler or preschooler in the preparations. After the baby arrives, one parent should arrange some time each day alone with the older child doing something special. They should anticipate some jealousy and allow the child to verbalize negative feelings about the new baby while setting firm limits on any hostile behavior.

Family Stressors

Two particular family types that are receiving much attention from professionals in several disciplines are the dual-career family and the single-parent family. Each of these family units experience unique stressors that can affect the health and well-being of the children.

Dual-career families are identified as those in which both parents work. Time constraints and energy limitation require the members of this family pay particular attention to developing ways of meeting the needs of *all* individuals in the family. Leisure time and time spent together is at a premium and often must be scheduled. These parents report they must defer or deny themselves a certain amount of adult socialization in order to spend time together as a family. Communication and joint problem solving is particularly important in these families.

The adult in a single-parent family also experiences a shortage of available time and energy for meeting the needs of self and the children. An active social support system is particularly important to the single parent in order to provide some relief time from the continual demands and responsibilities of rearing children alone

(Norbeck, 1981). Single parents may be especially stressed, as they usually lack adequate financial resources to support a family and spend much energy prioritizing spending needs. Preventive health care may not be a primary priority.

COPING MECHANISMS

Health Beliefs and Behaviors

There has not been much research and investigation into the health beliefs and practices of toddlers and preschool children. However, researchers have found relationships between childrearing patterns, parents' health care practices, and the health behavior of school-age children that have implications for the developing beliefs and behavior of the younger child. Pratt (1973) found that parents who used a developmental pattern of childrearing (use of reason, reward, and autonomy) had children who demonstrated better health habits than children whose parents used a disciplinary pattern. There was also a positive relationship between the parents' health habits and that of the child. Although parents have a more direct control over the toddler's health behavior (nutrition, sleep, dental care), the preschooler is beginning to take some initiative for some selected areas of health habits. So, although parental influence is important, health education programs can effectively be directed at the preschool population. Health is a high-level and difficult concept for the young child to grasp; however, several investigators recommend beginning health teaching early on, especially with the inclusion of parents (Gochman, 1970; Lewis & Lewis, 1982).

Preoperational children (2–7 years) still continue to think in idiosyncratic and egocentric ways. They do not typically distinguish internal from external functions. They are unable to distinguish between structure and function and may talk about breathing without any conception of lungs or respiratory organs (Bibace & Walsh, 1981). Parts of the body are recognized, such as eyes, ears, and legs. Due to inability to identify functions of the various body interiors, the child feels little control over what happens inside of the body and will attribute any bodily dysfunction to outside causes. Preschoolers are unable to logically and systematically describe internal sensations or to use internal cues to signal recovery to themselves (Neuhauser et al., 1978).

Given an awareness of preoperational children's development, it is not difficult to understand why they find a Band-aid that will "plug up the hole and stop all the blood from running out" reassuring. The preschooler is unable to decenter long enough to accept the statement that an injection can be beneficial and cause pain at the same time. A nurse needs to understand how the young child thinks in order to plan effective assessments and intervention techniques. Asking a young child questions that the child is unable to comprehend will provide the nurse with little or no information about how the child thinks. In addition, interventions that are planned (i.e., preparation for a procedure, explanation of a treatment) must be geared to the level of the child's cognitive ability.

Young Children's Conception of Illness

If one were to ask a child how he or she got sick, the answer would be very age-specific. Bibace and Walsh (1981) describe the stages that children go through as their ideas about illness develop and how these stages closely parallel the child's developmental progression. The older child is more realistic, more complex, more process-oriented, and more aware of internal body cues to illness in his or her explanations than the younger child. The literature has not demonstrated any sex difference in children's understanding of illness (Campbell, 1975).

Toddlers and preschool children are still in a stage of prelogical thinking, and their explanations of how they became sick reflect this (Bibace & Walsh, 1981). Children 2 to 6 years of age are unable to explain how events cause an illness. Toddlers especially are likely to place blame on events occurring in the immediate environment such as wind, rain, sun, etc. When pushed for an answer to how, these children definitively state, "It just does, that's all!"

Preschoolers are more likely to use the concept of contagion in their explanation. The cause of illness is still not conceptualized as being located within the child, but rather is located in objects or people that are near to the child. Magic is often included in these explanations of the process.

Adaptive Responses

There have been several factors isolated in the literature as having an influence over the way a child responds to a stressful event (see Fig. 6–1). The factors have varying amounts of empirical support documented in the literature, but each needs to be considered when working with young children who are experiencing a stressful event.

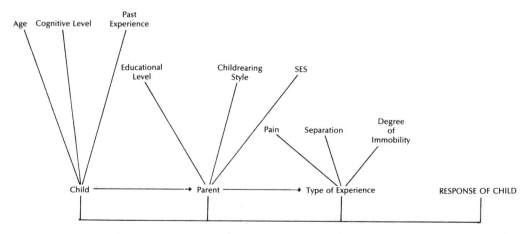

Figure 6–1. Factors Affecting a Child's Response to a Stressful Medical Experience

The cognitive level of the child is one of the most influential factors in how a child is able to deal with impending stress. This has been discussed previously, and the nurse must utilize his or her knowledge about how children at certain ages think when assessing responses and planning interventions. The parent–child relationship is also a critical variable in how children respond. Murphy (1974), Baumrind (1967), and White (1978) have all found that parents that are high in control and high in warmth have children who utilize cues and other people in their environment to gain needed information and/or support during a stressful period. Many researchers refer to these children as high in competence. Socioeconomic status and educational level of the parents can also influence a child's response. However, because these factors are highly correlated with childrearing style, it is difficult to separate out exactly how much influence they have.

Preparation for the stressful event has usually been found to decrease the degree of distress evidenced by children after stressful events (Wolfer & Vistainer, 1975). However, Broome and Endsley (1987) found that preparation for a finger stick did not significantly reduce the degree of reaction experienced and questioned whether the degree and type of stressor might not be important in whether preparation was effective. Those studies that have found a difference usually involve moderate to severe stressors such as hospitalization or surgery. More studies that investigate the degree of stress involved and timing of preparation need to be done.

The nurse needs to assess each child and family, individually exploring with them what their perception of the stressful event is and what types of support and/or assistance they feel they need. Generally, parents and children are unfamiliar with procedures, equipment, and illness course so that teaching and knowledge sharing on the part of the nurse can do much to decrease their anxiety.

Maladaptive Responses

It has been documented that the child from age 1 to 4 is most at risk after hospitalization for negative impact on growth and development (Vernon et al., 1965; Wolfer & Vistainer, 1975). The young child's dependency needs, undeveloped coping mechanisms, fantasy thinking, inability to understand the concept of cause, and lack of control over events all predisposed him to experiencing an inordinate amount of stress during hospitalization, medical procedures, and illness.

It is important not to identify responses to stress as either inherently adaptive or maladaptive. Individual differences in temperament, past history, cognitive development, and physical stamina will all influence how an individual responds. There are little empirical data available on long-term outcomes of stress in childhood that allow child experts to predict what responses are effective in reducing the effect of stressors.

Parental responses will vary, depending on many of the factors listed above. In addition, some studies have found that adults will recover at different rates depending on whether they cope better using denial or using methods to gain all available information about an event. Wolfer and Vistainer (1975) found that nursing support during stressful periods and hospitalization resulted in higher levels of parental satisfaction with care. Most parents will benefit from a caring nurse who provides the parent with support.

Some common responses of the young child to these stressful events such as hospitalization include aggression, regression, and withdrawal. The aggressive behaviors are generally observed first and are the child's attempt to gain some control over his situation and also to vent frustrations. Children rarely respond initially with passivity during strange and/or painful procedures (Caty, Ellerton, & Richie, 1984). It is only when they realize the total lack of control they have on the situation that they will submit. There is some difference of opinion among clinical practitioners as to where and when to (1) prepare the child for the event, and (2) allow the parent to be present during the procedure. The current research findings on both of these will be discussed shortly.

Regressive behaviors are commonly seen in young children when they are confronted with a stressful situation. The reversion to a more comfortable set of behaviors, particularly those dependency behaviors that will signal the parent to respond (crying, whining, bedwetting), are usually seen as temporarily healthy responses to stress in the young child. Withdrawal, however, especially for prolonged periods of time, is not generally thought to be a productive response, as it tends not to elicit helping behavior from adults for the child. Nurses should prepare parents for the appearance of regressive and aggressive behaviors and help them to decide how they will respond to the child. It is not likely that the behaviors will continue for a long time after hospitalization and/or stressful procedures (Vernon et al., 1965; Thompson, 1985). Parents who respond with firm guidance, warmth, and encouragement usually report their child has returned to pre-event behaviors after a short time.

NURSING ASSESSMENT

There are a number of structured assessment guidelines and tools available for the nurse to use when obtaining information about young children and their families. Those listed in Table 6–5 are just examples and are not inclusive of all those available. The advantage of using a structured and tested assessment tool include knowing what others using the tool found to be the norm and range of behaviors. Information that tells one how reliably (or consistently) the tool measures the behaviors is also provided with most measures.

Before choosing an assessment tool, one must consider the setting in which it will be used. Certain aspects of child and family life are better described by the families' perception of the event, while others necessitate actual observation. A combination of measurements (self-report and observation) is ideal. The nurse must also consider the cost of each assessment tool, the time needed to administer the tool, and the skill level required for administration. The nurse must use knowledge of adult development, marital interaction, and parent–child relationships in order to determine at what level a family is meeting their health needs. In order to make an accurate diagnosis and plan effective intervention, the nurse must spend adequate amounts of time listening to the family describe their perception of how healthy they are, what they perceive the major stressors in their life to be, and what measures they are taking to deal with these stressors. The nurse and the family must decide together what professional assistance they need in order to maintain their present health and

TABLE 6–5. ASSESSING THE FAMILY WITH A PRESCHOOLER

	Environmental Data
Provisions for care	Use of Home Inventory (Home Observation for Measurement of the environment) (Humenick, 1982) identifies and measures particular areas within the home that facilitate the development of children from birth to 6 years of age. After the assessment, the nurse can develop an intervention program to assist families in providing a positive environment in which their children can grow and develop.
Alternative caretakers	The "Quality of Day Care Instrument" (Endsley and Bradbard, 1981) provides the nurse with a tool to give parents guidelines to use when they choose a day care center. The tool assesses the safety, costs, physical arrangement, and stimulation of the day care environment.
	Communication Patterns
Child	The Denver Developmental Screening Test has a language and a social development section that can be used to assess the child 1–5 years of age for verbal abilities.
Between parent and child	Observe behaviors exhibited by parent and child during the health visit. How does the parent set limits? Is the child comforted by the parent when afraid? How does the parent relate to the child's expressed needs?
Among family members	Does one parent speak for both or the child during the visit? Do both parents ever attend the health visit? If the parents are divorced, do one or both see the child?
	Problem-Solving Skills
Decision-making abilities	The Family Dynamics Assessment by David Olsen (Humenick, 1982) was developed to quantify and
Support from significant others	empirically evaluate the degree of cohesion and flexibility a family has. It is theorized that a ba-
Societal interactions	lanced level of cohesion and flexibility promotes individual growth and effective functioning of families. Healthy families have a balance of family cohesion and interaction with the community and society. They are supportive to one another and make decisions as a group.
Health system	How accessible is the child health facility? Is cost a deterrent to use? Is well-child care sought?
	Life-Style
Role of child in family	Is this a dual-job (career) family? Is there enough time allotted for meeting the child's needs for parent interaction/nurturance? Are the parents planning more children?
Socioeconomic status	Estimated yearly income, financial assistance, direction of SES mobility, wage earner's feelings about status.

TABLE 6–5. *(continued)*

Family Roles	Traditional or nontraditional pattern, distribution, level of satisfaction with roles.
Work patterns	Wage earners in family, amount of work hours per day or week, anticipated job change.
Recreational patterns	Use of free time, amount of planned activities per month, amount of time spent in recreation/leisure by each family member, amount of group recreation.
Safety	Visible hazards (broken steps, exposed electrical outlets, glass in yard, etc.), use of safety features (car seats, latches on medicine cabinet, etc.), adult's knowledge of accident prevention, first aid, poison control.
	Potential Stressors
Conflicts in parenting	Parent(s) perception of parenting role, own recognition of conflicts, potential for unrecognized problems.
Interference with family tasks	Goals of family members, present health of family member.
Conflict of society	Incorporation of children and involvement with society, societal acceptance of family and children.
Family response patterns	Restructuring or reordering of goals, determining priorities, identifying realistic, practical approaches to meeting goals, changing family structure, or life-style. The Feetham Family Functioning Survey is a very useful tool when assessing the effect of either a maturational or situational event on the family (Humenick, 1982). The nurse uses this tool to ask the family to rate "what presently is" and "what should be." The difference between the rating and how important the individual says each item is contributes to the assessment of family functioning by providing an overall score. The 23 questions that comprise the survey assess household task division; health care; sexual and marital relations: interaction with family and friends; community involvement; and sources of emotional support on a 7-point scale. Administration time is 10 minutes.

promote higher levels of well-being. This will require an interchange of ideas on the nurse and family's part and a mutual respect for the other person's experience and knowledge.

Specific tools are used to enable the nurse to obtain a clearer idea of areas of concern or need the family has. For instance, if the adults in the family verbalize feelings of fatigue and depression, use of the Social Readjustment Scale (Humenick, 1982) will enable the nurse to better assess how much and what type of stress the family has encountered recently. After reviewing the couple's response to the scale with them, the nurse can help focus on areas needing adjustment and assistance to alleviate stress. Referrals to a social agency to assist with budget planning is an example. Most nurses find that reviewing an assessment tool with a family facilitates communication. Strengths as well as needs can be pointed out, which often serves to increase the family's self-esteem and confidence.

ALTERATIONS IN HEALTH

Acute Conditions

The toddler and preschool child are at risk for several particular threats to health. The most common include chronic otitis media, dental cavities, anemia, communicable diseases, and accidents and injury.

Otitis Media.   This is an infection in the middle ear that occurs most frequently during or after an upper respiratory infection. A large majority of young children experience at least one middle ear infection before they begin school (Nelson, 1979). Because the young child's eustachian tube, which connects the pharnyx and the middle ear, is shorter and more horizontal than the adult's, it becomes inflamed more easily and closes off. Fluid begins to build up in the middle ear because of the vacuum created by the blocked eustachian tube, which produces pressure. This fluid sometimes becomes infected. Although children will often run a fever, pull at their ears, refuse to eat, or become irritable, some do not evidence any symptoms at all. Chronic or untreated ear infections can lead to decreased ability to hear. Medical treatment consists of a 10-day course of antibiotics. Some children are also treated with a decongestant to decrease fluid buildup. Parents need to be aware of the symptoms of otitis media, and health professionals must remember to include an examination of the ear at every visit.

Dental Cavities.   The nurse should perform a basic review of each child's teeth during the physical examination to screen for dental cavities. A dental examination by a dentist should be performed at age 3. Children who have taken a bottle to bed or who have nursed on and off all night will present a characteristic appearance with the upper incisors (4–6 teeth) severely decayed, while other teeth are basically healthy (Nelson, 1979). It is recommended that parents discontinue the bottle when the child is between 10–12 months of age, never prop a bottle, and if the infant needs a bottle during the night, fill it with water so as to prevent the milk sugar from coming in contact with the teeth. Mothers should also be encouraged to properly brush their toddler's teeth twice a day with a soft toothbrush. The preschooler should begin to take responsibility for toothbrushing but will need adult supervision.

Anemia.   The diagnosis of iron-deficiency anemia is based on a blood determination of a hematocrit below 31 mg% (Nelson, 1979). Values between 31–33% are considered borderline. The most common reason for iron-deficiency anemia is inadequate intake. Toddlers and preschoolers are especially at risk due to their overall decreased intake, food fads, and growth needs. The nurse should discuss the child's dietary patterns with the parent at each visit, beginning with the 1-year-old well-child check. It is at this time that iron-fortified formula is discontinued, and more iron-containing foods need to be continued in or added to the diet such as dark green leafy vegetables and red meats.

Communicable Diseases.   After years of emphasis on immunizing young children, many communicable diseases have been drastically reduced and some virtually eliminated. These include smallpox, rubella, rubeola, diptheria, pertussis, and polio. The symptoms and incubation periods are listed in Table 6–6. Due to high immunization rates, rubeola and chickenpox are the only two common communicable diseases seen in most pediatric populations now. Treatment for these two illnesses is primarily symptomatic, and they are controlled at home. Treatment includes fever control, adequate fluid intake, respiratory isolation, and medication to decrease itching.

Accidents.   Accidents are the leading cause of injury and death in children under 14 years of age. The young child's high activity level, curiosity, inability to anticipate inherent danger, and impulsiveness makes him or her particularly vulnerable to potential injury in the environment. Motor vehicle accidents lead the list of accidents in children over 1 year of age (Ford, 1981). Use of infant car restraint systems needs to be continued until 4 years of age, when seat belts can be used. Many states have passed legislation in recent years *requiring* parents to use a restraining device with children under 4 years of age (Vaiden, 1983). In addition, doors should be kept locked when children are riding in the car to prevent inadvertent opening of doors and falling out. Toddlers should always be supervised when near roadways, as they are too young to understand how to cross roads safely. Preschoolers still require some supervision, although they can begin to learn about crossing a street and bicycle safely.

Other accidents that preschoolers are involved in include falls, burns, and poisoning. Although adult supervision will prevent or moderate some of these injuries, it is not possible for a parent to always be present with the child. As a result, it is recommended that parents assess their home and place all obviously dangerous objects out of reach or in an area that is locked. Such items include bleach, polish, oven cleaner, and gasoline. All parents should be encouraged to keep a bottle of ipecac in their medicine cabinet. Ipecac is an emetic (drug that causes vomiting), which is to be given a child when noncorrosive poisoning occurs. Common noncorrosive ingestions include aspirin, iron, and tylenol. Ipecac should *not* be used if the child ingests a corrosive or hydrocarbon such as gasoline, oven cleaner, or lye, as vomiting will increase the area burned or increase the change of aspiration. Parents should keep the nearest poison control center number at their phone and be instructed not to administer *any* treatment without calling the center first.

An assessment guide that can be used by the nurse to evaluate the safety hazards in the child's environment is in Table 6–7.

TABLE 6–6. COMMUNICABLE DISEASES

Disease	Incubation Period	Communicability Period	Causative Agent	Method of Spread	Clinical Manifestations	Treatment and Nursing Care	Complications
Chickenpox (varicella)	10–21 days	One day before onset to 6 days after first vesicles appear	Virus	Airborne droplets. Direct or indirect contact. Dry scabs are not infectious	Malase, slight fever, anorexia, headache, successive crops of macules, papules, vesicles, crusts. May all be present at the same time. Itching, generalized lymphadenopathy	Symptomatic Prevent scratching. Keep fingernails short and clean. Sedate PRN. Antibiotics or chemotherapy may be used with secondary infections	Secondary invasion of pathogenic organisms. Erysipelas, abscesses may occur
Measles	10–21 days	From 4 days before to 5 days after rash appears	Virus	Droplets. Contaminated dust. Direct contact	Fetus may contact rubeola in utero if mother has the disease. Coryza, conjunctivitis, Koplik spots: mouth, hacking cough, high fever, rash, enlarged lymph nodes. Rash: small reddish brown macules, changing to papules; fades on pressure. Rash behind ears, on forehead, on cheeks, progresses to extremities and lasts about 5 days	Symptomatic Keep in bed until fever and cough subsides. Dim lights. Keep hands from eyes. Tepid baths and soothing lotions relieve itching. Encourage fluids. Serum or gamma globulin may be given to modify illness and reduce complications	Vary with severity of disease: Otitis media; pneumonia, tracheobronchitis, nephritis, encephalitis may occur

156

Disease	Incubation period	Period of communicability	Causative agent	Mode of transmission	Symptoms	Treatment	Complications
Measles (rubella)	14–21 days	During prodromal period and for 6 days after rash appears	Virus	Direct contact, or by contaminated dust particles in air. From secretions of nose and throat of infected persons	Slight fever, mild coryza. Rash consists of small pink or pale red macules closely grouped to appear as scarlet blush, which fades on pressure. Rash fades in 3 days. Swelling of posterior cervical and occipital lymph nodes. *No Koplik spots or photophobia*	Symptomatic: bed rest until fever subsides	Chief danger of disease is a damaging effect on fetus if mother contracts infection during first trimester of pregnancy. Severe complications are rare, but encephalitis may occur
Mumps (infectious parotitis)	14–21 days	1–6 days before first symptoms appear until swelling disappears	Virus	Direct or indirect contact with salivary secretions of infected person	Salivary glands are chiefly affected. Parotid glands, sublingual and submaxillary glands may be involved. Swelling and pain may occur in these glands, either unilaterally or bilaterally. Child may have difficulty swallowing, headache, fever, and malaise	Local application of heat or cold to salivary glands to reduce discomfort. Liquids or soft foods containing acid may increase pain. Bed rest until swelling subsides	Less frequent in children than in adults. Meningoencephalitis, inflammation of ovaries or testes or deafness may occur

TABLE 6–6. COMMUNICABLE DISEASES *(continued)*

Disease	Incubation Period	Communicability Period	Causative Agent	Method of Spread	Clinical Manifestations	Treatment and Nursing Care	Complications
Rosela infantum	Unknown	Unknown	Virus	Incidence highest in spring and fall. Not contagious like measles, rubella, chickenpox	Temperature of 104–105°, without apparent cause. Convulsions are common. Anorexia, irritability, or listlessness. Temperature drops on 4th day, when rash starts. Maculopapular eruption appears first on chest, abdomen. May spread face and extremities. Last 2–3 days. Peasized, post-occipital lymph node swelling	Symptomatic ASA and tepid water baths for antipyretic effects	Convulsive seizures. Encephalitis rarely occurs

TABLE 6–7. INJURY RISK ASSESSMENT TOOL

Directions: Give each negative factor a −1 and each positive factor a +1. Add up points at end of each section and place in equation.

$$\underline{\quad\quad} + \underline{\quad\quad} + \underline{\quad\quad} = \underline{\quad\quad}$$

Agent + Host + Environment = Risk Potential

	Point	Check How Behavior Documented	
	Point	*Observed*	*Mother's Report*

AGENT (Substances)

Positive Factors

1. Ipecac left on premises.
Comments

2. Household cleansing agents/insecticides are kept in original containers.
Comments

Negative Factors

1. Medicines out on counter, tables, etc.
Comments

2. Medicines not currently prescribed are retained.
Comments

ENVIRONMENT (Home)

Positive Factors

1. Locks (child latches) on cabinets and storage containing poisons/household cleaning agents.
Comments

2. Poison control number available near phone.
Comments

3. Gate covers open stairway.
Comments

4. Mother uses approved car restraint system.
Comments

5. Matches are kept out of reach.
Comments

6. Adult supervision of play is provided.
Comments

7. Smoke detector outside bedroom area in operation.
Comments

TABLE 6–7. *(continued)*

	Check How Behavior Documented		
	Point	Observed	Mother's Report
8. Water activities (bath and swimming) are supervised.	_____	_____	_____
Comments			
9. Cribrails are less than 2⅜" apart.	_____	_____	_____
Comments			
Negative Factors			
1. Paint flaking off walls.	_____	_____	_____
Comments			
2. Play equipment in poor condition (broken swing, rusting, etc.).	_____	_____	_____
Comments			
3. Cords, pot handles hang over counter.	_____	_____	_____
Comments			
4. Loaded firearms kept in house.	_____	_____	_____
Comments			
5. Electrical outlet uncovered.	_____	_____	_____
Comments			
6. Family has recently moved into home.	_____	_____	_____
Comments			
7. Child (under 2 years) eats peanuts and raisins.	_____	_____	_____
Comments			
8. Child (under 3 years) plays with balloons.	_____	_____	_____
Comments			

From: Broome, M. and Weston, W. (1984). Injury Risk Assessment Tool. Medical College of Georgia.

Chronic Conditions

Chronic illness is an alteration in biopsychosocial functioning that persists over a long period of time, and usually produces some degree of deficiency in performance in a selected area. The incidence of chronic illness varies from 7 to 30%, depending on whether mental retardation, vision, speech, and hearing deficits are included (Matteson, 1972). Chronic illness has great potential for affecting individual and family development and requires the utilization of multiple coping skills to achieve positive adaptation. Chronic illness is also costly to society. Examples of chronic illness in childhood include:

Congenital Anomalies.   These include cardiac defects such as Tetralogy of Fallot, cleft lip and/or cleft palate, osteomyelitis, etc. Congenital anomalies vary in the degree in which they impair the development of the child. Some, such as cleft palate, are repairable but require numerous surgical procedures and hospitalizations. Cleft lip usually involves one or two surgical repairs and does not pose any major threat to health. However, due to the obvious facial deformity, many parents initially become more concerned than when cleft palate occurs alone. Other defects, such as tetralogy of Fallot, are threatening and require immediate and continuous monitoring. Growth potential is affected as well as available energy levels.

Genetic Disorders.   Phenylketonuria (PKU), sickle cell disease, cystic fibrosis, and Down's syndrome are just a few of the chronic illnesses that are identified as linked with some type of genetic transmission. Genetic disorders also vary in the degree to which they affect the child's functioning. However, parental guilt is most heavily evidenced in this group. Parents verbalize a sense of blame about the transmission, even when they were aware of the possibility.

Perinatal trauma.   This group of chronic conditions result from some insult experienced by the fetus during pregnancy or during childbirth and include cerebral palsy and congenital herpes. Nurses can play a major role in decreasing the incidence of these conditions through education and prenatal care.

Infections.   These include meningitis and rheumatic heart disease. The suddenness of these illnesses in a previously well child produces a dramatic effect on the family. After initial medical treatment is completed, the family may deny sequeale that occur or the need for follow-up.

Neoplasms.   As medical treatment for cancer has become increasingly sophisticated, children who are diagnosed as having bone and brain tumors, acute leukemias, and other malignancies are now living for years after diagnosis. In many cases, long-term treatment has yielded high 5-year survival rates, which are considered cures. However, the treatment itself is lengthy and very costly in both monetary and emotional energy for the family.

Sensory Deficits.   These include hearing and vision disorders. These can be present since birth or occur as a result of infection or medical treatment (drugs). A family with a blind or deaf child must learn new ways to communicate with their child. They often find that community resources (school systems) are not set up to provide quality experiences for their child. This frustrates many parents.

NURSING RESPONSIBILITIES

Preventive Measures

Toddler. Regular examinations in which the health status of the young child is assessed are crucial to the well-being and development of a child. The child from 1 to 3 years of age is the most difficult to examine of any age group. Due to an intense activity level, fear of separation, and intensity of attachment to the parent, the examination (especially developmental assessment) is best done without requiring the child to sit or lie on an examination table. Much of the exam can be carried out with the child on the mother's lap. The typical head-to-toe progression is altered so that the eye, ear, nose, and throat (EENT) exam is left to last. This will produce the least amount of upset in the small child in a strange environment.

Health assessments are recommended every 6 months from age 12 to 36 months. The physical examination consists of a history, an overview of the body systems, and vision and hearing testing. The history should include a report of the prenatal and birth experience, growth history, diet report (recall of 24-hour intake), allergies, hospitalizations, significant illnesses and injuries. Daily activities, including sleep patterns, are also recorded. The nurse will find it most helpful to have toys available for the toddler to play with during this time; otherwise it is difficult for the mother to accurately provide information with repeated interruptions from her young child. As the child plays, the nurse can also informally assess gross and fine motor skills. For example, according to the Denver Developmental Screening Tool (DDST), which will be discussed later, most children between the ages of 12 and 24 months will stack one cube block on top of another, walk alone, and scribble spontaneously with a crayon or pencil. All of these activities can be observed as the child plays with objects found in the examination room.

The physical examination consists of an assessment of pulse rate and regularity, respirations, and temperature. Most toddlers are unable to have their temperatures taken orally because of an inability to keep their mouths closed and breathe through their noses. However, placement of a rectal thermometer is upsetting to most young children; therefore, obtaining the temperature reading by an axillary placement is recommended.

Several immunizations are given to toddlers at the regularly scheduled health visits. These include a measles–mumps–rubella (MMR) vaccination at 15 months; the fourth diptheria–pertussis–tetanus (DPT) and the third oral polio vaccine (OPV) at eighteen months. In recent years an additional vaccine called HIB, haemophilus influenzae, has been recommended for children 18–23 months who are at risk. These include children in day care centers who interact with large numbers of young children and some chronically ill children.

Each body system is then inspected, palpated, percussed, or ausculated as appropriate (see Table 6–8). Any abnormalities are noted, and further follow-up is planned. Comprehensive vision testing is still difficult in the child aged 1 to 3 years. Most health professionals use the DDST to screen toddlers for gross vision problems. One uses the ball of red yarn to test for range of ocular muscle movement, and the gross ability of the child to see near objects can be assessed by placing a raisin on a white piece of paper in front of the child, who will attempt to pick up the raisin. Adequacy of hearing can be indirectly assessed by the level of the child's reported comprehension and verbal language ability. By the age of 14–15 months, 90% of children will say "Ma-ma" or "Da-da" to their parent and turn to the speaker when their names are called. If these abilities are not present, referral should be sought.

Nurses and other health professionals will find a toddler to be easier to examine if the approach to the exam is unhurried and each section is explained to both parent and child. Toddlers can be especially sensitive to their parent's anxiety. Any part of the exam that can be made fun and use of distraction techniques will promote cooperation in the child aged 1–3 years. An example

TABLE 6–8. PHYSICAL EXAMINATION OF THE TODDLER AND PRESCHOOLER

Body System	Primary Method of Examination	Normal Findings	Suspect Findings (Referral)	
Eyes, ears, nose, throat	Observation	Hearing and vision normal, no inflammation or drainage.	Eye:	Absence of red reflex, loss of vision.
			Ears:	Red tympanic membrane, foreign body.
			Nose:	Purulent discharge, consistent bleeding.
			Throat:	Injected tonsils, drainage.
Cardiovascular	Auscultation	Two heart sounds, no murmurs, good peripheral perfusion.	Murmur; extra heart sounds; cyanosis.	
Respiratory	Auscultation	Clear air passages over all lung fields.	Wheezing; rales; absence of sounds; shortness of breath.	
Musculoskeletal	Observation	Full range of motion, clear skin, adequate strength.	Limping.	
Abdominal	Palpation, auscultation	Soft, no masses, normal bowel sounds.	Mass; rigidity; distention; hypo- or hyper- bowel sounds.	
Central nervous system	Observation	Intact reflex, normal activity levels.	Hyper-reflexivity; hyporeflexivity; spasticity; flaccidity.	

would be the placing of a tissue in front of the child's face and asking the child to blow the tissue hard when listening for respiratory sounds. Allowing the child to hold and play with another stethoscope while performing the cardiac exam is also helpful. These few extra minutes spent establishing rapport with the young child will enable the nurse to perform a more accurate health assessment of the toddler.

Preschool Child. The growth and maturity of the preschooler is evident in the relative ease in which the health assessment proceeds. The child from 4 to 6 years of age more readily accepts strangers, separates more easily from the parent, and is better able to understand procedures. The preschooler's curiosity about instruments and the health examiner replaces the toddler's fears.

Health assessments are recommended yearly, and most parents find it most convenient if this is scheduled around the child's birthday. The final diptheria–pertussis–tetanus (DPT) and oral polio vaccine (OPV) immunizations are given between 4 and 6 years, usually around 5 years of age, due to the complete and up-to-date immunization status required for children entering kindergarten in most states.

The history and physical examination is very similar to that of the toddler (see Table 6–8). However, more emphasis is placed on the assessment of the child's ability to get along with other children and adults outside the home. The nurse can now use one of the two versions of the Snellen chart for vision screening. The Snellen chart is a wall chart that consists of 10 lines with letters on each line. For older children, different letters of the alphabet are used. For younger children who are not familiar with the alphabet, only the letter "E" is used and is placed in different positions so the child must indicate only which way the legs on the "E" point. The chart is placed on a wall from which the child can stand 20 feet away from the visual exam. The child calls out the letters of the lowest line he can read. This will indicate the vision acuity. Most preschool children have vision of 20/40 to 20/30. By age 7, 20/20 vision is attained.

Hearing assessment can be done using the audiometer with some young preschoolers and most 5-year-olds. This will require a soundproof room and a trained examiner. The child places a headphone over his or her ears that will emit a tiny "beep" from one earphone or the other. The child is asked to raise the hand that corresponds with the ear in which the "beep" is heard. The examiner manipulates the frequency levels. The hearing assessment should be done *after* the EENT exam so it can be determined that the child's ability to hear is not compromised by wax, foreign objects, or infection.

Once again, the DDST is used to screen for developmental progression. The behaviors that the majority (90%) of 4-, 5-, and 6-year-olds can perform are listed in Table 6–3. The DDST is fun for most preschoolers and can be administered prior to or after the examination.

Physical Examination. Most preschoolers can hold a thermometer in their mouths in order to obtain an oral reading of their temperatures. The reader is referred to Table 6–8 for the examination procedure and expected findings for each body system.

Nurses will find the preschooler to be generally excited over being the focus of attention during the exam and willing to cooperate with most requests. It is a good idea to direct several of the questions during the history and exam to the child. Children of this age are usually most interested in questions about their birth and experiences as babies and will enjoy providing the nurse with their perception of past experience. Most mothers will carefully validate the information the preschooler provides.

Health Promotion

One of the most important roles the nurse plays in health promotion of the young child and family is as an advocate. The nurse will be responsible for advocating for the young child and his family in their interaction with the health care delivery system. Family anxiety is usually high. They enter the system and need a concerned, caring professional to assist them. Other health professionals used to dealing with adults are uncomfortable working with children and families, and the child's nurse will need to help both parties to work with each other. For example, when a child is transferred to an intensive care unit (ICU) for adults, the ICU nurses appreciate the child's nurse communicating with them about the child's history and family preferences. The family appreciates the continuity of care provided by the child's nurse.

The nurse in the acute care setting is in a unique position to provide support for a family. Due to proximity and opportunity, the nurse can help decrease parental and child anxiety by explaining procedures, treatment, and the illness itself. The nurse can meet some of the parents' needs for attention by being available and talking informally when providing care to the child.

Illness prevention, health maintenance, and health promotion are major responsibilities of the child's nurse. Nurses have made major advances in illness prevention in administration of immunization programs, health education, and involvement in community health fitness programs. School nurses have been instrumental in teaching children effective health practices (Wold, 1981), and work is beginning at the level of young children in day care.

The provision of anticipatory guidance and education is a major responsibility of child nurses. Parents need to know more about normal developmental patterns; they can be informally taught these during the nurse's developmental assessment. Parents want to learn more about what their children will be doing and how to help them do it better.

Nurses can also influence the health status of young children and their families' through involvement in social policy making. Examples of this include nurses who were instrumental in making contraception available to adolescents, nurses involved in developing health screening programs for school systems, and nurses who administered programs in health screening and Early Periodic Screening and Detection Testing (EPSDT) programs. Social policy affects children as a whole. Individual nurses can influence these decisions by becoming involved in their local, state, and national professional organizations.

Anticipatory Guidance

Telzrow (1978) defines anticipatory guidance as "a discussion of ideas and opinions about normal child development and the normal parental responses to development." This discussion should include potential threats to the child's well-being that may result from natural developmental characteristics (i.e., injury from falls resulting from activity and testing of motor skills). Proper timing is important as well as inclusion of the opinions and perceptions of the parent (Telzrow, 1978).

Anticipatory guidance for children primarily involves four major areas with different subtopics to be covered. These are the physical self, cognitive self, emotional self, and social self. Parents will usually bring up concerns they have under each area if given time and opportunity and encouraged to ask questions. It is also very helpful to provide the parent with a written synopsis of the discussion and have a copy in the chart. The following is not meant to be a comprehensive discussion of all possible areas of consideration but guidelines for discussion.

Physical Self

1. *Growth patterns:* percentile range and any changes since the last visit; plotting of growth patterns.
2. *Nutritional status:* appetite and intake decreases; calorie requirements for growth decreases; milk intake needs to decrease and solid food to increase to meet the iron, vitamin, and mineral requirements; weaning from the bottle (to prevent dental cavities) should be encouraged during the second year of life.
3. *Activity level:* falls become increasingly common due to high activity level and lack of coordination and perceptual awareness; increasing motor abilities allow toddler to reach to areas to explore (pulling on cords on appliances, tipping over hot coffee, touching stoves; etc.); accidents are most common during the toddler and preschool years. Curiosity and oral needs also predispose this age group to poisoning. Parents should be encouraged to lock all poisons up and out of reach. Safety hooks are available (although relatively expensive) that make it more difficult for the young child to gain access to cabinets and drawers. Car safety should be emphasized during these years.

Toddlers are particularly verbal in their protests against being restrained in a car restraint device. Most toddlers respond well to consistent use and firmness on the part of the parents, and most eventually come to see "their seat" as a special place for them.

Parents of preschoolers need to provide supervision for young children while riding on tricycles and the newer motorized play vehicles. They should instruct their child in road safety when opportunities arise and encourage their preschooler to use a seat belt when riding in a car with friends.

Cognitive Self

The toddler is beginning to learn to express needs verbally, although the level of comprehension is greater than the level of verbal ability. Parents should be encouraged to stimulate the child by answering all questions and taking opportunities that naturally present themselves to teach their toddler and preschooler about the world around them. Overstimulation is to be cautioned against, as current findings indicate children who learn to read at very early ages are not any more advanced than those who learn during the preschool years and, in fact, may become confused in later years.

Emotional Self

Toddlers are prone to becoming frustrated and upset when presented with situations that exceed their ability to problem solve or control. They are often ambivalent about situations and become frustrated with their feelings. As a result, temper tantrums are frequent and puzzle parents. Ignoring the negative behavior is recommended by most authorities, and distraction is also often helpful (Powell, 1981). The toddler will also say "no" to requests as an attempt to differentiate the self and establish some independence. Parents should be encouraged to set firm guidelines and limits on behavior during this time.

The 3–6-year old begins to settle down emotionally and is much better able to understand and deal with situations that are ambivalent or demand self-control. The preschooler is better able to postpone the need for instant gratification and will share toys and activities with other children. The preschooler imitates those adults that are significant and wants to please them. Parents can capitalize on this by praising efforts at self-control and initiative taking. The parent can also give the preschooler small tasks to do to facilitate a sense of responsibility.

Social Self

Play with others is generally not cooperative, and solitary play is more common in toddlers. Fear of strangers prevails. Separations from parents are highly stressful, and hospitalization is an especially stressful experience. Appropriate counseling for parents during hospitalization will be discussed later.

The preschool child is much more active and outgoing in groups than the toddler and enjoys being with other children. Much role playing is carried out in groups of children in order to learn more about the self and the world.

Acute Caregiver

Acute injury and resulting hospitalization are very stressful experiences for the young child and family. The child's inability to understand certain events, inability to communicate needs, and immature coping resources make any new experience difficult, especially one involving certain degrees of separation and discomfort. Parents become very anxious when their child is ill and hospitalized. They fear the pain that may accompany the injury/illness, separation from the child, loss of control over what happens, and even the possible loss of their child. Studies (Wolfer & Visintainer, 1975; Thompson, 1985) have shown that support for parents during hospitalization will moderate parental perception of the stress and indirectly affect the child's response. This nursing support is usually given in the form of information about what will happen to the child, answering any questions they may have, encouraging discussion of their concerns and needs, and demonstration of caring and competence by the nurse as she administers care to the child.

The young child's ability to utilize environmental cues, such as preparation to decrease fear, is very dependent on cognitive level. The young toddler's greatest fear during hospitalization is of separation from the parents. This fear needs to be minimized by the nurse, encouraging parental presence and participation during hospitalization. Parents should be included during explanations and preparation periods. Preparation is best achieved if provided shortly before the event, using concise, clear explanation of what will happen. Use of puppets or dolls may be helpful, particularly for older toddlers.

The preschool child's imagination is exceptionally active, and this child needs a more detailed explanation of what will happen. Use of materials the child can manipulate (i.e., anesthesia mask, IV) are useful in helping the preoperational child to understand events. Several studies (Melamed, Meyers, Gee, & Soule, 1976) have effectively used filmed modeling techniques to prepare young children for preoperative injections and anesthesia induction. The children seemed to respond with less distress during the procedure if they had previously seen a film of a child similar to themselves undergoing the procedure.

The nurse is the health professional who has the most contact with a child and parents during hospitalization and the most opportunity to develop a relationship with them that can be used to decrease the stress during hospitalization. Nurses' awareness of developmental states, parental needs, and the stress of illness and hospitalization will assist them to effectively develop an individualized plan of care for each family and maximize their ability to adapt to the experience.

Role of Play in the Hospitalized Child.   Several theories have been developed to explain play and its critical nature in the development of children (Gellert, 1978; Petrillo & Sanger, 1980). They include:

1. *Surplus energy theory:* this states play is what children do when they have surplus energy
2. *Preparation theory:* suggests that children play to develop competencies and develop knowledge
3. *Relaxation theory:* states children use play to relax and rest
4. *Cathartic or psychoanalytic theory:* states the child acts out deep-seated feelings of tension, frustration, fear, confusion, and bewilderment
5. *Competence or effective motivation theory:* states that through explanation and interaction with the environment the child learns about self and begins to understand and cope with people and the world

Each of these theories explain partial reasons for children's play, but theory 5 was developed recently after much observation and research of children's play and is one of the most eclectic, useful, and applicable to nursing practice. There are several factors that inhibit play of normal children. Those that are inherent in hospitalization are:

1. *Immobility:* when a child is immobilized, outlet for behavior is limited and interaction with the world is limited. Immobilization can result from intravenous

therapy, traction, and casts in the hospital, and extensive use of cribs, strollers, and playpens in the home

2. *Dull or repetitive environment:* if the environment is dull, i.e., nothing to look at, listen to, manipulate, or investigate, the child may begin to make his or her own play, e.g., a baby pulls off the diaper and shreds it; a toddler dumps an ashtray with sand in it to play sandbox

3. *Overstimulating environment:* children need quiet times to reflect on what they have seen, heard, etc. A new environment, loud noises, or too many people may overstimulate the child and cause him or her to "freeze" or emotionally withdraw. Examples are a large crowded day care center, a busy doctor's office, or admission to hospital. It is estimated a child is exposed to 52 new people in the first 24 hours of hospitalization (Gellert, 1978)

4. *Fear:* response to strange, unknown situations that include a feeling of aloneness and decreased security. High degrees of anxiety or fear correlate with avoidance of anxiety-related objects and inhibition of exploratory behavior. Thus, the combination of separation and a strange environment is likely to induce fear and inhibit exploratory behavior until the fear is overcome. Examples are the child entering a new day care center

Illness and hospitalization constitute a crisis in the life of a child and family. Below is a comparison of a child's home and "hospital" life:

	Home	Hospital
Exposure to consistent nurturing persons	High	Low
Regular play with peers	High	Low
Changes in environmental stimuli	Low	High
School activities/day care	High	Low
Independence appropriate to developmental level	High	Moderate
Many family associations	High	Low
Threat of pain	Low	High

Hospital care primarily concerns itself with what is wrong with a child and works to correct the infirmity. It is very important for the nurse to remember what is right with the child and provide activities that will stimulate growth and development. Play can be used as a teaching tool, e.g., preparation for a painful experience or one that threatens body integrity (surgery). The child feels safe in play and will reveal fears and fantasies through this medium. Play can also be used to foster physical health, e.g., a post-operative child can blow bubbles through straw to aerate the lungs. The nurse needs to remember that play in isolation is not fun for children. Children are social beings who enjoy sharing their play with others.

To be effective, play needs to be age-appropriate. Infants respond best to brightly colored, moving toys such as mobiles and balls. Toddlers also like motion during their play or prefer toys they can begin to "operate" on, such as pull toys or stacking blocks. Preschoolers want to utilize their sense of initiative. They often need to work out some frustration. Toys best suited to a preschooler include picture books, simple games, and tricycles.

Working with Parents of the Hospitalized Child. Parents will all experience similar feelings when children have a chronic illness (Fortier & Wanlass, 1984). At diagnosis the first feeling is one of shock and disbelief. Parents will sometimes shop around with different physicians during this time in order to find one who will tell them the child is indeed all right. Even if the parents appear to accept the physician's diagnosis and explanation of the disease, they will ask that explanations be repeated over and over in the initial period. This need for repetition results from high anxiety levels and use of denial. The nurse will need to continually provide information about the child's illness and treatment plan.

The shock and disbelief usually lasts for a short period of time and is followed by feelings of guilt and anger. Parents will search for reasons and causes of the illness and often blame themselves and each other. Parents of children with congenital anomalies are particularly susceptible to guilt and blame. Parents of older children will often verbalize guilt and/or anger over their perceived inattention to early symptoms to the health care professionals. Anger and resentment at God, physicians, spouses, etc., is frequently voiced. Grief will follow this stage. Often parents of chronically ill children experience a "chronic grief" (Olshansky, 1962). The nurse can facilitate adaptation of these families by being available to listen to their anger and grief.

The physical appearance of a chronically ill child can influence how the child, family, and friends perceive the illness. It is not unusual for parents of an infant with an acyanotic cardiac defect to be less anxious about the severity of the defect than parents whose child is cyanotic, even though both may be equally serious. Children with cancer or handicaps have reported lower self-esteems when compared to well children (Darling & Darling, 1980). Some authors have inferred the low self-esteem results in part from appearances. The nurses can keep after the parent to encourage the child to develop strengths and maximize his or her potential.

Family coping styles and childrearing patterns can also moderate the effects of chronic illness on the child and family. Families who have developed effective communication patterns, who are able to utilize problem-solving techniques to make decisions, and are able to be flexible in their roles and power distribution will adapt most effectively to the demands of the illness.

Some of the most dramatic effects of chronic illness on the family include the strain on the marital and sibling relationships. Oftentimes, one parent (usually the mother) is responsible for the majority of the care and is away from home much of the time. She may have little time for her husband and other children, particularly during times of hospitalization. The nurse can be of great assistance by helping the parents to identify other support systems that can help them in meeting some of the ill child's needs in order to free time for each other and the remaining children.

The nurse's assessment and interventions with a family having a chronically ill child needs to be focused on assessing the strengths and resources of the child and family. The plan she develops needs to be arrived at after mutual goal setting with the family. The nurse is often the primary support from the health care team for the chronically ill child and family. The nurse provides this support by talking with the family about visits, being available by phone to answer questions and concerns in between visits, coordinating referrals and consultations, and preparing the family for hospital admission when it occurs.

The nurse in the acute care setting needs to be aware that the family brings much history, knowledge, and skills in dealing with the chronic illness, and needs to work with them to best meet the child's needs during the hospitalization. Parents of ill children have identified a caring attitude and competent manner as the most important characteristics of nurses. Chronically ill children and their parents will sometimes threaten health professionals when they make demands about medication scheduling, treatments, and dietary practices in the hospital. The nurse must realize the family has primary responsibility for decision making regarding these areas when their child is not in the hospital and that it is difficult (and many times unnecessary) for them to turn this control and responsibility over to someone else during hospitalization.

The chronically ill child and family present many challenges to the nurse. Facilitation of the child's growth and development should be the primary goal of nursing care in both the ambulatory and acute care settings. This is best accomplished when the nurse and family mutually plan goals and work toward them.

SUMMARY

The toddler and preschool years are an active period of development for both the individual child and family. Young children interact with nurses and the health care system frequently during routine health examinations as well as visits for minor illnesses. This chapter presented an overview of child and family development and discussed the critical role nurses can play in influencing the health and well-being of young children.

CARE PLAN FOR THE TODDLER/PRESCHOOLER WITH POTENTIAL FOR INJURY

Situation

John is an 18-month-old black male. His mother brings him in for his semiannual well-child visit.

John's head circumference is just above the 25th percentile. His height has been in the 75th percentile since birth. John is over the 95th percentile in height.

John's mother, Ms. B., reports that John has had only two or three colds since birth, usually occurring at the change of the seasons. His cold symptoms consist of rhinorrhea and irritability. His mother denies any fever. The colds resolved spontaneously without use of any medications.

At the age of 8 months, John had an ear infection, which was diagnosed at the physician clinic at the health department. The child was treated with antibiotics and returned to the clinic in 2 weeks for a follow-up visit. The infection had resolved by that time.

Ms. B. reports that all immunizations are current and administered by the health department. John has an appointment in two weeks for his diptheria-pertussis vaccination.

John's appetite has decreased markedly since his year-old checkup. However, his activity level has increased, and Ms. B. states he "is into everything." She does not have any locked cabinets, nor does she own a car seat.

Ms. B. also reported that John is "getting very difficult to make mind." She has attempted to toilet train him lately but has discontinued this temporarily.

Nursing Diagnoses

1. Potential injury for trauma and poisoning
2. Knowledge deficit related to toilet training procedures

SAMPLE CARE PLAN

Nursing Diagnoses	Goals	Intervention	Evaluation
1. Injury, potential for trauma and poisoning	Parents will become more safety conscious and take proper measures to decrease injury potential	Nurse will ask mother questions and/or visit home to complete Injury Risk Assessment Form (Table 6–8) to assess environment for risk and injury potential	Go over form with mother to validate nurse's perception
		Nurse will discuss with mother need for using approved car restraint system in terms of (1) statistics of child injuries/fatalities in automobile accidents and (2) convenience resulting from child's being limited to one location while car is moving	Follow-up with a call one week later to check if car seat is being used
		Nurse will demonstrate use of child restraint system, using model in office	Mother will place toddler in seat and restrain properly
		Nurse will provide mother with list of approved seats (including cost and location to buy) and/or rental possibilities	
		Nurse will discuss other areas identified as providing a risk potential for the toddler—encourage mother to (1) buy safety latches for	Mother will discuss specific measures she feels she will be able to take to increase safety in her home

SAMPLE CARE PLAN *(continued)*

Nursing Diagnoses	Goals	Intervention	Evaluation
		specific cabinets, (2) monitor child's activities while bathing, and (3) restrict child from eating nuts, popcorn, beans, etc.	
		Nurse will demonstrate Heimlich maneuver to mother as well as give her a pictorial handout describing the procedure	Mother will demonstrate for nurse how to do Heimlich maneuver, using her own child
		Nurse will instruct mother on where to buy ipecac syrup and provide handout materials that describe when and how to use it	Mother will measure and pour out ipecac in front of nurse and describe how she would get child to take it
Knowledge deficit related to toilet training procedures	Parents will assist child to learn self-toileting behaviors by 3 years of age	Nurse will describe readiness/maturity signs a child must have prior to beginning a toilet training program: 1. Neurophysiological maturation sufficiencies to control urethral and anal sphincters	
		2. Cognitive maturity sufficient to understand behavioral expectations and be able to communicate the need to void or defecate	Mother identifies specific behaviors of her child that will indicate readiness
		Nurse discusses techniques to use to assist toddler in learning self-toileting behaviors	Mother will: 1. Buy a potty chair for child to use 2. Discuss with child the expectations for toileting parents have 3. Mother/father will allow child to observe their toileting behaviors

SAMPLE CARE PLAN (continued)

Nursing Diagnosis	Goals	Intervention	Evaluation
		Nurse will discuss with mother ways to handle successful and nonsuccessful attempts toddler makes to use toilet	Mother will describe verbal (praises vs. ignoring) and nonverbal (hugs) methods to use with child

Review Questions

1. Cite specific examples of the reciprocal nature of developmental tasks of the toddler or preschool child and of his or her family.
2. Describe a plan of anticipatory guidance for a family with an 18-month-old to cover physical, emotional, social, and cognitive aspects of their child's development.
3. What considerations would a nurse have in mind when discussing day care options for a toddler and/or preschool child with the mother?
4. How do childrearing practices influence the development of competence in the young child?
5. Discuss changes in children's conception of illness and how those would affect the nurse's teaching plan.
6. Discuss how the nurse would differ in her approach to preparing a toddler and a preschooler and family for hospitalization. Why?
7. Describe common behaviors of families with a critically ill child.

REFERENCES

Baumrind, D. (1967). Parental control and parental love. *Children, 6,* 230–234.

Bibace, R., & Walsh, M. (1981). *Children's conceptions of health, illness and bodily functions.* San Francisco: Jossey-Bass.

Bowlby, J. (1969). *Attachment and loss.* New York: Basic Books.

Broome, M., & Endsley, R. (1987). Group preparation as a moderator of young child's response to a painful stimulus. *Western Journal of Nursing Research, 9*(4), 484–502.

Campbell, J. (1975). Illness is a point of view: The development of children's concepts of illness. *Child Development, 46*(1), 92–100.

Caty, S., Ellerton, M., & Richie, J. (1984). Coping in hospitalized children: An analysis of published case studies. *Nursing Research, 33*(5), 277–282.

Darling, R., & Darling, J. (1980). *Children who are different.* St. Louis: Mosby.

Endsley, R. and Bradbard, M. (1981) *Quality Day Care.* Englewood Cliffs, Prentice Hall.

Erikson, E. (1963). *Childhood and society,* 2nd ed. New York: Norton.

Flavell, J. (1963). *The developmental psychology of Jean Piaget.* New York: Van Nostrand.

Ford, A. (1981). Use of automobile restraining devices for infants. *Nursing Research, 29*(5), 211–224.

Fortier, L., & Wanlass, K. (1984). Family crisis: Following the diagnosis of a handicapped child. *Social Caseworker, 43,* 190–194.

Gellert, E. (1978). *Psychological aspects of pediatric care*. New York: Grune & Stratton.

Gochman, D. (1970). Children's perceptions of vulnerability to illness and accidents. *Public Health report, 85*(1), 69–73.

Hofferth, S. (1979). Daycare in the next decade: 1980–1990. *Journal of Marriage and the Family, 40*(3), 649–653.

Humenick, S. V. (1982). *Analysis of current assessment strategies in the health care of young children and childbearing families*. Norwalk, CT: Appleton-Century-Crofts.

Lewis, C., & Lewis, M. A. (1982). Determinants of children's health-related beliefs and behaviors. *Advances in Nursing Science, 2*, 85–97.

Matteson, A. (1972). Long-term illness in childhood: A challenge to psychosocial adaptation. *Pediatrics, 50*, 801–811.

Melamed, B., Meyers, R., Gee, C., & Soule, L. (1976). The influence of time and type of preparation on children's adjustment to hospitalization. *Journal of Pediatric Psychology, 1*(4), 31–37.

Millor, G. K. (1981). A theoretical framework for nursing research in child abuse and neglect. *Nursing Research, 30*(2), 78–83.

Murphy, L. (1974). Coping, vulnerability and resilience in childhood. In G. Coeholo, D. Hamburg, & J. Adams (Eds.), *Coping and adaptation*. New York: Basic Books.

Nelson, W. (1979). *Textbook of pediatrics*. Philadelphia: Saunders.

Neuhauser, C., Amsterdam, B., Hines, P., & Stewart, M. (1978). Concept of healing: Cognitive development and locus of control factors. *American Journal of Orthopsychiatry, 48*(2), 325–341.

Norbeck, J. (1981). Social support: A model for clinical research and application. Advances in Nursing Science, *3*(4), 43–61.

Olshansky, S. (1962). Chronic sorrow: A response to having a mentally defective child. *Social Casework, 43*, 190–194.

Petrillo, M., & Sanger, S. (1980). *Emotional care of hospitalized children*. Philadelphia: Lippincott.

Phipps, W., Long, B., & Woods, N. (1983). *Medical-surgical nursing: Concepts and clinical practice*. St. Louis: Mosby.

Powell, M. (1981). *Assessment and management of developmental changes and problems in children*. St. Louis: Mosby.

Pratt, L. (1973). Childrearing methods and children's health behavior. *Journal of Health and Social Behavior, 14*(3), 61–70.

Slattery, J., Pearson, G., & Torre, C. (1979). *Maternal and child nutrition*. New York: Appleton-Century-Crofts.

Steffensmeirer, R. (1982). A role model of the transition to parenthood. *Journal of Marriage and the Family, 44*(2), 319–333.

Telzrow, R. (1978). Anticipatory guidance in pediatric practice. *Journal of Continuing Education in Pediatrics, 7*, 14–27.

Thompson, R. (1985). *Psychosocial research on pediatric hospitalization and health care: A review of the literature*. Springfield, IL: C. Thomas.

Vaiden, L. (1983). The buckler. *Georgia Child Passenger Safety Association Newsletter, 2*(1), 1–4.

Vernon, D., Foley, J., Sipowica, R., & Schulman, J. (1965). *The psychological responses of children to hospitalization and illness: A review of the literature*. Springfield, IL: Thomas.

White, B. (1978). *Experience and environment: Major influences in the development of the young child*. Englewood Cliffs, NJ: Prentice-Hall.

Wold, J. V. (1981). *School nursing*. St. Louis: Mosby.

Wolfer, J., & Visintainer, M. (1975). Pediatric surgical patients' and parents' stress responses and adjustment. *Nursing Research, 24*(4), 244–255.

7

The Family with a School-Age Child 6–12 Years

Mary Thayer Wilson

Objectives

Upon completion of this chapter, the student will be able to:

1. Identify age-specific characteristics of the school-age child
2. Discuss the various developmental theories dealing with school-age children
3. Discuss the developmental tasks of the school-age child and family, and ways to promote healthy accomplishments of these tasks
4. Explain the effects parents and siblings may have on the development of the school-age child
5. Discuss the significance of peers and school on the school-age child, and their impact on the child's development
6. Discuss factors that can affect the outcome of stress and crisis situations in the school-age child
7. Identify potential stressors and health threats common to the school-age child
8. Identify adaptive and maladaptive coping mechanisms utilized by the school-age child
9. Discuss the impact of health alterations in the school-age child on the child and family
10. Identify factors to include in the assessment of a family with a school-age child
11. Discuss the role of the nurse in health promotion, maintenance, and crisis intervention

Concepts

Cognition: the act or process of the mind of knowing, which includes awareness, judgment, perception, thinking, and remembering

Industry: development of age-appropriate skills and behavior

Peer: one who is of equal standing with another; a classmate or age-related companion

School: an institution for the formal education of children

Socialization: the process of interaction of an individual with others, of relating to human society, and forming cooperative and interdependent relationships

The school-age stage of development begins when the firstborn is 6 years old and enters elementary school, and ends at age 13, when the adolescent stage begins. The growth and development during this time reflect the mastery of tasks of earlier stages, and are good indicators of what will occur during adolescence. During this period, children are absorbed in cognitive development and socialization. It is a time of active discovery of the environment and of themselves in relation to others.

Most families reach their maximum number of members, and, therefore, of relationships by the end of this stage (Duvall, 1977). The role parents play in their child's life decreases as the roles of other significant adults and peers increase. The child begins to have conflicting feelings, wanting to attain adult status and its benefits while retaining the privileges of childhood.

This phase of development is very important in that it marks the formation of habits that will continue throughout life. The foundation is being laid for future adult roles in the areas of work, leisure activity, and social interaction. Good health habits such as safety, diet, rest, exercise, and personal hygiene should be instilled at this time. This is the healthiest of all life stages, and the most ideal time to guide children into life-style behaviors that will support good health.

The school-age years cover a large span of development, and there is much variance among the different ages, as well as among individuals of the same age. Some generalized age-specific characteristics are outlined in Table 7–1.

The chief goals for nurses working with the school-age child and family are to assist them in establishing healthy life-styles, and in facilitating the child's optimal physical, intellectual, emotional, and social growth.

This chapter will focus on the school-age child and family in relation to individual and family tasks, common health and social stressors, and commonly utilized coping mechanisms. The role of the nurse in assessing the family and the nursing responsibilities in aiding the family to achieve health goals will be emphasized.

TABLE 7–1. AGE-SPECIFIC CHARACTERISTICS AND DEVELOPMENTAL MILESTONES OF SCHOOL-AGE CHILDREN

6-year-olds	7-year-olds	8-year-olds
High energy and activity level	More serious, quiet, pensive, and insightful	Expansive and gregarious
Egocentric		Opinionated and pragmatic
Boisterous and bossy	Activities become more cognitive	Defensive and resentful of criticism
Begin to enjoy verbal rather than physical agression	Increase in self-awareness and awareness of others	Vast curiosity, wants to know why
Talk in full sentences	Eager to please	Peers increasing in importance
Can count to 20	Seek approval	Relationships with opposite sex is a love-hate relationship
Play is rough and tumbling	Shy	
Have difficulty empathizing with viewpoints of others	Teasing tolerated poorly	Learns to write in cursive
Want instant gratification	Able to use symbols	Self-confident
Contacts with friends erratic	Tells time in hours	Beginning understanding of present, past, and future
Prefer same-sex friends	Enjoys collecting	
Does not know when to stop before getting hurt	Becoming aware of family roles and responsibilities	
	Better able to take care of self	

9-year-olds	10-year-olds	11-year-olds
Increase in self-confidence	Happy, cooperative, and relaxed attitude	The storm
Increase in peer involvement		Mood swings
Increase in group activities	Very peer-oriented	Critical of adults
Capable of responsibility	Want to belong	Resent being told what to do
Play and work hard	Intense peer loyalty	Desire unreasonable independence from adults
More interested in friends than family	Form secret clubs with strict membership	Organized and competitive games become common
Females begin to show interest in clothes and fashion	Increased ability to use logic and reasoning	Peer relationships even more intense
Males disdainful of fashion and cleanliness	Enjoy privacy	Highly moralistic
	Enjoy reading	Beginning interest in opposite sex
	Congenial and more affectionate with parents	
	The calm before the storm	

12-year-olds
On the verge of adolescence
Less self-centered
More self-disciplined and tolerant of others
More ethical and able to resist temptation
Able to foresee consequences of actions
Interest in sports increases
Able to carry on adult conversations
Cooperative and friendly
Increased interest in the opposite sex
Learn quickly
Concerned with appearance
Female height and weight gain at a peak

FAMILY TASKS

Each person in a family is working on his or her own developmental tasks, just as the family as a whole attempts to fulfill its tasks. Most of the family's activities at this time revolve around the school-aged child's world. The developmental tasks of the school-age family include:

1. Meeting the physical needs of the family
2. Expanding family communications and activities
3. Maintaining marital satisfaction
4. Socialization and education of the children
5. Developing the potential of all individual family members
6. Communicating effectively with all family members

Meeting the Physical Needs of the Family

It is frequently difficult to reorganize and continually meet the changing needs of the school-age family. The school-age child needs space for play and activities, while at the same time, parents may desire privacy. This is often the time that a family will consider moving into a larger home, or adding onto their present one. Such a change and other changes during this period cause family costs to escalate. In order to meet the needs of school and extracurricular activities, the family must make decisions concerning finances and how to live within their economic means.

Maintaining financial solvency may necessitate alterations in roles and responsibilities for some or all family members. The majority of school-age children have mothers who work, either by choice or necessity. Fathers often moonlight or work extra hours to bring home more money. Mothers who previously stayed at home may begin working outside the home. Many school-age children begin working in some capacity to supplement their allowances, especially in the summer, when school is out of session. Children in the middle years of childhood are also expected to become more involved in sharing household responsibilities.

Expanding Family Communications and Activities

The school-age child is beginning to emerge from the home to the outside world. The community begins to play a larger role. As the child's world expands, so does the family's. Parents become involved in activities that relate to their child's interests and needs. These include PTA, athletic groups, clubs, religious, and scout activities. Families mature together as they broaden their community involvement (Duvall, 1977).

As the child expands his or her world, it is also a time for the family to accept the child's relationship with outsiders. Peers, teachers, coaches, and other adults begin to play a significant part in the child's life. The child is exposed to a variety of new people and learns to communicate and interact with those outside the home. It is often difficult for parents to accept the child's seemingly decreased dependence on them, but socialization should be encouraged.

Maintaining Marital Satisfaction

Parents need to continue to satisfy each other as married persons. For parents, the school-age period is a time for increased involvement with children and decreased privacy and time together. Marital satisfaction appears to be significantly lower during this period of family development than during any other time in the childrearing years (Rollins & Feldman, 1970). In a study by Burr (1970), middle-class parents of school-agers indicated decreased levels of satisfaction with sex, companionship, finances, task performance, and relationships with their children.

Maintaining marital satisfaction is important for the healthy development of children. A healthy marriage free of significant marital discord will enhance a child's feeling of love and security.

Socialization and Education of the Children

The socialization and education of children are the most significant tasks of the family during this period and occupy most of its time. These two major milestones form the foundation for a healthy transition to adulthood.

Stimulating cognitive development and promoting school achievement are important in assisting the child to develop a sense of adequacy. The family can promote this development by stimulating a desire for achievement and offering experiences for growth. This is essential in the child's developing a sense of industry. The higher value a parent places on education and intellectual achievement, the more likely there will be encouragement by the parents, as well as interest in these by the child.

Parents are the primary agents of socialization in that they have longer and more intense interactions with the child than do others. However, as the child is introduced into society, primarily to school and peers, socialization makes its major thrust.

Developing the Potential of All Individual Family Members

Each individual family member needs to continue to develop to his or her fullest potential. Just as the family remains strong in the school-age child's development, so must the family work to assist other members in achieving their competencies. There may be other children in the family who need time and attention with their individual developmental tasks. All family members need to be fulfilled.

Parents may have to readjust their own lives. Many mothers return to work, revive old interests and hobbies, or join clubs. Parents must also learn to deal with letting go of their children. They need to allow them to make some of their own decisions, as long as safety is not compromised, so that they can learn from these experiences and take responsibility for their own actions. Their decisions may not always be the best ones, but children do learn from their mistakes. Parents who have other interests outside their children find it much easier to make the gradual separation. When parenting is the central and only significant role in their lives, the separation may be painful and resisted.

Communicating Effectively with All Family Members

Communication difficulties may come to surface at this stage within the family (Koch, 1960). Sibling rivalries may result in competition for family resources. Finding time to spend with each child is helpful for parents to ensure their children's feelings of importance in the family.

Communicating with relatives outside the nuclear family is part of this developmental task. As families get busier and schedules get tighter, it is often difficult to find the time to spend with family members outside the home. School-age children are now old enough to take responsibility for letter writing, sharing, and communicating with others without constant supervision.

INDIVIDUAL TASKS

The school-age child is confronted with a variety of new developmental tasks. Duvall (1977) has done extensive work in identifying these tasks. The primary tasks of the school-age child include:

1. Developing and maintaining healthy growth patterns
2. Learning basic fundamental skills
3. Mastering age-appropriate physical skills
4. Developing a realistic understanding of the use of money
5. Becoming an active, responsible, and cooperative member of the family
6. Learning to relate effectively to peers and adults outside the family
7. Continuing to learn appropriate ways to handle feelings, emotions, and impulses
8. Learning age-appropriate sex behaviors and adjusting to body changes
9. Developing self-awareness, self-respect, and a healthy self-concept
10. Developing a conscience with loyalties to religion and moral values

Developing and Maintaining Healthy Growth Patterns

A major task of the school-age child is to grow and develop physiologically. Physical growth in preceding years has been rapid. The school-age years are a time of more gradual growth, with steady and more even progress, before the prepubescent growth spurt, which will be discussed in Chapter 8. The approximate gain in height is 2 to 3 inches per year, and in weight is 5½ pounds per year. Boys are usually taller and heavier than girls in the early school-age period, but girls eventually pass their male classmates in height between ages 10 to 14. Although many school-age children begin sexual maturation toward the end of this period, discussion of this will be deferred until Chapter 8.

The school-age child begins to appear slimmer than the preschooler. Posture improves, and coordination increases. Bones continue to ossify and become harder and longer (Chin, 1974). The skull and brain grow very slowly, and by age 12 the brain reaches adult size (Murray & Zentner, 1985).

The heart grows slowly and is smaller in relation to the rest of the body than at any other time. For this reason, strongly competitive sports such as tackle football and extreme physical exertion are not encouraged. This is difficult for children to understand and accept, particularly males. Exercise and physical activity should be encouraged, however, and opportunities to participate in sports that do not require such extreme exertion should be made available. Sports such as tennis, swimming, soccer, ballet, gymnastics, and tee ball provide a means for positive social interaction, exercise, and feelings of accomplishment.

Twenty-twenty vision is usually well established by age 10, and the sense of hearing is well developed. Screening for hearing and vision difficulties should be a part of routine physical exams. Problems with sight or hearing are often identified by teachers in the classroom before the child recognizes the problem.

The young school-age child generally needs 11 to 12 hours of sleep per night. This gradually decreases to 9 or 10 hours per night by age 12, with the child usually seeking the necessary amount of sleep required to meet his or her needs.

The school-age years are noted for relatively few nutritional problems. Until the prepubertal growth spurt, nutritional needs are fairly stable. There is a slightly increased need for calories (quantity) rather than quality of food, though caloric needs are not as great as they were in infancy. A balanced diet is, however, necessary for adequate growth and development. The reason for the increase in caloric needs is that the school-age child has an increase in physical activity and basal metabolic rate (Vaughn & McKay, 1975).

During the school-age years, the loss of all 20 deciduous teeth is completed, with gradual replacement of 30 permanent teeth (excluding wisdom teeth). Because of this, school age is an ideal time to institute good dental health practices. Regular dental hygiene and prevention of dental caries are an important part of health supervision during these years. Children should be taught correct brushing technique as soon as they are capable of brushing their own teeth (during the preschool years), and it should be reinforced. The role that diet plays in the development of dental caries should also be emphasized. Regular dental supervision, with checkups twice a year, is an essential part of overall health maintenance (Whaley & Wong, 1987).

School-age children have definite food preferences. They enjoy snacks, eating with peers, and seem hungriest after school. Many parents find it difficult to believe the amount of food their children can consume. With more mothers at work, children select foods without supervision, which can result in an excess of sugar, fat, and starch consumption. Magazine and television commercials also influence eating habits. The school-age period is the best time to instill lifelong eating habits of nutrition, manners, and a balanced diet.

Learning Basic Fundamental Skills

Piaget (1961) described children's progress through stages of cognitive development in sequential order. He maintained that assimilation and accommodation are the processes that enable children to adapt and progress. *Assimilation* means to incorporate new ideas, experiences, or stimuli into a presently familiar cognitive schema. *Accommodation* means to change or organize a presently existing schema to solve a more difficult task and allow new ways of thinking to occur, in order to form a new schema. Understanding of new experiences is based on all relevant prior experiences (Maier, 1978).

The school-age years are in Piaget's stage of concrete operations. This stage encompasses the years from 7 to 11, or 6 to 12, but the ages are only approximate. The child becomes increasingly logical during this stage. The beginning of this stage is marked by inductive logic, but by the end, the child's thinking is deductive (Maier, 1978). Children in this stage are capable of classification, sorting, ordering, and developing a sense of conservation. This brings the realization that measurements such as volume, weight, and numbers can remain constant, even if outward appearances are changed. The child begins to deal with various aspects of a single situation simultaneously. Children in this stage still think in concrete ways and do not have the capability to deal in the abstract.

As play is the work of toddlers and preschoolers, acquiring knowledge, skills, and abilities is the work of the school-age child. The accomplishment of this developmental task is strongly affected by successful school experiences and academic achievement. The school-age child is learning to read, write, and develop rational approaches to problem solving. The child begins to develop concepts necessary for day-to-day living. As the child begins to grow in thinking, language, and imagination, ability to understand the world expands (Hymovich & Chamberlin, 1980).

Mastering Age-Appropriate Physical Skills

The school-age child is learning how to control his or her body. The refinement in neuromuscular development makes the school-age child more physically capable in both fine and gross motor skills. The increase in coordination allows children to pursue games, sports, and activities. Both males and females increase in strength and physical capabilities. This strength, however, can be misleading. The school-age child's bones are still ossifying; muscles are still relatively immature, and cannot tolerate a great deal of pressure and pull. This makes school-age children more prone to injury from excessive exercise and physical activity than adolescents and adults.

The school-age child is learning self-care skills, including personal hygiene and good safety habits. The child is now better able to assume responsibility for household chores, such as taking out the garbage, washing dishes, housecleaning, and keeping one's room neat, as well as responsibility for oneself.

Developing a Realistic Understanding of the Use of Money

School-age children are beginning to learn about money—how to get it, save it, and spend it. They are able to learn acceptable ways of getting and earning money, such as helping with household duties, mowing lawns, babysitting, and doing odd jobs for others. Many children receive allowances and must learn to budget their own money. School-age children may find it necessary to reconcile the differences between desires and available resources, and also to accept the fact that other children and their families may be richer or poorer than they (Duvall, 1977).

Many parents encourage their children to save money in a bank savings account rather than a piggy bank. This is often not easy. Having money in a bank account, out of sight, makes the money seem less real. Teaching children how to be responsible for their own money and how to save it and not spend it indiscriminately is an important task.

Becoming an Active, Responsible, and Cooperative Member of the Family

School-age children are beginning to become less egocentric. They realize they are not the only ones with needs. They are better able to participate in family discussions and decision making, and should be included in these, particularly when the decisions affect them.

Relationship with Parents.   Although other people are beginning to have an increased influence on the school-age child, parents remain the most influential persons in the child's life. Children usually identify with the same-sex parent and thus, learn their appropriate social roles.

Although school-age children are striving for increased independence, they are not yet ready to give up total parental control. Children need and actually want restrictions placed on their behaviors, even though they may protest loudly about these restrictions. Children feel secure in knowing there are adults on whom they may rely. They sense love and concern in their parents when reasonable and consistent controls are placed on their behaviors. Children need a stable and secure strength provided by parents, especially during times of stress (Whaley & Wong, 1987).

Relationship with Siblings.   Approximately 80% of children in the United States have siblings. Through interactions with them, children learn patterns of helpfulness, loyalty, protection, conflict, domination, and competition. These may be carried over into their relationships with others. The number of siblings a child has, his or her birth order, and the relationship between siblings constitute an important aspect of a child's learning and behavior. Sibling influence is usually most keenly felt when the child is between 2 and 10 years of age (Mussen, Conger, & Kagan, 1979).

Learning to Relate Effectively with Peers and Adults Outside the Family

The school-age child is increasing in communication skills at a fast pace. Articulation skills continue to develop, and the child is better able to see things from another's point of view. Ability to carry on a meaningful conversation increases.

The child is developing a social awareness of people and things outside the home, and an awareness of being a member of different groups such as family, school, church, neighborhood, and the world. School-age children's social networks expand as they move into school and the outside world. Peers, teachers, and other adults begin to have an increasing influence on their behavior. School-age children usually prefer relationships with same-sex peers. They become less dependent on the family for interaction and satisfaction. This may be difficult for parents to accept, but should be recognized as a normal and healthy part of the child's development and maturity.

Continuing to Learn Appropriate Ways to Handle Feelings, Emotions, and Impulses

The school-age child is becoming better able to cope with frustrations. He or she is growing in maturity and in expressing feelings in an appropriate manner. Ways of releasing negative emotions and feelings are learned. Temper tantrums fade, and constructive modes of expressing impulses and emotions are utilized. Physical activity, rechanneling energies into positive and worthwhile accomplishments, and calm, rational discussions are all ways in which the school-age child may now handle strong feelings and frustrations.

Learning Age-Appropriate Sex Behaviors and Adjusting to Body Changes

School-age children have learned gender identity, and their sex role is usually well established when this stage of development is entered. They continue to come to terms with their sex role, and begin to see it in future terms as well. They begin to learn what is expected of males and females, and what is appropriate behavior for each. Parents are the major role models in gender identity, as are older siblings and significant adults such as teachers and favorite relatives.

In the past, examples of traditional female roles were those of homemaker, teacher, nurse, waitress, and secretary. The female has traditionally been seen as nonassertive, nurturing, caring, and subservient. Some examples of traditional male roles were those of head of household, doctor, lawyer, mechanic, engineer, and sportsman. The male has traditionally been seen as aggressive, assertive, the breadwinner of the family, strong, protecting, and of superior intelligence.

Major activities are still often segregated into masculine and feminine roles, although society is seeing a gradual change from this. Many women are entering into more traditional male occupations, as are men into women's. There is a trend toward less stereotypical sex roles and more equality between genders. This is significant in that it opens more doors for children of both sexes and allows them to make choices based on interest and ability rather than sex.

Freud termed the school-age years the *latency period*. These years represent the tranquil period of sexuality between the earlier oedipal period and the eroticism of adolescence. During this period, the child turns attention away from sexuality and focuses upon the tasks of socialization and education.

School-age children are also faced with adjusting to body changes brought on by the prepubertal growth spurt. They need anticipatory guidance concerning body size, form, functions, and the nature of sex and reproduction. This will be discussed in more detail in Chapter 8.

Developing Self-Awareness, Self-Respect, and a Healthy Self-Concept

The school-age child is growing in self-confidence, and is continually establishing his or her own individuality. The body changes encountered in the later part of this stage are accompanied with changes in body image and self-concept. Recognition by the opposite sex begins to become important. Children derive their self-concept by seeing themselves as others do. Acceptance by peers also contributes to their sense of self-worth, while lack of acceptance decreases their self-esteem and sense of worth. The family remains the greatest influence over the child's development of self-esteem and plays a key factor in fostering a healthy body image and self-concept in the child.

The crisis of the school-age years is that of industry versus inferiority, with mastery as the major theme (Erikson, 1963). Children want and need achievement. They are determined to master tasks, and spend a great deal of energy in the drive to succeed. They also feel incapacitated by the very fact of childhood, and may fear failure despite actual competence. The drive for success always includes some sense of threat of failure. Children do generally have some protection against these feelings of inferiority. They maintain a certain cognitive deceit that serves to maintain a sense of adequacy, despite actual adult superiority (Hymovich & Chamberlin, 1980).

A certain degree of success in personal relationships and academic achievement is necessary for successful resolution of this developmental crisis. Parents can assist the child in developing a sense of industry by not expecting perfection, not comparing their child negatively to peers or siblings, and not setting unrealistic standards for behavior. Peer activities and home responsibility should be encouraged, with recognition given for accomplishments. All children have positive traits, and parents should build on these.

Developing a Conscience with Loyalties to Religion and Moral Values

The school-age years are crucial ones for learning moral values, obeying rules, learning about religion, and developing a conscience. School-age children begin to learn appropriate social and moral codes and are becoming more accepting of others' views. They acquire principles of right or wrong and apply them in a variety of situations. They also acquire principles of cause and effect and choice with accountability. This means that they must learn to take responsibility for their decisions and actions.

Lawrence Kohlberg is considered the leader in the development of theory concerning moral development. He views moral development as being closely correlated to cognitive development, and sees increasing cognition as enabling the child to make more mature moral judgments (Kohlberg, 1971).

Kohlberg (1968, 1971) has identified three stages of moral development, with a total of six substages. These are based on the child's abilities to make moral judgments, and the reasons used to make decisions (Appendix 2).

The early school-age child is in the preconventional stage of moral development, but gradually moves into the conventional stage. He or she begins to be capable of judging an act by the intentions that promote the act, rather than the consequences that result afterwards, such as punishment of a wrongdoing.

Children are beginning to learn more about religion. The family religion and place of worship plays the major role in this, but there is also peer influence. Children are exposed to a variety of different religions, and may begin to question and search for what is meaningful to them.

A healthy conscience in a child is facilitated if the parents' own conscience and moral values are mature, reasonable, not overly harsh and rigid, and if the child adopts the parents' standards based on positive identification and modeling (Mussen, Conger, & Kagan, 1979).

Successful accomplishment of the developmental tasks of the school-age child depends upon available opportunities in the home, school, and community, and gives the child a strong foundation for the upcoming tasks of adolescence.

POTENTIAL STRESSORS

It is inevitable that children will be confronted with various stressful situations throughout their lives. These may be physical stressors, social-emotional stressors, or some conflict with family tasks. As a nurse working with children affected by these stressors, it is important to keep in mind three things: (1) the seriousness and intensity of these stressors will vary from child to child, (2) each stressor has multiple causes, and (3) prevention of problems is the best approach (Tackett & Hunsberger, 1981).

The stressors most commonly encountered in the school-age child are those associated with separation and the hazards accompanying the child's exposure to the world outside the home. Most parents will experience some degree of anxiety upon letting go of their child as he or she enters school. Also, the broader social exposure that school creates forces families to have to cope with attitudes of prejudice and potential threats to the child's safety while away from home.

Social-Emotional Stressors

School itself is a potential stressor. As a child enters first grade, it is often the first time he or she has spent any length of time away from home and family. This separation and exposure to new people and activities lends itself to conflict for the child. Maladaptive responses to school-related problems will be discussed later in this chapter.

Prejudice.   A child entering school and a new world of people may encounter prejudice for the first time. Once away from home, parents are no longer able to protect their child from ugly and hurting remarks or behaviors from others that may be made because of the child's color, ethnicity, size, appearance, beliefs, family social status, or place of residence. Children are brutally honest and often cruel. They say whatever they think, often not intending to be malicious, but hurting someone just the same.

True prejudice is not innate, but is learned with parents as the primary teachers. Children listen to their parents and frequently repeat what they hear. Imitation is common among school-age children, and if they hear adults talking in a prejudicial manner, they think it is all right for them to do the same. In the same respect, when children are confronted with prejudice, they will most likely react as their parents have in similar situations. Parents should learn to handle prejudice in positive ways. It is not easy, but a calm, forceful approach is probably the most effective. Parents need to help build their children's self-confidence and ability to relate tolerantly to others who may show prejudice against them (Brown, 1977). Parents should be honest with their children and help them to understand that being different does not lessen their worth. Exposing children positively to different kinds of people will help them appreciate rather than develop disrespect for others.

Latchkey Children.   Ideally, both parents are involved in child care. Realistically, however, the mother is usually the primary caretaker. When the mother works, child care often becomes a problem. It may result in children coming home to an empty house after school, using their own front door key (latchkey). These children have been called "latchkey" children.

Approximately 10 million elementary school students are latchkey children, and the number is on the rise. Fifty-eight percent of all school-age children have mothers who work, and one out of six children lives in a single-parent household. Economic problems make it necessary for many parents to work, and after-school programs are often too expensive for many families to afford (Long & Long, 1982).

Many secondary problems have been associated with latchkey children. Bronfenbrenner (1977) has associated academic and behavioral problems, reading difficulties, high dropout rates, drug use, and juvenile delinquency with these children.

Latchkey children are frequently given responsibility beyond their developmental capabilities. Many are expected to clean the house, do laundry, prepare dinner, and care for younger siblings. This results in a decrease in time spent on school-related activities. Excessive demands made on them may result in a passive attitude toward life, and depression is not uncommon. In a study by Long and Long (1982), two major characteristics of latchkey children were identified. These were loneliness and fearfulness. It is apparent from their study that the fears of these children are not without reason, and that in addition to loneliness and fearfulness, they have a vulnerability to danger. Many of these children experience obscene phone calls, medical emergencies, and neighborhood crime, and many do not have the knowledge needed to cope with these dangers.

Two options available to working parents are (1) to provide adult supervision after school until an adult gets home, and (2) to teach the child how to become more responsible, how to cope with potential problems, and what to do in case of an emergency. Limits must be set for these children in order to enhance their safety, and they need to understand the reasons for these limits.

Family Disequilibrium.   Family disequilibrium or disturbed family interactions may cause overwhelming stress for a child. The family is the primary social reinforcer and influence in a child's life and continues to influence the child from infancy to adulthood. Among the factors affecting many families that may cause stress for the school-age child are mobility, variance in family structure, marital stress, poor role modeling, genetics, and a poor life-style.

The mobility of families is on the rise. Job security, income, and employment responsibility often require a family to move in order to maintain employment and keep the family together at the same time. Changing schools, breaking and making relationships, and resocializing to new places can be a hardship on children. Many withdraw or become reluctant to establish new friendships, for fear they may lose them again.

Family structure is an important variable affecting the adaptation of children. An increasing number of children live in what is considered a nontraditional family (Wold, 1981). Sussman (1978) states that 16% of households are headed by a single parent, and many children live in a foster, adoptive, or combined family. Many children adapt to these nontraditional families, but they do have a significant impact on the child and are a great potential for stress.

Marital stress and divorce can be just as stressful and painful for children as for parents. Children of parents in marital discord commonly worry that they may be the cause of the problem. Complaints of illness and academic-related problems frequently arise in an effort to distract the parents, and hopefully keep them together.

Parents are key role models in their children's lives. It is through imitation that children often learn and pattern certain aspects of their lives. Brothers and sisters and other relatives and friends also serve as role models. It is important for these key figures to set good examples and foster positive development. A poor role model gives negative reinforcement, and may result in maladaptive behaviors in the child.

Life-style patterns begin to be established in early childhood. Diet, exercise, hygiene, sleep, and recreational habits greatly affect health. Families can assist one another in forming healthy life-style habits. Role modeling by parents plays a significant part in this. Children of parents who are overweight, out of shape, and practice poor health habits will likely follow suit. Children learn by example. It is unfair to children to set them into habits that are harder to break the longer they are practiced. Poor nutritional habits, lack of exercise, and poor hygiene can lead to chronic problems later in life. By setting healthy examples, parents can foster positive life-style habits that will assist their children to achieve and maintain optimal health.

Some other ways parent–child relationships and interactions may cause stress for a child are pressure on the child to achieve, lack of child's involvement in family decisions, and failure of parents to let go. Parents often place unrealistic expectations on a child to achieve beyond the child's capabilities. This only causes frustration, anger, feelings of inadequacy, low self-esteem, and resentment. Parents should foster achievement within the child's abilities. Many decisions that a family makes will have an impact on the child. Decisions on household duties and responsibilities involve the child. Allowing the child input, listening to his or her opinions, and treating those opinions with respect aid in helping the child learn self-respect and ways of mature decision making. Parents frequently hesitate in letting their children grow up. They want to keep them young and babies. As children age, they need to be allowed to grow emotionally and socially. Stifling the growth of children may result in immaturity, excess dependence on parents, and difficulty in socialization.

Child Abuse. Although child abuse is commonly thought of as a physical stressor for the child, it is also a rapidly growing area of social concern. State laws and definitions of abuse vary, but an abused child is generally considered one who has sustained nonaccidental injury through acts of commission or omission by parents or legal guardians. Abuse occurs in children of all ages and in all socioeconomic classes. Major categories of child abuse include nonaccidental injury, neglect, sexual abuse, and emotional abuse.

It is believed that two million children are moderately or severely abused each year in the United States, but only one million of these cases are reported. Eight hundred thousand are neglected children, two hundred thousand physically abused, and sixty thousand to one hundred thousand sexually abused. Approximately four thousand cases result in death, and six thousand in permanent brain damage (Shyne & Shroeder, 1978; Gray, Culter, Dean, & Kemp, 1978; Fontana, 1979).

The exact cause of child abuse is not known and probably varies among individuals. Stress within three types of characteristics, however, seem to be necessary in order for a child to be abused. These are parental, child, and environmental characteristics. Abusing parents typically have a low self-esteem and self-image, lack of knowledge of parenting skills, little concept of normal developmental expectations, and were frequently abused themselves as children. A child who is abused is often illegitimate, unwanted, hyperkinetic, and brain-damaged. This is, however, not always the case. The child's temperament, ordinal position in the family, activity level, additional needs if ill, and sensitivity to parental needs all contribute to why a child escapes from or fosters abuse. The environment of an abusing situation is typically one of stress, including problems with finances, divorce, extramarital relations, unemployment, poor housing, alcoholism, drug abuse, and lack of support systems. The cumulative effect and interaction of these factors all have an impact on the etiology of child abuse.

Nurses are in a position to contribute to the identification and treatment of abused children. It is not necessary for a nurse or health care professional to know with certainty whether or not abuse has occurred. A nurse who suspects that child abuse has occurred is required by law to report this suspicion to the police or protective child care service agency. Failure to do so may result in a misdemeanor charge, or worse, further injury to the child.

Prevention of child abuse is, of course, the ultimate goal. Nurses may aid in this through careful assessment of parents and families, and in preventive education. Abusing parents were very often abused children. Children may be reluctant to admit abuse for fear of further abuse, or fear of losing their parents. Nurses working with these families must be perceptive to verbal and nonverbal cues and able to identify both the negative factors and positive resources of the family.

Physical Stressors

Illness. Illness poses another obvious stressor on the school-age child, whether it is illness of self or of significant others in his or her life. Accidents are the number one killer of children, and much primary prevention is needed in this area. Both acute and chronic illnesses cause change and the need for adaptation in family life, and will be discussed later in this chapter.

COPING MECHANISMS

Health Beliefs and Behaviors

In working with school-age children and their families, the nurse must be aware of varying health beliefs and behaviors among different cultures, classes, families, and individuals. It is important to understand basic health practices and beliefs in order to assess and plan health care. There are seven areas of assessment identified by Wold (1981) that the nurse should utilize in individualizing health care for children and their families. These are (1) definitions of health, (2) beliefs concerning the cause and prevention of disease, (3) illness behaviors, (4) accessibility to the health care system, (5) communication patterns, (6) culturally determined sex roles, family living structure and roles, and (7) beliefs about death.

The school-age child's health beliefs and behaviors will be primarily influenced by his or her family, and will vary according to culture, religion, age, income, family structure, and family values. Setting health goals must be a cooperative effort between the nurse and family, with appropriate interventions planned according to individual beliefs.

Responses to Stressors

When a child encounters a potentially stressful situation, there are several factors that determine how he or she reacts and deals with it. Caplan (1964) and Wold (1981) have identified six factors that affect the outcome of stressful situations. These are the child's (1) developmental stage, (2) previous experience, (3) perception of the problem, (4) culture, (5) support system, and (6) number and chronicity of stressors. The nurse working with children should be alert to these influencing factors.

Adaptive Responses.   The school-age child uses a variety of adaptive mechanisms in dealing with stressors. These mechanisms aid their adjustment and emotional development and are learned behavioral responses (Murray & Zentner, 1985). The adaptation process enables the child to maintain a balanced organization and deal effectively with the environment. The increasing development of competence enables the school-age child to better deal with stress. New coping mechanisms are learned, and the child's maturity and experience all increase the ability to handle stressful situations.

A healthy parent–child relationship plays a significant part in the school-age child's adjustment and response to stressors. Such a relationship gives the child security and enables the child to feel comfortable in seeking parental help when a situation arises that is beyond his or her control.

There are several adaptive mechanisms used by the school-age child. The most commonly used include ritualistic behavior, reaction formation, undoing, isolation, fantasy, identification, regression, malingering, rationalization, projection, and sub-limation.

Ritualistic behavior means consistently repeating an act as a means of warding off imagined harm and increasing the feeling of control (Murray & Zentner, 1985). Many call behavior such as this *compulsive behavior.* Examples of this are repeated handwashing and not stepping on cracks in sidewalks. It is important not to be critical of a child's ritualistic behavior. While it may seem quite silly to an observer, the behavior has very real meaning to the child.

Reaction formation is the direction of one's behavior or attitudes in the opposite direction of the underlying impulses. These impulses may be conscious or unconscious (Rowe, 1975). This is most often used by children who are dealing with hostile feelings that cause discomfort. A child may resent a younger sibling, but overtly be a loving, cheerful babysitter.

Undoing is "unconsciously removing an idea, feeling, or act by performing certain ritualistic behavior" (Murray & Zentner, 1985). Many children have certain chants or ritualistic motions that will undo or reverse expected but unwanted consequences. For example, children in gangs or clubs may have chants required of members who break promises or break secret codes before the member will be allowed to return.

Isolation is the unconscious separation of emotion from an act or idea. This occurs when the emotion associated with the act or idea is too difficult to handle. A child may use isolation to deal with moving to a new city and leaving close friends by talking very objectively about the move and displaying little emotion.

Fantasy involves a fabricated series of mental pictures or sequence of events (Rowe, 1975). Children found to be frequently daydreaming may be fantasizing. This is also frequently seen in children who have imaginary friends. Fantasy may be used as a compensatory mechanism for feelings of inferiority or inadequacy. It is closely related to creativity, and need not be discouraged unless used excessively. In reasonable amounts, fantasy can be an enjoyable and even productive experience.

Identification is the wishful adoption of the identity of another who possesses qualities the child envies or admires. This frequently takes the form of hero worship of teachers, friends, movie stars, or someone whom the child respects and tries to emulate.

Regression is the return to a previous level of development or emotional adjustment, in which the child feels more at ease and more capable of handling the environment. It may aid children in handling stressful situations. Children who are hospitalized often regress to earlier patterns of behavior such as bedwetting or baby talk.

Malingering means to feign illness as an avoidance of an unpleasant or intolerable alternative. A classic example of this is when a child stays home from school because of illness on the day of a big test.

Rationalization, or giving excuses, is frequently seen in school-age children. It allows them to do what they want when they should not. It also aids them in accepting themselves when they have not lived up to goals or expectations. One of the most serious consequences of this is self-deception. Children should be encouraged to accept the truth about their motives and behaviors, painful though it may be (Bailey & Dreyer, 1977).

Projection is attributing one's own feelings or behaviors to another (Wold, 1981). Blaming someone else for one's own actions or feelings is common. A child may be angry at his or her parents for punishment received, and shout, "You hate me," placing the blame for the punishment on the parents.

Sublimation is when the child channels unacceptable impulses into socially acceptable behavior. A physically aggressive child who becomes active in athletics is one example of this.

These adaptive mechanisms are all normal when used in moderation. When overused, they may result in maladaptive behaviors.

Maladaptive Responses.   Children may respond to stressors or potential stressful situations with maladaptive responses and behaviors. These behaviors are often benign and are the child's way of coping. They become truly maladaptive when they interfere with the achievement of developmental tasks. These maladaptive responses may be precipitated by a number of circumstances, but most often an unhealthy parent–child relationship is the underlying factor. Some commonly seen maladaptive behaviors in school-age children include school phobia, antisocial behaviors, tics, obsessions, compulsions, and a variety of fears and phobias.

School phobia is relatively common. It is a fear, which may approach panic, of leaving home and going to school. The child will do absolutely anything not to go to school. School phobia can occur at any age, but peaks around age 11. These children are usually of average or above intellect, and the frequency of this phobia is equal among boys and girls (Leventhal & Sills, 1964).

Children resisting school attendance may manifest actual physical signs of illness such as vomiting, diarrhea, headache, or nausea. The cause of the illness is fear of going to school, but the physical manifestation of the problem is very real.

The cause of the child's resistance to school must be determined before the problem can be dealt with effectively. Two theories have been proposed as to the etiology of school phobia. The first is that it is a form of separation anxiety (Nadar, Bullock, & Caldwell, 1975). The anxiety may be the child's, the parent's, or both. Often the child is overdependent and the parents are overprotective. The child may not be afraid of school as much as afraid of what will happen at home while he or she is away. For instance, a child may feel that a younger sibling at home is usurping the parent's attention while he or she is at school.

A second theory explaining school phobia is that children may have an unrealistic view of their abilities (Leventhal & Sills, 1964). They may overestimate their capabilities, and when others do not support this view, feel threatened and embarrassed. Their self-image may be so damaged that they resist going to school.

Because school phobia is usually only partially the child's problem, the entire family may need counseling in order to resolve the situation. After it has been established that the child is free of any physical illness that would prohibit school attendance, the child should, as a rule, be forced to attend. This firmness will help to prevent other problems, such as failure in school, peer ridicule, or repeated patterns of avoidance of difficulties (Pilliteri, 1981). Many children may need a gradual program of school involvement, such as going to school for an hour or two a day, until the child can stay all day, every day. These families will need much support and guidance. Parental needs should not be neglected, as parents may have many anxieties regarding their child.

Stealing, cheating, and lying are common aspects of *antisocial behavior* manifested by school-age children as they attempt to test right and wrong and are developing their moral codes. If properly managed, the child working through these temptations will develop a conscience. These behaviors are overwhelming to parents when their previously well-behaved child suddenly manifests such behaviors so contrary to societal norms. They may get angry, frustrated, or disturbed, and need assistance in managing their feelings and the child's behavior.

School-age children are at a stage where they are beginning to observe and judge the behavior of others, particularly parents and significant adults in their lives. They are cognizant of situations in which others do not behave honestly, and it is confusing to the child who has been constantly admonished to be truthful and honest to notice inconsistencies in what parents say and do.

It is important to be aware of family behaviors and communication patterns when dealing with families of children with antisocial behavior. An assessment of the type of restrictions and expectations placed on the child, the child's interests and activities, and discipline measures utilized by parents should all be explored. Anticipatory guidance relating to these issues may help to prevent these behaviors.

Tics are commonly observed symptoms of psychological stress in children. They are involuntary, repeated, and seemingly purposeless motor responses, usually of the face, neck, and head, of which the child is unaware. Tics may include rapid blinking, facial grimacing, coughing, throat clearing, or shoulder shrugging. They are most frequently symptoms of repressed needs and conflicts, and commonly seen in tense children with strict parents who put too much pressure on their child. It is important not to scold or correct the child with a tic. Instead, efforts should be made to discover the underlying cause for stress and alleviate it. If tics persist or become severe, psychiatric evaluation and counseling may be necessary (Mussen, Conger, & Kagan, 1979).

NURSING ASSESSMENT

When working with children, regardless of the setting, nurses must incorporate the family into their plan of care. It is imperative to have an understanding of the child as an integral part of a family system in order to provide appropriate care.

One value of a family developmental framework is in its utilization by nurses in assessing needs and planning appropriate interventions. According to Duvall (1977), there are three basic areas of assessment useful in determining whether or not a family is developing in a healthy fashion. These are (1) achievement of short-term goals, (2) achievement of society's goals, and (3) achievement of developmental tasks.

Nurses need to be aware of the family's present stage of development and its stage-critical tasks. They also need to help the family understand this stage and its tasks, and offer support and encouragement as the family moves through the various stages of the life cycle. Lastly, nurses are in a position to provide anticipatory guidance so that the family will know what to expect and how to plan and manage forthcoming tasks and potential crises (Wold, 1981).

An example of a format that could be used in assessing the family with a school-age child is shown in Table 7–2. Some additional specific questions that the nurse could ask to elicit data during an assessment are listed in Table 7–3. The assessment should tell the nurse about the presence of any stress, potential health hazards, and the child's coping abilities. Any problem areas need to be more thoroughly assessed.

TABLE 7–2. ASSESSING THE FAMILY WITH A SCHOOL-AGE CHILD

	Environmental Data
Provisions for care	Who is major caretaker?
	How many and who are living in the house together?
	What are provisions for child care after school?
	What type of school does child attend?
	Communication Patterns
School-age child	What is level of child's language development?
	To whom does child communicate needs?
	How does child communicate with peers?
Between child and caretaker	How do caretaker(s) and child communicate?
	Is there reciprocal communication between child and caregiver(s)?
Among family members	What are methods of communication in family? (Constructive, nonconstructive level of participation by each member.)
	How do child and sibling(s) communicate?
	Problem-Solving Skills
Decision-making abilities	How are major decisions made; does caretaker make any decisions independently from other adults in household; roles of family members during decision making/implementing?
Use of health care system	When instituted and for whom, location, accessibility, cost, purposes as perceived by family?
Support from significant others	Viewed as positive or negative by major caretaker, by child, areas of strongest support, areas of weakest support (as viewed by caretaker, and as viewed by nurse)?
Societal interactions	Use of public agencies (welfare, crippled children, school, etc.), ability of caretaker to deal with or circumvent "the system" when appropriate, business communicative skills?

TABLE 7–2. ASSESSING THE FAMILY WITH A SCHOOL-AGE CHILD (continued)

	Life-Style
Role of child in family	What is family structure? How many siblings? What are family and personal responsibilities of child?
Socioeconomic status	Estimated yearly income, financial assistance, direction of SES mobility, wage earner's feelings about status.
Family roles	Traditional or nontraditional pattern, distribution, level of satisfaction with roles.
Work patterns	Wage earners in family, amount of work hours per day or week, anticipated job change.
Recreational patterns	Use of free time, amount of planned activities per month, amount of time spent in recreation/leisure by each family member, amount of group recreation.
Safety	Visible hazards (broken steps, glass in yard, etc.), use of safety features (seat belts), adult's knowledge of accident prevention, first aid, poison control.
	Potential Stressors
Conflicts to parenting	Parent(s) perception of parenting role, own recognition of conflicts, potential for unrecognized problems.
Interferences with family tasks	Goals of family members, present health of family members.
Conflict with society	Incorporation of child and involvement with society, societal acceptance of family and child.
Family response patterns	Restructuring or reordering of goals; determining priorities; identifying realistic, practical approaches to meeting goals; changing family structure, or life-style.

TABLE 7–3. SPECIFIC QUESTIONS TO ASK TO ELICIT DATA DURING AN ASSESSMENT WITH A SCHOOL-AGE CHILD

Tell me what you think about coming here.
What did your parents tell you about coming here?
Some people who have this problem think. . . ; does that make sense to you?
Tell me about your family.
What sort of things do you do with your brothers and/or sisters?
Do you like school? What are your favorite subjects?
Does your school have a health service and a nurse? What does the nurse do?
Do you belong to a group or club?
What do you do for fun?
Who are your best friends?
How do you feel about yourself?
Do you think it's harder for you to do certain things than for other children? If so, why?
What do you usually eat in one day?
What sort of exercise do you enjoy most?
Have you had any cavities? How many? How often do you brush your teeth?
What do you do when you're upset? To whom do you talk and confide?

The Social Readjustment Rating Scale (SRRS) developed by Coddington (1972) is a tool that can be used in assessing life changes that result in stress for school-age children (Table 7–4). An adaptation of a tool originally developed for adults by Holmes and Rahe (1967), it lists life events requiring social readjustment regardless of the desirability of the event. A numerical weight or Life Change Unit (LCU) is assigned to each event, with the higher value of LCU given to events with a greater degree of impact on the life change.

TABLE 7–4. LIFE CHANGE UNIT VALUES FOR ELEMENTARY SCHOOL CHILDREN

Rank	Life Event	Life Change Units
1	Death of a parent	91
2	Divorce of parents	84
3	Marital separation of parents	78
4	Acquiring a visible deformity	69
5	Death of a brother or sister	68
6	Jail sentence of parent for 1 year or more	67
7	Marriage of parent to stepparent	65
8	Serious illness requiring hospitalization of child	62
9	Becoming involved with drugs or alcohol	61
10	Having a visible congenital deformity	60
11	Failure of a grade in school	57
12	Serious illness requiring hospitalization of parent	55
13	Death of a close friend	53
14	Discovery of being an adopted child	52
15	Increase in number of arguments between parents	51
16	Change in child's acceptance by peers	51
17	Birth of a brother or sister	50
18	Increase in number of arguments with parents	47
19	Move to a new school district	46
20	Beginning school	46
21	Suspension from school	46
22	Change in father's occupation requiring increased absence from home	45
23	Mother beginning to work	44
24	Jail sentence of parent for 30 days or less	44
25	Serious illness requiring hospitalization of brother or sister	41
26	Addition of third adult to family (i.e., grandmother, etc.)	41
27	Outstanding personal achievement	39
28	Loss of job by parent	38
29	Death of a grandparent	38
30	Brother or sister leaving home	36
31	Pregnancy in unwed teenage sister	36
32	Change in parents' financial status	29
33	Beginning another school year	27
34	Decrease in number of arguments with parents	27
35	Decrease in number of arguments between parents	25
36	Becoming a full-fledged member of a church	25

From Coddington, R.D. (1972) The significance of life events as etiologic factors in the diseases of children. I. A survey of professional workers. Journal of Psychosomatic Research 16(1), 14.

To determine the overall magnitude of the changes confronting the child during a given time period, the LCUs are totaled. The degree of crisis is determined as follows:

- 0–149 = no life crisis
- 149–199 = mild life crisis
- 200–299 = moderate life crisis
- 300 or more LCU = major life crisis

Research indicates that the higher the total LCU score, the more likely the individual will experience a change in health (Williams & Holmes, 1978).

To assess physical and mental development of the school-age child, there are many available tests, serving several purposes. The Goodenough–Harris Drawing Test assesses overall development, and provides an index of self and social awareness. The Peabody Picture Vocabulary Test (PPVT), the Wide Range Achievement Test (WRAT), and the Developmental Test of Visual-Motor Integration (VMI) are useful in identifying sensory, perceptual, and learning disabilities. The Denver Developmental Screening Test (DDST) and the Slosson Intelligence Test (SIT) are used to assess developmental delays. The Verbal Language Development Scale (VLDS) serves as a tool to assess language and language age (Jones, Lepley, & Baker, 1984). Plotting a child's height and weight on appropriate growth charts provides a means of comparison with normative growth rates.

ALTERATIONS IN HEALTH

Acute Alterations in Health

Temporary and acute alterations in health are a potential stressor in any age person. Although school-age children are relatively healthy individuals, there are many conditions, both preventable and nonpreventable, that are more prevalent during these years. These specific illnesses and problems will not be discussed in detail in this book.

Accidents remain the leading cause of death and injury in children aged 6 to 12. Their energy, inquisitiveness, and increased time away from adult supervision all serve to make children susceptible to accidents. Motor vehicles are the leading cause of accidents. This includes those accidents with children riding in cars, hit by cars while on bicycles, go-carts, or skateboards, or hit as pedestrians. Falls, drowning, suffocation, and burns are also common accidents. Most accidents can be prevented. Safety measures including anticipatory guidance to both parents and children should be emphasized early in order to avoid these often life-threatening, but preventable, accidents.

A *fracture* is a break in the continuity of a bone. Because of their activity, curiosity, and often immature judgment, children are particularly susceptible to fractures. They are most frequently the result of accidents such as falls and motor vehicle accidents. Children's bones heal more rapidly than adults and usually heal without complications. Unless the fracture necessitates traction, most children do not require hospitalization. They are often casted and taught to care for the cast at home, including modifying clothing to fit over the casted area.

Dental cavities and malocclusion are the most common dental problems during the school-age years. Dental cavities usually can be prevented with careful dental hygiene, sound nutritional practices, use of fluoride in toothpaste, and regular visits to a dentist. Malocclusion is usually corrected with braces. This can be difficult for a child who is beginning to be concerned with looks and attractiveness. Although it is a temporary situation, having braces may seem endless and catastrophic to the child.

Acute glomerulonephritis (AGN) is an inflammatory disease of the kidney, primarily involving the glomeruli. It is characterized by hematuria, edema, and hypertension, and most frequently follows an infection caused by group A beta-hemolytic streptococcus. The majority of children require a short hospitalization with follow-up. Most children, although acutely ill for a period, recover without sequelae. In severe cases chronic renal glomerular disease may develop.

The child with *osteomyelitis,* an infectious process of the bones, appears very ill. The area over the involved bone is usually painful, warm, and swollen, and the child has an elevated temperature and pulse. Osteomyelitis requires a lengthy hospitalization of 3 to 6 weeks for antibiotic therapy and immobilization of the affected extremity. This is often difficult for the child, particularly after he or she is feeling well. Bedrest is boring and frustrating, and activities allowing creativity while maintaining immobilization need to be provided.

Appendicitis is inflammation of the vermiform appendix, or blind sac, at the end of the cecum. The treatment is surgical removal of the appendix, and therefore necessitates hospitalization. An inflamed appendix is relatively minor, with a length of stay of only 3 to 5 days. A ruptured appendix, however, requires more extensive treatment and a hospital stay of 7 to 10 days.

Precocious puberty is the development of puberty, or physical sexual development, before the expected age of onset. The cause is usually unknown. Treatment primarily involves psychological support to the family and child. It is hard for children to accept looking different from their peers. Parents need to be aware that although their child's heterosexual behavior is usually appropriate for their age, the child is able to reproduce. Their awareness is essential in the event the child becomes sexually active and needs proper counseling on appropriate birth control methods.

Childhood obesity results from an increase in caloric intake that consistently exceeds body requirements and expenditure. A variety of factors may be involved, such as genetics, metabolic and endocrine factors, cellular structure, caloric equilibrium, social and cultural factors, and simply increased intake. Obese children often have a vulnerable personality, low self-concept, poor body image, and periods of depression. The primary complication with obesity is its persistence into adulthood and the associated dangers such as diabetes and cardiovascular disease. Treatment is difficult, long-term, and frequently unsuccessful. It requires a change in everyday eating habits and life-style. Without motivation from the child, efforts are futile. Prevention of obesity is, of course, an area to which nurses should be attuned.

Ramifications for the Family.   When a child becomes ill, the entire family may be affected. The family must be seen as an interdependent unit. Any disturbance in one member will result in a disturbance of the family functioning as a whole (Teung, 1982). Family functions may be upset by financial burdens, hospitalization, and change in routines due to visits to doctors or treatment regimes. The interpersonal family interactions may also be disrupted because of worry, fear, or guilt.

Parents of an ill child may have anxiety concerning the diagnosis, prognosis, and treatment of their child. Their emotional reserves center on the ill child and the threats confronting his or her situation. Normal routine family activities are altered in order to provide time and attention for the ill child. The parents focus on their ill child (Teung, 1982).

If there are siblings in the family, the situation may be seen quite differently. Guilt, fear, and jealousy are common feelings of brothers or sisters. They may harbor guilt feelings because they think they may have caused the illness. They may be jealous of the attention given the sick brother or sister, and feel neglected by their parents (Teung, 1982). Siblings may have misconceptions concerning the illness, their parents' feelings, and all that is involved. The nurse may serve to correct these inaccurate ideas and also assist parents to realize what their other children may be feeling.

Ramifications for the Child.   The school-age child with an acute health alteration may be affected in any area of development—physical, cognitive, or social-emotional. School may be interrupted, which could disrupt learning experiences and peer activities. The school-age child may become angry due to forced dependency on others. If a change in physical appearance accompanies the illness, there may be interferences with development of self-concept. Any limitations or confinements placed on the child have the potential to interfere with the child's development of industry. Creative means to release energy should be provided in order to facilitate the development of industry and decrease the child's frustration.

The nurse serves an important role in assisting the child and family to cope with health alterations and all the accompanying ramifications. When support, education, and anticipatory guidance are offered, the child's health and normal family functioning may be more quickly resumed.

Response to Hospitalization.   Hospitalization is a stressful experience and a potential trauma for a child and family. Although school-age children are better able to deal with the threats of hospitalization than younger children, due to their increased intellectual and emotional development, nurses must remember that the potential for trauma still exists.

The perceived threats of hospitalization for a child are multifold, and include (1) fear of bodily harm, injury, pain, mutilation, or death; (2) separation from parents and peers; (3) fear of the unknown; (4) perception of hospitalization or illness as punishment; and (5) loss of control (Teung, 1982; Wolfer & Visintainer, 1975). All of these are potential problems for a child; however, the predominant fears of the school-age child are those of pain, bodily injury, and the loss of control.

Because of all the intrusive procedures associated with hospitalization, and of the school-age child's increasing concern over his or her body, the fear of pain and bodily injury may be paramount. Younger children may have grave misconceptions about surgery and procedures that are not verbalized. Older children may worry that their illness or operation may make them different, and this will be a threat to their body image. School-age children's understanding of hospitalization and all that goes on concerning their illness is most likely to be incomplete or incorrect.

Careful questioning and assessing by the nurse is essential in order to reveal misconceptions and clarify misunderstandings. Games, projective techniques using drawing, puppets or toys, and acting-out situations may aid the nurse in picking up on the child's perception of the hospital and of the illness. The school-age child's developing cognition makes reasoning and factual explanations feasible. Educating the child about his or her illness and/or surgery may alleviate fears and inaccurate ideas. The school-age child is also becoming more modest. The nurse must appreciate and respect this when working with the child, and make every attempt not to impinge upon this modesty.

School-age children have achieved body control and are constantly striving for more independence. Hospitalization imposes some degree of immobility and dependence upon children. Bedrest, the use of wheelchairs, bedpans, restrictions on activities, and lack of knowledge make them feel a loss of self-control. Things are often done to children, rather than with them. They may feel powerless and vulnerable. Activities to express aggression and release energy should be allowed and planned for these children. Play therapists are excellent resources when available. Allowing choices within the realm of safety will serve to increase a sense of control over a potentially frightening and frustrating situation.

Because of their newly developed consciences, young children may view hospitalization as punishment for a past misdeed, or a misfortune thought to occur because it was willed by God or their parents as a retribution for a past wrongdoing (Waechter & Blake, 1976). This is the concept of *immanent justice*. Children may not verbalize these feelings, but harbor them internally. Nurses need to be aware of this, and assure children that this is not true, and not the reason for their pain and condition.

The school-age child may experience separation anxiety from their parents while hospitalized, especially during traumatic procedures; but the older school-age child is more likely to miss peers and peer-related activities. Allowing visitation, phone calls, and encouraging letters from classmates will aid in alleviating these feelings.

Research supports the theory that a parent's emotional state may be transmitted to a child, and that parents who are emotionally upset are often unable to assist their child in coping with stress. The basis for this is the *emotional contagion hypothesis* (Campbell, 1957; VanderVeer, 1949). The child may see worried expressions on parents' faces and create a fantasy of explanations, which are often more frightening than the truth. The child and family must be seen as a dynamic unit in the planning of care. When the nurse works with both parent and child, they all learn from one another in the three-way transaction.

The manner in which a child reacts to and copes with hospitalization depends on several factors. These include the child's age and stage of development, family relationships, duration and severity of illness, prior experience with hospitalization, prior stresses, parents' anxiety levels, type and frequency of intrusive procedure, and preparation for hospitalization (Smith, Goodman, Ramsey, & Pasternack, 1982).

Nursing Goals. The nurse's primary goal in working with a child and family with an acute health deviation is to resolve the child's health problem, assist in restoring family functioning, and prevent any similar crisis from occurring. Follow-up after a prolonged hospitalization may be necessary to assist the family in handling any residual effects of the hospital experience. Hospitalization is a temporary situation and can be a positive learning experience for the child and family if handled properly. It is not possible to eliminate all of the threats hospitalization imposes, but they can be minimized and made less stressful when the nurse works with the child and family together, always keeps the child's developmental stage in mind, and finds creative outlets for expression by the child.

Chronic Alterations in Health

Chronic illnesses in children constitute a major area of concern for health care professionals. It has been estimated that approximately 10% of all school-age children in the United States have some sort of chronic illness. If mental retardation, behavioral, sensory, and learning disorders are included, the figure is estimated to be between 30 and 40% (Battle, 1977).

Chronic illnesses are distinguished from others in that they are long-term, rather than acute. The duration may be months, years, or a lifetime. The degree of disability in children also varies. Many children are able to live quite normal lives with little interruption, while others may be severely incapacitated and in frequent need of medical assistance and hospitalization. A person with a chronic illness has been defined as one who has a disorder "with a protracted course which can be progressive and fatal, or associated with a relatively normal life span, despite impaired physical or mental functioning. Such a condition frequently requires intensive medical care" (Mattson, 1972, p. 801).

When speaking of chronic illness, it is important to distinguish among the terms *illness* or *disease, disability,* and *handicap* (Pless & Pinkerton, 1975). Many persons use these terms interchangeably, but there is a difference. Disability and handicap can be conceptualized as results of the disease. A chronic illness or disease is a primary pathophysiological process underlying a child's condition. Examples of this are diabetes, epilepsy, asthma, and sickle cell anemia. Disability refers to the behavioral manifestations or limitations in function as a result of an illness, such as shortness of breath or walking with a limp. Handicap refers to organic and functional limitations, as well as socially determined limitations such as being unable to compete in athletics (Hymovich & Chamberlin, 1980; Battle, 1977). Frequently it is the degree of disability and handicap, and not just the disease process itself, which interferes with the development of the child and requires adjustment of activities and life-style.

Approximately six million school-age children in the United States are thought to have *handicaps*. All too frequently in the past, handicapped children were not given the opportunities to develop their abilities and talents to the greatest potential. To ensure that these opportunities would be available and accessible, regardless of family financial status, Congress enacted Public Law 94-142, the Education for All Handicapped Children Act, in 1975. This piece of legislation mandates a "free appropriate education" for all handicapped children between 3 and 21 years of age. One of its components also mandates that handicapped children be placed in the "least restrictive environment." This means that handicapped children will be placed in as normal an educational environment as possible.

This so-called *mainstreaming* of handicapped children into regular classrooms opens an area of concern for nurses. Besides the educational concerns of these children, health needs are also a key issue. School nurses, in particular, are becoming more involved as educators, counselors, and children's advocates, as well as carrying on their usual and more traditional roles of health care providers and managers.

The most commonly seen chronic health alterations affecting school-age children include diabetes mellitus, bronchial asthma, cerebral palsy, sickle cell anemia, and neoplasms.

Diabetes mellitus is an endocrine disorder primarily involving carbohydrate metabolism characterized by a deficiency of the pancreatic hormone called insulin. It causes metabolic adjustments or physiological changes in almost every body system. Approximately 1 out of 600 school-age children are affected by diabetes. There are several classifications of diabetes. The type typically having onset in childhood is called *insulin-dependent* diabetes mellitus, or Type I. This type necessitates the use of daily insulin injections. Diabetic children must often follow careful patterns of diet, exercise, and urine and/or blood testing. The life span of a diabetic is estimated to be two-thirds that of a nondiabetic person. This adds to the already existing psychological burden of the affected child and family. Life expectancy in the diabetic child is lengthened, however, if the body is maintained in as normal a physiological state as possible. Promotion of good health, good nutrition, a balance of rest and exercise, and close management of the disease will allow the child to live as long as, if not longer than, the nondiabetic person who may not develop these healthy habits (Whaley & Wong, 1987).

Bronchial asthma is a reversible obstructive process manifested by labored breathing, bilateral wheezing, prolonged expiration, and a tight cough caused by a reduction in the diameter of the airway. The mechanisms responsible for the obstructive symptoms are mucosal edema, increased mucus gland secretion, mucus production, and constriction of the smooth muscle of the bronchi and bronchioles decreasing the caliber of the bronchioles. Children with asthma may have frequent exacerbations requiring hospitalizations, and some require daily medication at home. Chest physical therapy and breathing exercises help to prevent overinflation of the lungs and to improve the strength of respiratory muscles. Moderate exercise is advised, as vigorous physical activity is frequently followed by an asthmatic attack. Parents of asthmatic children are often overprotective. This results in peer alienation and isolation. Children and parents need to be taught to live within the confines of the illness. In some cases, children outgrow the disease as they get older.

Cerebral palsy is a nonspecific term applied to impaired muscular control resulting from an abnormality in the pyramidal motor system. The etiology, clinical features, and course are variable. The primary disturbances are abnormal muscle tone and coordination. Cerebral palsy is the most common permanent physical disability of childhood. The goals of therapy are to promote optimum development so that the child may develop full potential within the limits of existing brain dysfunction. Much physical therapy, parent teaching, and education is required. Children with cerebral palsy are frequently rejected by others, because this condition is often frightening and unpleasant. Many view them as being socially unacceptable and retarded. Not all children with cerebral palsy are mentally retarded. In fact, one-third of these children have normal intelligence. Education of the public regarding this condition is an important nursing goal (Whaley & Wong, 1987).

Sickle cell anemia is an autosomal recessive disorder that is a disease of hemoglobin. It primarily affects the black population. The pathological changes from sickle cell anemia are mainly the result of increased blood viscosity and increased red blood cell destruction. Eventual tissue ischemia and necrosis may result, with pathological changes in almost every body system. Acute symptoms of the disease occur during periods of exacerbation called crises. The clinical manifestations vary in severity and frequency. There is no cure for sickle cell. The nursing objectives are primarily directed toward the prevention of sickling, the management of the child's pain, and assisting the child and family to live with a chronic, hereditary, and potentially fatal disease.

Neoplasms are abnormal formations of tissue, such as tumors. Malignant neoplasms are also known as cancer. The most common sites of childhood neoplasms are the central nervous system and the lymphatics. Therapy consists of surgery, chemotherapy, irradiation, and/or immunotherapy. The treatment, clinical manifestations, and prognosis depend on the type and location of the disease. Nurses have a significant role in aiding families to understand the various therapies and prevent or manage side effects. The knowledge that one's child has cancer is devastating for a family and requires much support and understanding. For more detailed information on childhood cancer, refer to a general pediatric nursing textbook.

Ramifications for the Family.   Although a child with a chronic illness is the one with a physical disorder, nurses must remember that the entire family is affected and needs assistance. Besides the obvious additional financial burden, family members are placed at greater risk for stress in many other ways.

Parents must adjust and accept their child's condition, and often have feelings of shock, denial, guilt, grief, depression, and resentment. Anger is a common response, and is often directed toward nurses, doctors, and God. Couples may become angry at each other and harbor feelings of resentment or blame for their spouses.

Parents often feel overwhelmed at the thought of all the care that the child will require at home. They may feel incapable and frightened and have difficulty integrating these new treatment regimes and routines into their normal household activities.

Parents often become overprotective of a child with a chronic condition. This may occur because of guilt, fear of the child's death, genuine love, or a combination of these. Overprotection often results in a child who is spoiled, dependent, and lacking self-control.

Siblings of a chronically ill child are also at risk for potential problems. They may resent the attention given their brother or sister by their parents, be afraid or embarrassed to have friends home with them, have increased somatic complaints, or show a deterioration in school achievement (Pless & Pinkerton, 1975).

A family of a child with a chronic illness is always at risk for a crisis. The psychological effects are often more devastating and difficult to cope with than the physical condition itself. The nurse must continually assess the family in order to effectively plan and intervene. To ensure the family's optimal adjustment, long-term support is needed. The nurse may need to assist the parents in anticipating sibling responses, and in recognizing the benefits and/or potential problems with their own behaviors. The nurse is also the one to serve as a family advocate. The nurse may need to intervene in order to prevent the illness, treatment, and other health care personnel from disrupting the family unit (Whaley & Wong, 1987). The nurse is in a position to coordinate treatments, ensure consistency, and serve as a liaison with other members of the health care team.

Ramifications for the Child.   The school-age child with a chronic illness is at a particular risk for conflict in achieving many developmental tasks. Four areas of greatest concern are (1) relationships with peers, (2) adjusting to school, (3) increasing independence, and (4) fulfilling a sense of industry (Tackett & Hunsberger, 1981).

Peers are of increasing importance to the school-age child, and an integral part of the development of self-esteem and identity. A chronic illness may impose separation and restrictions on a child that cause time away from friends and social activities. Many children feel self-conscious about their condition, fear being thought of as strange or different, and isolate themselves as a protective mechanism. Parental support and education of others, particularly classmates and teachers, will greatly influence the child's adjustment to illness and decrease the stigma often attached to chronic illness.

Absences from school due to illness, appointments, and hospitalization may hinder the education process for many children. Children with a chronic illness may fear going to school because of embarrassment or adverse reactions of others, such as fear of contagion of the illness. School phobia is common with these children. When a child is unable to attend school, a homebound teacher should be arranged. When able to attend, the child should do so. Nurses may serve as liaisons between the child and family and the school. Teachers should be made aware of the child's condition, and any necessary information regarding its management or emergency measures that may be needed while at school should be given. The nurse can also educate teachers and students about the child's illness and dispel any myths or misconceptions that may be held.

The school-age child strives to become more independent of adults. Limitations placed on the child secondary to illness may cause a forced dependency and serve to decrease the feelings of self-control. The child may become frustrated and withdraw, or react in the other direction and take risks that are not warranted. Nurses should assess the child's environment for any unnecessary restrictions in order that the child may function as independently as possible and as much as his or her condition permits.

As discussed earlier in this chapter, the school-age child is trying to fulfill a sense of industry. The child with a chronic illness may feel unable to do many things, and feel handicapped by the physical illness. These feelings may or may not be realistic. The chronically ill school-age child should be given tasks and challenges he or she is able to master. Patience is often required on the part of the child, parents, teachers, and significant others. Every child, no matter what the illness or handicap, is capable of certain accomplishments, and should be encouraged to make an effort to succeed in dealing with challenges.

The School-Age Child's Concept of Death.   Before age 6, children generally view death as something that happens to others. They may see it as punishment for bad thoughts or deeds. As the child gets older, however, death is seen as a more personal event (Nagy, 1978). Most young school-age children relate death to old age, and conceive it as being the result of some external agent and not of a physiological breakdown. Death is usually associated with bodily injury and mutilation. Older school-age children begin to understand the universality and irreversibility of death. They begin to understand that death is the cessation of bodily life and conceptualize it as an inevitable process. By the end of the school-age period, most children have a fairly mature and adult view of death, but may still have difficulty comprehending it as an event occurring to anyone close and significant to them (Hostler, 1978; Kastenbaum, 1967).

Nursing Goals.   The three main nursing goals in working with a child with a chronic illness are to (1) treat the handicap/disease itself by correction of the defect, control of symptoms, and/or arrest of progress; (2) prevent the disease process, treatment regime, and various people involved from interfering with the child's development; and (3) prevent the illness, treatment regime, and various people involved from disrupting family functioning (Yancy, 1972).

The nurse must foster family involvement in the child's care. Child and family counseling should be made available. The nurse is also an educator, and should help the child and family understand the nature of the illness and all that may be entailed in its course and treatment. Limits may need to be set for the child's safety. The nurse should see that these are realistic and reinforce them while the child is in the hospital. The nurse should also assist the parents in reorganizing their home life, in order to make it as normal as possible.

NURSING RESPONSIBILITIES

Nurses have a vital role in the health care of children. Not only do they play a significant part in the care of acutely and chronically ill children, but also in the health maintenance and promotion of well children. The goals of nursing care for school-age children include the following: (1) to facilitate optimal biopsychosocial growth and development, and (2) to aid the child in the acquisition of knowledge and the establishment of behaviors necessary as a foundation for a healthy life-style.

In carrying out these goals, the nurse has several roles. Many of these are interchangeable and interdependent. The primary roles of a nurse working with school-age children are as a child advocate, health educator, counselor for the child, family, schools, and significant others, manager of health care for the child and family, and deliverer of health care services.

Health maintenance and promotion are vital to the optimal development of the school-age child. A major thrust of this for the nurse involves anticipatory guidance and education of the child and family in areas such as nutrition, dental care, sexual development, and safety. Health values, habits, and behaviors begin to be established in the school-age years, and it is essential for healthy life-styles to be encouraged at an early age. The desired outcome is for children to be able to maintain their health, prevent illness from occurring, and know what to do, where to go, and from whom to seek assistance if they should become ill or be faced with a potential crisis situation (Wold, 1981).

There are three levels of crisis prevention: primary, secondary, and tertiary. Primary prevention is aimed at the prevention of crises. The goal of secondary prevention is early detection of crises and prevention of maladaptive behaviors. Tertiary prevention involves the prevention of further maladaptive behaviors, and the restoration of adaptive behaviors, after a crisis has already occurred and precipitated maladaptive behaviors (Wold, 1981).

Health promotion and maintenance require attention to nearly every facet of the child's life. Areas that the nurse may be involved in are:

1. Assessing health status through regular health examinations, including immunizations, screening, dental care, nutrition assessments, and growth and developmental appraisals
2. Safety education
3. Sexuality awareness and sex education
4. Anticipatory guidance for parents concerning their child's development
5. Education on substance abuse
6. Personal hygiene

Prevention and early detection of problems are the goals. A cooperative effort among the child, family, and nurse will facilitate the child's optimal development and enhance a healthy lifetime life-style.

Safety is an area of particular concern for nurses working with school-age children. These children are particularly vulnerable to accidents because of their curiosity, increased ability to explore outside the home, a relative lack of caution and inexperience with potential hazards. Children must learn to be responsible for their actions. Education of children and their families regarding safety hazards and risk taking must be introduced and reinforced whenever possible.

Sex education is also an area of great concern in working with school-age children. Many school-age children begin to reach physical maturity in the latter part of this stage. This and the child's curiosity about sex and sexual development prompt questions and concerns for the child and parents. Nurses are in an ideal situation to provide information on human sexuality to both children and parents. This will be discussed in greater depth in Chapter 8.

School nurses have a vital role in promoting and safeguarding the health of school-age children. More and more schools are utilizing nurses in their health programs. The basic functions of school health programs can be incorporated into three areas. These are (1) provision of a safe and healthful school environment, (2) implementation of an ongoing and effective health education curriculum, and (3) delivery of health services to students and staff (Wold, 1981). School nurses are often thought of as being only responsible for the first aid of students. Looking at the above functions, however, it is easy to see the many facets and multiple roles involved in this job. For example, school nurses are often responsible for health appraisals, screening, emergency care and safety, communicable disease control within schools, counseling, direct instruction on health education, and serving as student advocates in areas of safety, nutrition, and physical education. Often the school nurse is the first person who picks up on health needs of a child and family. Although the preparation, qualifications, and utilization of school nurses vary throughout the United States, it is a role receiving more widespread recognition and importance.

SUMMARY

This chapter has outlined and discussed the many aspects of the school-age child's development and health needs, and the nurse's role in the health care of the child and family. It is impossible to give complete care to a child without also being involved with the family. The two are interdependent, and must be recognized as such. The child's family assists the child in assuming responsibility, and provides necessary motivation for the achievement of personal goals.

School-age children differ in their patterns and stages of development, and each child should be viewed as a unique individual when planning care. These formidable years are very important in the outcome of their long-term development, and healthy life-style patterns should be instilled as early as possible.

REVIEW QUESTIONS

1. What are the major developmental tasks of the school-age child and his or her family, and how can the nurse promote healthy accomplishment of these tasks?

2. What are the two major milestones of the school-age years?

3. How do parents and peers differ in their impact on the school-age child's development of industry?

4. What are some common school-related stressors, and how can parents help their children cope with these?

5. What impact does chronic illness have on the socialization and education of the school-age child?

CARE PLAN FOR THE SCHOOL-AGE CHILD WITH A KNOWLEDGE DEFICIT

Situation

A. W. is an 11-year-old white male who is beginning sixth grade. He is an only child. His father lost his job last year and is now working for a considerably lower salary. His mother, who has not been working since A. was born, has returned to work to supplement the family income. A. gets home from school at 3 PM, but Mrs. W. does not get home until 5:15 PM, and Mr. W. even later. Mr. and Mrs. W. cannot afford to pay a babysitter every day, and have tried to make other arrangements for A. after school, but these do not always work. As a result, there are often afternoons when A. is home alone after school. A. has never before been left home alone, and his parents are very worried about him being alone and taking care of himself. These concerns and worries were voiced to the nurse this past summer, while A. was getting a physical for camp. They asked the nurse how they could best prepare A. for being alone. They do not feel he knows all he should about taking responsibility for himself. A. says he is not afraid to be alone and is ready to learn how to take care of himself and be responsible.

Nursing Diagnoses

The two primary nursing diagnoses identified by the nurse relating to this family are:

1. Knowledge deficit of responsible behavior to expect of A. W. while home alone related to lack of information

2. Alteration in family process related to change in family roles and tasks

The following care plan addresses the primary diagnosis of knowledge deficit.

SAMPLE CARE PLAN

Nursing Diagnosis	Goals	Interventions	Evaluations
Knowledge deficit of responsible behavior to expect of A. W. when home alone related to lack of information.	A. W. will describe 8 measures of safe, responsible behavior when home alone.	Give 5 simulations to Mr. and Mrs. W. to review with A. Discuss appropriate action for each (e.g., toilet overflows, electricity goes off, doorbell rings). Encourage Mr. and Mrs. W. to sit down with A. W. and discuss and decide very specifically what he can and cannot do while home alone (such as: he can do homework; which snacks he can eat; he can watch TV, but not cook or leave the house); and whom he can and cannot have at home with him. Identify adult resource person in neighborhood. Encourage Mr. and Mrs. W. not to place too much responsibility on A. while he is home alone (such as being responsible for major housework and cooking supper). Discuss with Mr. & Mrs. W. safety rules A. should know: Locking door behind him Not opening door to strangers	A. W. will verbalize what he is to do and not to do while home alone. A. W. will verbalize safety rules of which he should be aware. A. W. will know telephone numbers of parents at work and other emergency numbers. Mr. and Mrs. W.'s worries (not concerns) about A. W. being alone will decrease.

SAMPLE CARE PLAN *(continued)*

Nursing Diagnosis	Goals	Interventions	Evaluations
		Not telling anyone on telephone his parents are not at home (teach him to say that his mother/father cannot come to the phone right now and could he take a message)	
		Have Mr. & Mrs. W. call A. at a special time every day to make sure he arrived home safely and is okay	
		Basic first aid	
		Emergency telephone numbers	
		Telephone numbers of parents at work and/or other adults he could call if needed	

REFERENCES

Bailey, D. S., & Dreyer, S. O. (1977). *Therapeutic approaches to the care of the mentally ill.* Philadelphia: Davis.

Battle, C. U. (1977). Disruptions in the socialization of a young, severely handicapped child. In R. P. Marinelli & A. E. Orto (Eds.), *The psychological and social aspects of physical disability.* New York: Springer.

Bronfenbrenner, U. (1977). The changing American family. In E. M. Hetherington & R. D. Park (Eds.), *Contemporary reading in child psychology.* New York: McGraw-Hill.

Brown, K. (1977). How parents can best fight prejudice. *Family Circle,* December *13,* 52.

Burr, W. R. (1970). Satisfaction with various aspects of marriage over the life cycle: A random middle class sample. *Journal of Marriage and the Family* (32), 29–37.

Campbell, E. H. (1957). *Effects of mothers' anxiety on infants' behavior.* New Haven: Yale University Press.

Caplan, G. (1964). *Principles of preventive psychiatry.* New York: Basic Books.

Chin, P. (1974). *Child health maintenance: Concepts in family-centered care.* St. Louis: Mosby.

Coddington, R. D. (1972). The significance of life events as etiologic factors in the diseases of children. I. A survey of professional workers. *Journal of Psychosomatic Research, 16*(1), 14.

Duvall, E. M. (1977). *Marriage and family development* (5th ed.) Philadelphia: Lippincott.

Erikson, E. H. (1963). *Childhood and society* (2nd ed.). New York: Norton.

Fontana, V. J. (1979). Child abuse: An attack every two minutes. *Pediatric Consult*, January 2.

Gray, J. D., Culter, C. A., Dean, J. G., & Kemp, C. H. (1978). Prediction and prevention of child abuse and neglect. In M. L. Lauderdale (Ed.), *Child abuse and neglect: Issues on innovation and implementation* (Vol. 1) (Pub. No. 78-30147). Washington, D.C.: Department of Health, Education and Welfare (CHDS), pp. 246–254.

Holmes, T. H., & Rahe, R. H. (1967). The social readjustment scale. *Journal of Psychosomatic Research, 11*(2), 213–218.

Hostler, S. L. (1978). The development of the child's concept of death. In O. J. Sahler (Ed.), *The child and death*. St. Louis: Mosby.

Hymovich, D. P., & Chamberlin, R. W. (1980). *Child and family development, implications for primary health care*. New York: McGraw-Hill.

Jones, D. A., Lepley, M. K., & Baker, B. A. (1984). *Health assessment across the life span*. New York: McGraw-Hill.

Kastenbaum, R. (1967). The child's understanding of death: How does it develop? In E. A. Grollman (Ed.), *Explaining death to children*. Boston: Beacon Press.

Koch, H. L. (1960). The relation of certain formal attributes of siblings to attitudes held toward each other and toward their parents. *Monographs of the Society for Research in Child Development, 25*, 1–124.

Kohlberg, L. (1968). The child as a moral philosopher. *Psychology Today, 2*(4), 24–30.

Kohlberg, L. (1971). *Recent research in moral development*. New York: Holt, Rinehart, & Winston.

Leventhal, T., & Sills, M. (1964). Self-image in school phobia. *American Journal of Orthopsychiatry, 34*(July), 685–695.

Long, L., & Long, T. (1982). What are the special problems of latch-key children? *Instructor*, May, 39–41.

Maier, H. W. (1978). *Three theories of child development*. New York: Harper & Row.

Mattson, A. (1972). Long-term physical illness in childhood: A challenge to psychosocial adaptation. *Pediatrics, 50*(11), 801–811.

Murray, R. B., & Zentner, J. P. (1985). *Nursing assessment and health promotion through the life span* (2nd ed.). Englewood Cliffs, NJ: Prentice-Hall.

Mussen, P. H., Conger, J. J., & Kagan, J. (1979). *Child development and personality* (5th ed.). New York: Harper & Row.

Nadar, P. R., Bullock, D., & Caldwell, B. (1975). School phobia. *Pediatric Clinics of North America, 22*(3), 605–617.

Nagy, M. (1978). The child's theories concerning death. *Journal of General Psychology*, 73, 3.

Piaget, J. (1961). *The growth of logical thinking from childhood to adolescence*. New York: Basic Books.

Pilliteri, A. (1981). *Child health nursing, care of the growing family* (2nd ed.). Boston: Little, Brown.

Pless, F. B., & Pinkerton, P. (1975). *Chronic childhood disorder—promoting patterns of adjustment*. London: Henry Kimpton.

Public Law 94-142 (1975). Education for All Handicapped Children Act of 1975. Washington, D. C.: U.S. Government Printing Office.

Rollins, B. C., & Feldman, H. (1970). Marital satisfaction over the family life cycle. *Journal of Marriage and the Family, 32*, 20–28.

Rowe, C. J. (1975). *An outline of psychiatry*. Dubuque, IA: Brown.

Shyne, A. W., & Shroeder, A. G. (1978). National study of social services to children and their families. (Pub. No. 78-30149). Washington, DC: National Center for Child Advocacy, U. S. Children's Bureau, Department of Health, Education, and Welfare.

Smith, M. J., Goodman, J. A., Ramsey, H. L., & Pasternack, S. B. (1982). *Child and family: Concepts of nursing practice.* New York: McGraw-Hill.

Sussman, M. (1978). The family today. *Children Today, 7,* 32–36.

Tackett, J. J. M., & Hunsberger, M. (1981). *Family-centered care of children and adolescents.* Philadelphia: Saunders.

Teung, A. G. (1982). *Growth and development, a self-mastery approach.* E. Norwalk, CT: Appleton-Century-Crofts.

VanderVeer, A. H. (1949). The psychopathology of physical illness and hospital residence. *Journal of Child Behavior, 1,* 55–71.

Vaughn, V. C., & McKay, R. I. (Eds.) (1975). *Nelson's textbook of pediatrics.* Philadelphia: Saunders.

Waechter, E. H., & Blake, R. G. (1976). *Nursing care of children.* Philadelphia: Lippincott.

Whaley, L. F., & Wong, D. L. (1987). *Nursing care of infants and children* (2nd ed.). St. Louis: Mosby.

Williams, C. C., & Holmes, T. H. (1978). Life change, human adaptation, and onset of illness. In D. C. Longo & P. A. Williams (Eds.), *Clinical practice in psychosocial nursing: Assessment and intervention.* New York: Appleton-Century-Crofts.

Wold, S. J. (1981). *School nursing: A framework for practice.* St. Louis: Mosby.

Wolfer, J. A., & Visintainer, M. A. (1975). Pediatric surgical patients' and parents' stress responses and adjustment. *Nursing Research, 24*(4), 248.

Yancy, W. S. (1972). Approaches to emotional management of the child with a chronic illness. *Clinical Pediatrics, 11*(2), 64–67.

8

The Family with an Adolescent 13–19 Years

Mary Thayer Wilson

Objectives

Upon completion of this chapter, the student will be able to:

1. Discuss the developmental tasks of the adolescent and family, and means to promote healthy accomplishment of these tasks
2. Explain the significance of peers in adolescent development
3. Discuss the physical changes of puberty
4. Discuss the sexual maturation and the accompanying emotional responses of adolescents
5. Discuss the role parents play in the nurturing of an adolescent into a mature and responsible adult
6. Identify potential stressors and health threats common to adolescents
7. Identify positive coping mechanisms utilized by adolescents
8. Identify maladaptive responses to stress common to adolescents
9. Identify areas of importance to include in the assessment of the family with an adolescent
10. Discuss the impact of health alterations on the adolescent and family unit
11. Discuss the role of the nurse in health promotion, maintenance, and crisis intervention

Concepts

Identity: a sense of self; the feeling that one is a specific unique person

Independence: not requiring or relying on others

Peer: one who is of equal standing with another; a classmate or age-related companion

Puberty: the stage of development when reproductive organs begin to function and secondary sex characteristics develop

Sexuality: one's feelings and behavior as a male or female

For the purposes of this book, adolescence begins at age 13 and ends at 19. A more accurate definition of adolescence would be that its beginning is marked in biology, with puberty, body, and sexual changes; and its ending is marked in culture, with physical and psychological maturity and the development of identity. It is hoped that by the end of this stage, the adolescent is ready to assume adult responsibilities and be self-sufficient.

Adolescence is a period of physical growth, when the body reaches the size and structure at which it will remain for a long time. The general good health of adolescents tempts them to abuse their bodies through poor nutrition, inadequate rest, and as many health violations as they can get away with to their unknowing parents. They will experiment and rebel and try many things they have been told to avoid, such as cigarettes, alcohol, drugs, and sex. As adolescents try to prove things to peers, act grown up, experiment, and prove their sexuality, they come across many health hazards and are a high-risk age group for potential stressors.

Adolescence is a time of frequent parental conflicts. Many see these years as a recycling of the growth and development of earlier years—in particular, the terrible twos.

This chapter will explore the developmental tasks of the adolescent family and the adolescent as an individual. Potential stressors and coping mechanisms will be identified. Nursing assessment of the family and the adolescent and nursing responsibility in health maintenance and promotion will also be discussed.

FAMILY TASKS

While each family member must work through his or her individual developmental tasks, the family as a whole must also try to accomplish its developmental tasks. These family tasks have been identified as (Duvall, 1977):

1. Allowing for and providing for individual differences and needs
2. Working out a system of financial and family responsibility
3. Refocusing the marriage relationship
4. Maintaining open communication among family members
5. Widening the horizons of adolescents and their parents
6. Maintaining family ethical and moral standards

Allowing for and Providing for Individual Differences and Needs

Each family member is at his or her own stage of development and will have different needs. Adolescents are becoming more active and varied in their activities. Females become more concerned about home appearance as they begin to date and have friends over. Males tend to demand more time for their hobbies and activities. Both are beginning to want more privacy, and this is typically the time when an additional telephone is purchased for the household. More and more adolescent activities are outside the family focus, involving school and peers.

While the adolescent is concerned with dating, recreation, and job pursuits, younger siblings may be a part of the family, and their interests and needs must also be considered. They may envy the freedom allowed their older brother or sister. They may also resent the activities and interests that take the adolescent away from them and signal the end of their years of playing together.

At the same time, parents continue to need time alone together, and time to pursue their individual interests. Trying to meet the many demands for adequate time and space of all family members during these years is a big chore. Many adaptations and compromises on the part of all family members are necessary.

Working Out a System of Financial and Family Responsibility

Adolescents are quite capable of taking responsibility for household functions. Families in this stage of development often work out a division of labor and responsibility to include the children. Adolescents often become partly responsible for meal preparation, cleaning the house, taking care of the yard, and caring for younger siblings. Adolescents are still accountable to their parents, but are becoming progressively more able to assume responsibility for the family's well-being, as well as their own behavior (Duvall, 1977). It is important for parents to recognize and commend the contributions the adolescents make to the family. This recognition will serve to increase their self-esteem, and hopefully encourage mature, responsible behavior.

Families with adolescents may also become acutely concerned about money. Ever-increasing costs of social activities and education (both high school and post-high school) add a particular financial burden to many families. This is an important time to incorporate the meaning of money to children. Involving adolescents in family decisions regarding the budget is one way to help them see that there is a limit to income and what can be spent on non-necessities. Many adolescents are given set allowances to use for their personal activities and have to learn to budget them.

This is also a time when many teenagers obtain part-time jobs in order to earn extra money. They often do such jobs as yard work, work in garages or groceries, on golf courses, as babysitters, sales clerks, or in restaurants. It is important for these jobs not to interfere with schoolwork.

Refocusing the Marriage Relationship

At this time in a family's development, the marital relationship is of major concern. Many couples have been so all-consumed with the demands of parenthood that their marriage has taken a back seat. Both spouses often spend a great deal of time away from home, absorbed in work, and pressured by careers as well as domestic responsibility. These activities leave little time or energy for their spousal relationship. As a result, the marital relationship may weaken.

This stage can, however, be a time when parents have more of an opportunity to take time to be a couple. The demands of parenthood are not lessened, but are of a different nature. The adolescent's involvement in activities outside the home and ability to be left in charge of the home for short intervals leaves parents time to be alone or get away for an occasional evening together. This provides the couple the chance to regain the initiative to be attractive to each other. Keeping a marriage alive rests on the eagerness of both parties to attract and to be attracted by each other (Duvall, 1977).

Parents who take pride in and enjoy each other usually enjoy their children. It is important for adolescents to see love between their parents. They need parents who model love as a rewarding and satisfying experience (Satir, 1972). This role modeling sets the stage for healthy heterosexual relationships for adolescents.

Maintaining Open Communication Among Family Members

Living successfully with an adolescent requires open communication. Communication breaks between generations in many families. Teenagers may interpret parental interest and suggestions as intrusions and attempts to control. Parents often find it difficult to discuss personal issues with their children. This is partly because their concern is so great and partly because of embarrassment.

According to Duvall (1977), there are two factors in parents' ability to communicate with adolescents. These are their willingness to listen and their ongoing acceptance and affection. Successful communication involves active listening. Anything not understood should be clarified through questioning. When parents complain that they are not able to get through to their children, it is often because they do not let the adolescents come through to them (Wahlroos, 1974).

This period in a family's life is a busy one with much to do and little time for family interactions. It is not enough for parents just to feel love for their children. They must also be able to show it by treating adolescents' opinions as important and by discipline that makes them feel valued and enables them to achieve their full potential.

Parents also need the love, confidence, and respect of their children. They may feel threatened when their children disagree with them. These disagreements should not lead to arguments. Parents must insist that differing views be expressed in a respectful manner. Parents gain and maintain the love and respect of their children when they meet, day by day, the developmental needs of their children. Teenagers do need parents, and realize this most of the time.

Widening the Horizons of Adolescents and Their Parents

The teenage years are characterized by a widening of interests and activities among family members. As mentioned earlier in this chapter, many adolescents work. Jobs strengthen self-confidence and independence, and provide valuable experiences.

Social development takes on great significance during these years. Friendships with members of both sexes and activities involving dating and emotional involvement become more predominant. Peers are particularly important to teenagers. It is in peer relationships that many decisions are made, skills developed, confidences shared, and values weighed. Parents who are not prepared to release their children often feel threatened by these outside influences. Accepting their children's friends and activities as a normal part of growing up makes it easier for both parents and children to learn and grow.

Teenagers begin to get involved in more and more activities. They join clubs, teams, and various groups. Life is really opening up before them, and they want to try it all. Parents who accept these adventures without feeling unnecessarily afraid or threatened are able to join in exploring and evaluating new ideas and ways of looking at things, and gaining the flexibility that modern times require (Duvall, 1977).

Maintaining Family Ethical and Moral Standards

The teenage years find adolescents searching for their own beliefs and values. Parents must defend and adhere to sound principles and standards of conduct. Protecting adolescents from harm and life's disasters is as important as giving them enough room to grow, even if in the process mistakes are made. Families with teens may have to deal with many problems, both real and potential, such as delinquency, irresponsibility, drugs, friends of questionable reputation, and confusions about love, sex, and marriage.

Moral development during the adolescent years is no longer automatic, based on parental standards, but is based on understanding. Social order is examined, justified, and hopefully preserved and supported.

Parents and their children can learn from one another during these times. The family serves as a mediating link between adolescents and groups, and is a stable force to which they can turn for value development (Bengston, 1975). The anxieties parents have concerning their children in the areas of drugs, drinking, alcohol, sex, and other risk-taking conduct are often calmed when the family can openly discuss matters and reveal adolescents' emerging values.

As children grow, parents can teach by doing rather than preaching. Their imprint on their children has already been made. Families teach adolescents trust by trusting, values by valuing, and love by loving (Duvall, 1977).

All of the above developmental tasks of the family with an adolescent serve to accomplish the overall family goal of this period. This goal is to allow the adolescent greater freedom with balanced responsibility in preparation for the emancipation of a mature young adult into the world.

INDIVIDUAL TASKS

Adolescents are entering a period of change and face many developmental tasks. The primary tasks of this stage are:

1. Accepting one's changing body and learning to use it effectively
2. Consolidating a satisfying and socially accepted identity

3. Establishing mature relationships with peers of both sexes
4. Gaining emotional independence from family members
5. Selecting and preparing for an occupation and economic independence
6. Developing adult intellectual skills and concepts
7. Preparing for marriage and family responsibility
8. Becoming socially responsible and developing realistic values and moral codes
   (Duvall, 1977; Havighurst, 1972)

Accepting One's Changing Body and Learning to Use It Effectively

The physical and emotional changes brought on by puberty have a major impact on adolescent development and encompass a major developmental task. Adolescents mature at different rates, but this stage is characterized by a progression of physiological changes that require an adaptation of body image. These physical changes require adolescents to adjust to their new appearance and feel comfortable with it. They must also learn to cope with the emotional and social pressures that accompany these changes. These events may be overwhelming, or they may be useful as a foundation for learning healthy adaptive behaviors.

Puberty is the term used to refer to the maturational, hormonal, and physical development that occurs when the reproductive organs begin to function and the secondary sex characteristics develop. Puberty ends with the ability to reproduce. For girls, this is with the establishment of ovulation some time after the onset of menarche. For boys, this is when spermatogenesis is established some time after the first nocturnal emission.

Freud terms this period the genital stage (Appendix I). He maintains that at puberty, sexual impulses break through, and the genital zone is of primary concern (Teung, 1983).

This developmental task is so major and involved that for discussion, it will be broken into areas of physical development, male and female sexual maturation, and male and female responses to puberty.

Physical Development.   The physical changes of puberty are primarily the result of hormonal activity under the influence of the central nervous system. Growth and change are more dramatic and visible during this period than at any other in life. Particularly noted are the increase in physical growth and the appearance of secondary sex characteristics. *Primary* sex characteristics are the internal and external organs that carry on reproductive functions, while *secondary* sex characteristics are those characteristics that externally distinguish the sexes from each other, but play no direct part in reproduction (Whaley & Wong, 1987). Examples of secondary sex characteristics in females are hip development, growth of pubic and axillary hair, and body contour, and in males voice changes and growth of facial and pubic hair.

During puberty, both males and females attain the final 20 to 25% of their linear growth. Most of this occurs during a growth spurt that lasts from 2 to 3 years. This spurt begins earlier in girls. Although the beginning age is variable, it is from 10 to 14 years of age for girls, and 12 to 16 years for boys. During their growth spurt, boys average approximately an 8-inch gain in height, while girls, whose spurt is slower and less dramatic, gain an average of 5 inches. At age 18, more than 99% of growth has occurred in most people, with about one inch in height left to be gained.

Skeletal changes are dramatic during adolescence. Skeletal mass doubles, which accounts for the significant weight gain during this period. Lean body mass (muscle) and nonlean (primary fat) double during puberty. Muscles increase in both number of cells and in size in males, while in females, they increase in size only. This may account for the presence of generally greater strength in males. By the end of puberty, females average twice as much body fat as males. Total body fat in males actually decreases during puberty.

Growth in the length of extremities and neck precedes that in other areas, and often the adolescent's hands and feet appear larger than normal. Following this is an increase in hip and chest breadth, followed by an increase in shoulder width. This is then followed by an increase in trunk length and chest depth.

Adolescents have already achieved normal adult vision and hearing. Pulse, respiration, and blood pressure values reach adult norms by age 15 or 16. Sebaceous glands become extremely active at this time, which is important in the pathogenesis of acne, a common and often devastating problem for adolescents.

Sexual maturation, involving the development of primary and secondary sex characteristics, includes hormonal changes. These hormonal changes occur in males and females and are not a matter of either/or, but of proportion. Both sexes secrete masculinizing and feminizing hormones, but not to the same degree.

The chemical substances that trigger adolescent physical development are the hormones secreted by endocrine glands. The *gonads* (ovaries and testes) are stimulated by gonadotropic hormones from the anterior pituitary gland to secrete estrogen, progesterone, and testosterone. Androgens (primary testosterone) are the masculinizing hormones responsible for rapid growth changes, increased thickness and darkening of skin, and body hair. These are produced primarily in the testes. Estrogen, produced primarily in the ovaries, is the feminizing hormone. This hormone is responsible for the development of secondary sex characteristics. Progesterone is the hormone that prepares the uterus to accept a fetus and maintain a pregnancy. The small amounts of progesterone that are present in both sexes before puberty originate in the adrenal glands.

Female Sexual Maturation. Female sexual development involves an increase in the size of breasts and reproductive organs, an increase in axillary and pubic hair, and the onset of menarche (first menstrual period). There is a usual sequence of maturational changes, but it should be remembered that these are average, and will not occur in this order in every female. This usual sequence is:

1. A noticeable increase in height and weight
2. Breast development
3. Increase in pelvic girth
4. Pubic hair
5. Axillary hair
6. Menarche
7. An abrupt deceleration of linear growth

Menarche seems to occur earlier with each generation. The reasons are not clear, but it is thought to be from the effects of environment, nutrition, and better health care. The normal age range of menarche is presently 10 to 15 years of age, with the average age being around 12 years. The first menstrual period usually occurs about the time the growth spurt slows. The onset of menstruation does not occur simultaneously with ovulation. Most girls are irregular in their periods at first, with the first mature ova cycling in about 1 to 2 years.

Adolescent Female Responses to Puberty. Adolescent girls become very body-conscious as they begin physical maturation. They may feel embarrassment as they grow taller than their male classmates in the early stages of puberty. There is normal fat deposition accompanying puberty, which they may perceive as evidence of obesity, and they may try to diet at a time when their bodies need essential nutrients.

Most girls are very interested in their changing bodies. They see their developing breasts as a sign of maturity and femininity. Many observe and compare their progress with that of their friends. They also begin to wear bras, which can be a major landmark for many girls.

The development of some of the secondary sex characteristics may not be as pleasing to girls as to boys. The growth of body hair may seem a nuisance to many, because our culture prefers smooth skin, and this necessitates shaving of legs and underarms. Adolescent females are becoming increasingly conscious of beauty and fashion during this period of development. They spend hours playing with makeup and experimenting with hairstyles before the mirror. This provides a narcissistic outlet that is similar to that of boys while shaving.

Menstruation is the most significant feature of puberty for females. It is a positive sign of womanhood and the ability to reproduce. Most females are prepared for menarche and look forward to it. Others find it distressing and frightening. If one is not prepared for the onset of menstruation, it can be a very traumatic experience.

Females generally become interested in their attractiveness to males before males become interested in females. This is a time of great concern over body image and looks, and the slightest uncomplimentary remark may be devastating, just as a compliment can send the spirits soaring. Fathers play an important role in adolescent females' self-concept, and it is from paternal attitudes that much of their self-esteem is established. As girls mature, fathers may feel it is not appropriate to be as close to their daughters as they once were, and draw away. This can be interpreted as rejection and cause a great deal of pain. This is a dilemma that calls for much tact and understanding on the part of parents.

Sexual feelings in the adolescent female are not usually centered in the genital region, as they are in the male. Her feelings are more generalized and associated with romance and feelings of love. The female reproductive organs are not as obvious as those in the male, and thus do not account for as much of her sexual awareness as they do in the male. The adolescent female does not feel the urge for self-stimulation as strongly as a male, and when masturbation is practiced, it is usually combined with fantasy.

Sexual maturation is an area where much anticipatory guidance is necessary. Adolescents need to be prepared and knowledgeable about their maturational changes before they occur. Most will hear things from peers, but to assure accuracy, they should hear about sexual maturation from a knowledgeable adult. A healthy mother–daughter relationship is conducive to a healthy transition from childhood to puberty to adulthood, but many parents are not comfortable discussing these issues. Nurses can provide the information and education necessary for both parents and children.

Male Sexual Maturation.   The sexual development of the adolescent male involves genital growth, the appearance of pubic and body hair, voice deepening, sperma- togenesis (process of the formation of sperm), and seminal or nocturnal emissions. As with females, there is a usual sequence of these maturational changes. The usual sequence is:

1. Increase in weight
2. Enlargement of testicles and scrotum (the testes, epididymides, and prostate increase their prepubertal size seven times)
3. Rapid weight increase
4. Growth of body hair (pubic hair appears about 2 years before facial hair)
5. Voice changes, which usually occur concurrently with penile growth
6. Seminal emissions
7. Abrupt deceleration of linear growth

Nocturnal emissions, commonly called wet dreams, are reflex ejaculations of seminal fluid that occur spontaneously during sleep, with or without sexual stimula- tion. They usually occur at intervals of approximately 2 weeks, when there is a buildup of seminal fluid in the genital ducts. These often persist into adulthood. Just as females are not usually fertile with their first period, viable sperm are not normally produced until about 1 year after the first ejaculation. Nocturnal emissions are often a source of concern for adolescents. They should be assured that these ejaculations are a normal part of development, so as not to develop conflicts of good and bad concerning their bodies. Like menarche, this is an area where anticipatory guidance is vital. Knowledge beforehand makes for a much healthier transition into puberty.

Adolescent Male Responses to Puberty.   Adolescent males eagerly await their growth in height and muscle, particularly because they have lagged behind their female classmates. The development of their secondary sex characteristics has much psychological and social meaning. The growth of facial and body hair is closely associated with feelings of masculinity, and shaving at the slightest evidence of facial hair growth is a means of validating their sexual role. It also gives an excuse to look in the mirror and admire their changing bodies.

Penile and testicular growth often create some problems for adolescent males. Their reproductive organs are readily visible and very sensitive to sexual stimulation. Their sexual feelings are centered in the genitals, and their desire is urgent; thus, they seek quick relief from pressure and tension through ejaculation. Their sexual feelings are related to the sex act itself, and not so much with love as with females. Males' sexual desires generally peak a year or two after puberty.

Adolescent males are frequently not well prepared for the onset of puberty.

Spontaneous ejaculations can be confusing, bothersome, and embarrassing. When preparation has not been received beforehand, they may not feel comfortable going to their parents for explanations. They often obtain information from peers or reading materials, or puzzle about things in silence.

There are few legitimate outlets for the gratification of these genital urges. Our culture frowns upon premarital sexual involvement, and if it is practiced, it is often compounded with many problems. Homosexual practices are also condemned by our society. As a result, adolescents resort to masturbation. As stated previously, this practice is more prevalent in males than females, so it will be discussed here.

Masturbation for males is the manipulation of one's own genitals for the purpose of ejaculation. It is normal activity, and most boys do practice this, alone or in the company of the same sex. Masturbation may be associated with guilt and stress, and there are many misconceptions concerning it. Many believe it is evil, morally wrong, and results in things such as acne, epilepsy, blindness, insanity, or impotence. It is, however, normal, and aids pubescent males with information concerning how their bodies work sexually. The greatest harm that can be attributed to masturbation is the worry, guilt, and self-condemnation adolescents may experience because of poor sexual guidance.

All of the physical changes of adolescence require an acceptance of one's body. The adolescent needs to develop a realistic self-concept and body image, and deal with all the erratic and dramatic changes he or she is experiencing. Adolescents must learn to make mature decisions concerning sexual activity and maintaining a healthy body.

Consolidating a Satisfying and Socially Accepted Identity

This developmental task includes sex-role mastery. By age 3, most children know what sex they are. Sex behaviors are reinforced since birth. By school age, children usually accept and begin to imitate a sex-role preference. Relationships with same-sex peers helps reinforce that preference and continue shaping sex-role identity. During early adolescence, these relationships intensify, and provide opportunity to refine male/female roles and function and learn peer group expectations regarding heterosexual relationships. By midadolescence, teenagers test out sex-role behaviors in heterosexual socialization, and by late adolescence the prominent social relationships usually involve one person of the opposite sex (Tackett & Hunsberger, 1981).

The adolescent faces the emotional crisis described by Erikson (1963) as identity versus role confusion. The adolescent must find out who he or she is, a purpose for existence, and how he or she fits into the world. Forming an identity means that the adolescent has an "internal stability, sameness, or continuity, which resists extreme change and preserves itself from oblivion in the face of stress or contradiction" (Murray & Zentner, 1985). Erikson (1963) identifies three types of identity, which comprise identity formation. These are: (1) personal identity–what one believes oneself to be; (2) ideal identity–what one would like to be; and (3) claimed identity–what one wants others to think one is. Role confusion results when one's sense of identity is not established.

The search for identity leaves adolescents open to many influences, both con-structive and detrimental. They may identify with politicians, religious leaders, movie stars, athletes, teachers, gang leaders, or family members. Having parental and adult support from those with a stable identity who uphold sociocultural and moral standards of behavior enhances adolescents' own identity formation (Josselyn, 1975).

An adolescent also needs love, guidance, and discipline. Responsibility should be geared to individual development. Opportunities should be used to help the adolescent feel good about the self. Recognition should be given by providing positive verbal feedback and by displays of affection and approval.

If there is role confusion, the adolescent may feel insecure, powerless, self-conscious, and confused. He or she may have difficulty making decisions and de-laying gratification. As a defense mechanism, the adolescent often appears brazen and arrogant. Adolescents also frequently have difficulty at work or school, with peers, and in intimate relationships. A real danger is that the adolescent may take on antisocial behavior.

Hopefully, successful resolution of this developmental crisis occurs with social roles defined and articulated, a stable body image and gender identity, and a solid sense of self-esteem.

Establishing Mature Relationships with Peers of Both Sexes

Part of the emancipation process of adolescence involves the development of rela-tionships outside the family. These relationships are essential to the socialization process. Adolescence is seen as a time of intense sociability and often a time of equally intense loneliness (Whaley & Wong, 1987).

Peers begin to assume a much more significant role in adolescence than in earlier years. Peers and peer groups provide strong support, a sense of belonging, and a feeling of strength. Peer group relationships in early adolescence are mostly with the same sex. Friendships become more intimate. These young adolescents are curious about members of the opposite sex but are confused as to how to approach them.

Adolescence is characterized by beginning contact with the opposite sex. The telephone becomes extremely important, because it helps avoid embarrassment of being observed while talking with a member of the opposite sex. Teenagers begin to explore sex appeal and the feelings of falling in love. Peer groups begin to consist of both sexes, rather than one, and social activities are more group parties than one-on-one dating. Late adolescence is a time when teenagers usually begin dating, and peer groups become less important than that one significant boyfriend or girlfriend. This increase in heterosexual relationships is a natural outgrowth of the physical matura-tion that is taking place. Adolescents turn toward the opposite sex, not motivated by a need to find a permanent partner, but as a means to enhance their sex-role identity (Whaley & Wong, 1987).

Involvement with peers of both sexes helps adolescents learn how to get along with a variety of people. It also aids in the development of skills in inviting and refusing, solving problems and resolving conflicts, making decisions, and evaluating experiences (Duvall, 1977). It is a vital factor in social integration.

Gaining Emotional Independence from Family Members

Independence from the family is a major developmental struggle for adolescents. As a result, this is often a low point in parent–child relationships. Teenagers continually test their parents and demand more freedom. They typically complain that their parents give them too little freedom and do not trust them. Parents, in turn, often feel that the freedom and trust they do offer is abused. This is exemplified by the frequent struggles concerning curfews for teenagers.

As adolescents learn how to be autonomous persons, capable of making decisions, parents begin to have less influence. This developmental task involves growing out of the dependence of childhood and the impulsivity for which early adolescents are known, and evolving into mature, interdependent young adults. Older adolescents usually find it easier to consult their parents than they did in earlier years. They are now able to satisfy their need for affection and intimacy outside the home as well as within, to take responsibility for their choices, and to construct their values out of a sense of self rather than from rebellion, so that they no longer perceive their parents as threats to their autonomy (Tackett & Hunsberger, 1981).

Selecting and Preparing for an Occupation and Economic Independence

Adolescents are becoming more aware that their dependence on parents will soon terminate. They begin to appraise their potentials, abilities, and interests regarding careers. Planning for the future becomes a paramount concern. Teenagers need feedback and reinforcement concerning their capabilities and skills. They may seek counsel and specific knowledge about various fields of work that are in line with their interests, abilities, and opportunities. In this area, parents exert more influence than peers, as role models and by persuasion. It is important for parents not to force their children into a particular career for which they have no desire or talent. Teachers also play a significant role by the kind of feedback and reinforcement they offer about the student's skills and capabilities.

Preparation for a chosen occupation requires training or education. More and more adolescents are attending college. Whether they live at home or away, this may necessitate a change in family economics. Teenagers must learn to budget money and live within their means.

Developing Adult Intellectual Skills and Concepts

The development of adult intellectual skills and concepts is related partly to the adolescent's cognitive stage and partly to experience. Progression in the realm of cognition culminates in what Piaget (1961) terms formal operations (Appendix I), and is characterized by the capacity for abstract thinking.

Formal thinking involves two major aspects: (1) thinking about thoughts, and (2) separation of the real from the possible. At this stage children are able to use abstract logic and scientific reasoning. They can examine relations, construct hypotheses, and manipulate multiple categories of variables at the same time. This change in thinking also enables adolescents to argue logically with adults. They are capable of examining issues and values from others' viewpoints. They can realistically plan for their future.

Although there are not overall differences between male and female adolescents' intellect, females generally show greater verbal skill, while males are better in quantitative and spatial problems. These differences may be the result of interest, societal expectation, and training rather than a difference in innate abilities (Whitehurst & Vasta, 1977).

The achievement of adult intellectual skills and concepts gives adolescents an awareness of human needs and the ability to deal more effectively with problems. They develop concepts of law, politics, human nature, and social organization that enable them to become socially responsible.

Preparing for Marriage and Family Responsibility

Marriage and family responsibility follow social responsibility and involve more than just the capacity for intimacy, although that is one component. The preparation for this responsibility involves learning to love others as much as oneself. Parents can assist their teenagers in gaining a perspective for family responsibility by including them in activities such as babysitting, family budgeting, and decision making.

Adolescents are learning to distinguish between infatuation and lasting forms of love. Dating, going steady, and becoming involved with a member of the opposite sex are part of the process of developing mutually satisfying relationships. They begin to learn what they desire in a marriage partner.

Many adolescents enter into marriage during this stage, but statistically, teen marriages are unstable, often ending in divorce. The current trend for both males and females is to wait for marriage until young adulthood when education and career choices have been made.

Becoming Socially Responsible and Developing Realistic Values and Moral Codes

Becoming socially responsible means being accountable to oneself, one's family, and also one's community. More thought is given to how one's behavior affects others.

Moral development is closely associated with teenagers' cognitive functions. As adolescents mature into formal thinking, their morality changes, taking postconventional characteristics (Appendix 2). They are now able to make decisions based on internalized principles and individual conscience. Their behavior is determined by what is perceived as humanly and personally right (Kohlberg, 1969).

The change from conventional to postconventional morality is characterized by adolescents' seriously questioning moral values, particularly when they see contradictions in existing social and value structures. Whereas younger children blindly accept the view of their parents or other adults, adolescents need their own set of moral codes and values. Parental standards are usually maintained, but not with blind faith. Adolescents need internalized moral principles enabling them to make decisions involving moral dilemmas consistent with their ideals. According to Erikson (1963), without an internalized moral code, adolescents will either develop a weak ego or search for a deviant group to which to be faithful. By developing their own set of values and morals and assuming social responsibility, adolescents are able to achieve behavioral, emotional, and value independence.

POTENTIAL STRESSORS

Adolescence is often considered a more difficult and stressful period in development than the school-age years, both for adolescents and their parents. G. Stanley Hall (1905), founder of the American Psychological Association and studier of adolescence, described this period as a time of great storm and stress along with a great potential for physical, mental, and emotional development.

The reason adolescence is characterized by such turbulence and stress stems from this being a period of changes—physical, psychological, sexual, cognitive, and social. Adolescents are experiencing new feelings, emotional upheavals, and pressure from peers and other outside sources. Many are able to pass through this stage with only minor problems, whereas others may experience many traumas. Limited experiences, feelings of indestructibility, and an incomplete sense of self lead many adolescents into situations and activities that may have serious or devastating consequences.

Families play an important role during adolescence. Positive role modeling by parents and maintaining a high sense of self-worth by the adolescent are crucial. Families must strive to encourage the adolescent to grow and work through stressful periods while maintaining a sense of identity and self-esteem.

Physical Stressors

Illness. Illness is, of course, a potential stressor in any age group. Whether an illness is acute or chronic, it causes family disruption and requires adaptation. Accidents, with motor vehicle accidents heading the list, are the number one cause of death among adolescents. Much anticipatory guidance concerning illness and nursing responsibilities will be discussed later in this chapter.

Social-Emotional Stressors

Family Disequilibrium. Although peers become increasingly important during this period, parents still remain a primary source of influence. Any sort of family disequilibrium can jeopardize healthy adolescent adjustments. Many of these family situations are discussed in Chapter 7. Table 8–1 provides the common causes of family disequilibrium. Most families are able to cope with one of these situations. It is when a combination of these occurs that the stress is compounded and frequently results in maladaptive behaviors.

TABLE 8–1. COMMON CAUSES OF FAMILY DISEQUILIBRIUM RESULTING IN STRESS
DURING ADOLESCENCE

Divorce	Illness
Communication difficulties	Financial difficulties
Poor parental role modeling	Sibling hostility
Death of family members	Frequent Parental Absence
Blended families	Frequent family relocation
Substance abuse	Insufficient discipline

Peer Influences. As stated previously in this chapter, peers become increasingly more important in the adolescent's life, exerting influence on feelings and behaviors. This is a period when the adolescent especially needs to feel liked and accepted by contemporaries. Peers become the standard-setters.

Adolescents are very susceptible to peer approval and demands. They behave in a manner that will ensure acceptance into their desired group. To be ignored, criticized, or left out creates feelings of inferiority, inadequacy, and overall poor self-esteem. Problems arise when adolescents follow others who are poor role models. Because of peer pressure, many youth are tempted by and succumb to the use of drugs, alcohol, sexual misconduct, and other hazardous activities.

Parents are often concerned over their child's selection of friends and naturally desire quality friends who exert a positive influence. Exposure to a variety of friends and friendships can be healthy. Parents must recognize the adolescent's need to make friends and encourage it, while fostering independence. It is when they see the adolescent selecting friends of questionable reputation and developing unhealthy behaviors that they must intervene to prevent what could be lasting difficulties.

Abuse. Child abuse includes various forms of mistreatment, including physical abuse, sexual abuse, and neglect. This is generally thought of as a problem in younger children; however, it is also a problem among adolescents. Manifestations of abuse tend to appear less dramatic in adolescents due to body maturation and an increased ability to flee from an abuser. Whether the abuse is physical or emotional, it is traumatic and has long-term implications.

As noted previously, adolescence is a potentially stormy period. Conflict between parents and the adolescent is common as the youth seeks to accomplish the developmental tasks of this period and establish identity and independence. Peer influence increases, and parental standards are often challenged. In most cases, the standards and moral codes of parent and child will eventually coincide, but when they do not, conflict may emerge.

Parents also face crises during these years. They may experience such stresses as midlife crisis, career crisis, marital discord, health problems, jealously or resentment toward a child, or difficulty letting go of a child. This, compounded with the crisis of adolescence, can create a potentially volatile situation. Families with no history of abuse may develop a problem. It is usually an accumulation of factors, rather than an isolated reason, that is responsible for adolescent abuse.

It is difficult to identify the victim of teenage abuse because most teens live with it rather than report it, due to fear of future abuse (Remsberg & Remsberg, 1977). The social stigma attached to sexual abuse and incest also contributes to the lack of reporting. Noninvolved family members are frequently aware of sexual abuse within their family, but choose not to face it because of guilt, shame, or denial (Tackett & Hunsberger, 1981). The sequelae of abuse also vary. There may be physical evidence, emotional problems, or cognitive delays from school absenteeism and poor motivation to succeed.

Sexual abuse produces few physical signs. Adolescents may not attempt to halt sexual contact due to their emerging feelings of sexuality. Adults who sexually abuse adolescents frequently blame the victims as being seductive. Although sexual abuse and incest occur among males and females, it is more common among adolescent females (Lempp, 1979). The sexual involvement occurs with family members, acquaintances, or outsiders.

Health care workers have little contact with abused adolescents unless a major injury results. Rehabilitative efforts concentrate on mental health and must involve the entire family. Most efforts presently involve treatment rather than prevention, but prevention of abuse is an area where nurses must begin to place increasing effort. Public education is another step necessary in the attempt to fight this problem. Unless cases of suspected abuse are reported, health care workers and law officials are hindered in their efforts to resolve this horrendous problem.

Sexuality. Sexuality and sexual development are common causes of adolescent stress. The physical changes of puberty and the associated emotions and feelings often cause confusion and anxiety.

Adolescents who are slow to mature are under particular stress. Those who lag behind their peers in physical development are acutely aware of their differences. Females whose breasts have not developed or who have not yet menstruated feel cheated and out of place. Males who are behind in muscular development and whose voices are still high feel weak and rejected. Both males and females observe others, see variations in development, and compare themselves to others. This can result in poor self-concept and poor body image when they are not able to cope with the differences in development, particularly when they receive negative feedback. These adolescents need support and reassurance that they are not abnormal, and will, in time, develop as their peers have.

Sexual experimentation is common among adolescents. Most experiment in petting, and more and more are experiencing intercourse. Statistics indicate that approximately 40% of females and 80–95% of males experience coitus by the end of adolescence. The reasons for their sexual relationships and experimentation are numerous, including the need to satisfy curiosity and sexual drives, to express affection, and the inability to withstand peer pressure to conform (Whaley & Wong, 1987).

Homosexual experimentation is not uncommon, especially in early adolescence. It is usually a result of curiosity and experimentation rather than actual homosexuality. As teenagers move into adulthood, it is probable that heterosexual life-styles will be chosen (Kappelman, 1981).

Sexual experimentation makes adolescents prime candidates for stress. Some pass through these years with relatively few problems, while others will be guilt-ridden, become pregnant, or contract venereal disease.

One of the most significant consequences of adolescent sexual impulsivity and experimentation is pregnancy. There are approximately one million teenage pregnancies in the United States every year, with an additional thirty thousand occurring in girls under 15 years old (Tackett & Hunsberger, 1981). These teens present a group at risk medically, socially, economically, and educationally. Morbidity is high among teenage pregnancies. Adolescent girls and their unborn infants are at greater risk for complications, both prenatally and during delivery. The most common complications are premature labor, low-birth-weight infants, toxemia, neonatal mortality, iron-deficiency anemia, fetopelvic disproportion, and prolonged labor. There may also be a competition for nutritional needs between the growing fetus and the growing teenager. Those who have not completed their own growth and become pregnant are at greatest risk. Adolescents whose growth is completed and who have achieved physical and reproductive maturity are not as much a biological hazard as those who are still developing. The most essential factor in a healthy pregnancy is the provision of quality, comprehensive prenatal care (Whaley & Wong, 1987).

Teenage pregnancy is also one of the primary causes of school dropout. This can lead to educational and social problems. The decision of marriage may also become an issue. Many pregnant teenagers choose to marry, but these marriages are generally unstable. The highest divorce rate is among couples married in their teens.

The pregnant teen who does not marry must decide whether to continue or terminate her pregnancy. This is never an easy decision, and is even more difficult for an immature adolescent. If a girl chooses abortion, it is not without risk, physically or psychologically. The girl who decides to carry to term also faces the dilemma of whether or not to keep her child. This is a difficult and painful decision, and requires much thought, guidance, and support.

Teenage pregnancy forces the adolescent girl to cope with several developmental tasks simultaneously—adolescence itself, pregnancy, marriage, and motherhood. The need for dependency caused by pregnancy is in conflict with the adolescent's need for independence. The father of the child, usually a teenager, is faced with many of the same conflicts, and is often a neglected person in this crisis (Whaley & Wong, 1987).

The most important goal in nursing care for a pregnant adolescent is to ensure that she obtains early prenatal care. This is imperative for the welfare of both the adolescent and the infant. Options must be made clear, and decisions supported.

It is important to prevent all sexual problems, but public education for adolescents and their parents is of paramount importance. Teenagers need to be aware of the consequences of early sexual activity. Parents need to be aware of the realities of adolescence and to be able to discuss sex and their feelings about sex with their children in a healthy manner. Many parents withhold information regarding sex, thinking that avoiding the issue will prevent experimentation. This is not true. Parents may need assistance in feeling more comfortable discussing sexual issues with their children (Tackett & Hunsberger, 1981).

Teenagers are eager to learn about themselves, their bodies, and sexual issues. Nurses are in an ideal position to identify potential and actual problems, and can provide teenagers with factual information concerning their bodies and clarify misconceptions concerning puberty, sexual development, and sexual issues. Nurses must be able to take a nonjudgmental attitude and gain the confidence and trust of adolescents in order to be effective caregivers and counselors. Adolescents need someone with whom they feel free to express their feelings and fears.

COPING MECHANISMS

Health Beliefs and Behaviors

Nurses working with adolescents and their families must be aware of the various health beliefs and behaviors among individuals. Family structure, religion, culture, and income level all play a part in adolescents' health beliefs and should be considered before appropriate interventions are planned. The seven areas of assessment that nurses should utilize in individualizing health care for children and their families are outlined in Chapter 7. These apply to adolescent families as well as school-age families.

Responses to Stressors

When an adolescent is confronted with a stressful situation, disequilibrium results. The adolescent deals with the stress in either an adaptive or maladaptive manner. In order to deal successfully with stress, Wold (1981) identified *counterbalances* that assist the adolescent to adapt. These include a realistic perception of the stressful event, an adequate support system, and previous successful coping mechanisms. Wold also identifies three methods of dealing with stressors. These are successful in overcoming of the stressor, avoidance, and coexistence, or learning to live with it.

Adaptive Responses.   In this discussion of adaptive responses to stress, concentration will be on the psychological, rather than physiological aspects. It is through adaptation that one is able to constructively cope with conditions imposed internally or externally. Adaptation permits the adolescent to cope by reducing or eliminating the effects of discord, deviance, or adverse forces that accompany change. Adaptation should be accomplished without extreme physical illness, loss of long-range goals or values, or disruption of one's overall social functioning (Murray & Zentner, 1985).

Adaptation is achieved through that part of one's personality called the *ego*. The ego is the part of the personality that interacts with the outside world. It is also responsible for the use of adaptive functions. The presence of a strong ego is vital to the accomplishment of the developmental tasks of adolescence.

Psychological stress results when there is failure to satisfy needs or reconcile conflicting value systems. Three basic causes of psychological stress are: (1) loss of something valuable, (2) actual or threatening physical or emotional injury, and (3) frustration of drives (Murray & Zentner, 1985). Different people respond differently to similar situations, and this accounts for the variety of possible adaptive or maladaptive behaviors.

Most people, including adolescents, are able to resolve frustrations and conflicts by conscious and deliberate coping mechanisms. Most complex stressful situations, however, are dealt with through unconscious defense or adaptive mechanisms. Adaptive mechanisms allow adolescents to cope while maintaining a sense of self and identity. They are not harmful unless overused to such a degree that they distort reality. These adaptive mechanisms are automatic, not planned behavior, with the purpose of preventing anxiety (Rowe, 1975).

The adaptive mechanisms used in adolescence are the same ones used in previous developmental stages, although they may be used in different ways.

The adaptive ability of adolescents is largely influenced by inner resources built through parental love, esteem, and guidance. Adolescents with parents who demonstrate healthy adaptive patterns may still have difficulties, but the chances for acceptable adaptive responses to stress are more likely if parents are a positive example.

Maladaptive Responses and Behaviors.   Adolescents often deal with stress and frustration with maladaptive responses and behaviors that interfere with the achievement of their developmental tasks. There are certain characteristics that help to identify those adolescents at risk for maladaptive behaviors (Table 8–2). No single pattern of behavior may result in difficulty, but a combination of these is indicative of a potential hazard in terms of adjustment. There are numerous maladaptive behavioral responses to stress. The main ones affecting adolescents that will be discussed are sexual misconduct, depression, runaways, delinquency, substance abuse, school attendance problems, suicide, and eating disorders.

Early physical and emotional maturation, along with changing cultural norms for acceptable sexual behavior, have led many adolescents into *sexual relationships*. Their relative immaturity and ignorance regarding sexual activity often results in stressful situations. Pregnancy, social isolation, guilt, rejection, or venereal disease may be the outcome. This issue has already been introduced under "Potential Stressors" and will be dealt with further later in this chapter.

TABLE 8–2. CHARACTERISTICS OF ADOLESCENTS AT RISK FOR MALADAPTIVE BEHAVIOR

Poor body-image/self-concept	Substance abuse
Low self-esteem	Sleeping problems
Prolonged grief	Severe mood swings
Communication difficulties at home	Antisocial behavior
Poor peer role models	"Loner" behavior/decrease in verbalizing
School problems	Premature or late puberty

It is generally expected that American teenagers graduate from high school. State laws make school attendance compulsory until age 16. Although educational expectations fluctuate with the time and vary among socioeconomic levels and families, education beyond high school has become the expected norm for many, and if often a prerequisite for job security.

Problems with school attendance can be categorized into the following areas: (1) dropouts—students leaving the educational system electively prior to graduation, (2) truants—students enrolled but absent from school without permission, (3) expulsions—students forced to leave a school by the educational authorities, and (4) those who have never attended school due to lack of opportunity or successful avoidance of authorities by parents.

Those who do not regularly attend school are deprived of the very important education and socialization that school offers. Not attending school also hinders opportunities in the job market. It often results in idle time, no sense of direction, poor choice of activities, and confrontation with the law.

Families play a significant role in school attendance patterns. Parents who place little value on education may not enforce attendance. Parents need to realize the impact of their encouragement on their children's progress in school. Being sensitive to the strengths and weaknesses of their children can enable them to negotiate the system to ensure a more meaningful educational experience. Students need to be instilled with values that allow them to realize the importance of education and give them the desire to attend school.

Children leaving home without notice is nothing new. Nearly two million youth leave home or disappear every year. It may be for a short period of time, an extended period, or forever. The average age of a runaway youth is 15 years. Most *runaways* are female (67%) and Caucasian (70%) (Jarvis, 1983). Although many people do not realize it, it is against the law to run away, and parents or guardians may press charges or have a warrant issued for the runaway's arrest. It is often difficult to enforce this, due to problems in locating runaways, but arrests can be made. This should be a last resort, however, when all other strategies to prevent running away have failed.

There are many reasons why adolescents run away from home. These include family strife such as divorce, death, physical and sexual abuse, or discipline problems. Teenage runaways characteristically have a poor self-concept, are anxious, defensive, full of self-doubt, and have difficulty relating to others (Wold & Brandon, 1977).

Runaways usually go to one of two places after they leave home. Many go to the home of a friend, whose parents may not realize the situation. These teenagers usually do not stay away longer than a few days. The second place runaways often go is a large city. Frequently adolescents have not made any preparation for survival and will have little money and no place to live. After their money is gone, they may try to find a job, but are usually limited due to poor qualifications. Their plight is often recognized by panderers, drug dealers, pimps, and other undesirable persons. They may become involved in illicit activities and be placed in jeopardy with the law. The day-to-day difficulties and emotional turbulence compound their feelings of desperation (Tackett & Hunsberger, 1981).

Prevention lies in recognition of problems before the adolescent feels unable to cope. Nurses, school nurses in particular, can be of assistance with this problem. Knowledge of normal behaviors and awareness and sensitivity to deviations in developmental behaviors can alert nurses to those who need early intervention and counseling.

Delinquency has been defined by Fredlund (1970) as "antisocial behavior that is beyond parental control and therefore subject to legal action." As reported in "Upsurge in Violent Crime" *(U.S. News and World Report,* 1978), juveniles between the ages of 7 and 18 are the groups most prone in the United States to commit a crime. Juvenile delinquency has serious ramifications for society, such as school safety, costs to citizens financially, child abuse potential, and future health and life-styles of the delinquent. Delinquency is a problem of epidemic proportion and continues despite efforts to diminish it.

Peer pressure frequently influences delinquency. Delinquent acts are often the work of gangs or several individuals. Rehabilitation of these youth is possible. "The Youth Crime Plague" *(Time,* 1977) reported that only 10% of juvenile delinquents are incorrigible offenders. The solution, however, lies in prevention. The identification of stressors is the first step. Child abuse is highly correlated with delinquency, and its prevention is in curricular programs, such as teaching problem solving, teaching parents about care and expectations for their children, and providing adolescents with classes on vocational choices and opportunities, family living, and sex education (Wold, 1981). Ultimately, it is hoped that delinquent-prone behaviors can be recognized, and help provided before the adolescent's actions become aberrant.

The widespread misuse of drugs by adolescents puts a great deal of pressure on youth and their families. Drug or substance abuse encompasses a variety of substances such as alcohol, tobacco, marijuana, and so-called hard drugs. Hard drugs include narcotics such as heroin and cocaine, stimulants such as amphetamines, and hallucinogens such as mescaline, PCP, and LSD.

There is often confusion and misunderstanding regarding terms applied to drug use. In order to clarify between drug abuse and drug misuse, the following definitions serve:

- *Drug abuse:* the regular use of drugs for other than accepted medical purposes, and to the extent that physical or psychological injury results, and/or in a way that is detrimental to society.
- *Drug misuse:* the overzealous use of drugs or the using of poor judgment in their use (Whaley & Wong, 1987).

Statistics on teenage drug use are staggering. One out of two 14- to 15-year olds has smoked marijuana. Approximately 90% of high school students have had some experience with alcohol, and there are over a half million alcoholics in their preteen and teen years in the United States (National Institute on Drug Abuse, 1980). Alcohol is the most widespread substance abuse problem among adolescents, and its use is closely related to the drinking behavior of their parents.

There is no single cause for substance abuse. Several possible causative or motivating factors are curiosity, boredom, escape from anger or depression, family problems, peer pressure, the need for peer acceptance, poor self-concept, and the availability of drugs. An adolescent abuser usually exhibits one or more of the danger signals of which parents and others should be aware. These are denial, ignorance of common drugs of abuse, the need to gain control of the environment, and the need to convince others (particularly peers) of his or her power. The adolescent also is generally one who does not fit in well with others, has a poor school record, and difficulty dealing with authority. An adolescent abuser also frequently uses significantly more coffee, cola drinks, aspirin, tobacco, and alcoholic beverages (Tackett & Hunsberger, 1981).

Many parents have sought to prevent teenage drinking by teaching that it leads to personal disaster. Hoping that teaching the serious health consequences of drinking will make adolescents afraid to use alcohol is, unfortunately, a false hope. The goal of teaching about alcohol is to prevent irresponsible drinking. Responsible drinking will vary among individuals. Some are able to partake of an occasional drink with no harmful effects, while others cannot, and must abstain.

Despite the factual information concerning tobacco use, cigarettes are still widely used among adolescents. There is a steady decline in the proportion of smokers in the general population, but there is an increasing proportion of teenage female smokers. Adults serve as poor role models where smoking is concerned (and alcohol also). Health care personnel who smoke are in a very poor position to counsel others concerning this practice. Adolescents are very aware of incongruities in others, and advice against smoking, given by smokers, will not likely be heeded. Assertiveness classes about not smoking should begin early, in sixth or seventh grade.

Smokeless tobacco, often used by male teenagers, is frequently viewed as "safer" than cigarettes. It can, however, be associated with oral cancer. Early detection of oral cancer is important, and any person with a mouth lesion that does not heal within 2–3 weeks should seek medical care.

The drug marijuana is an illegal form of cannabis considered fairly safe by most adolescents. It is not tobacco. Data regarding this substance are incomplete, and the effects of its use on the unborn children of its users is still not well understood. It should not be considered a harmless drug. Parents should be aware, however, that there is a tremendous difference between its occasional or experimental use and its habitual use.

Cocaine is an increasing drug problem. This drug can be administered by a variety of methods. It can be sniffed, infused, and even smoked. Crack, a cheap, highly addictive, and smokable type, is becoming epidemic among youth. Parents must be alert to symptoms of its use, such as weight loss, chronic hoarseness, a drop in grades, constant talking, mood swings, and new and inappropriate friends.

The effects of substance abuse are many. The mind-altering effects from the use of many drugs can lead to irresponsible behaviors such as sexual experimentation and reckless driving, and in some cases the ultimate outcome is death. Those who become addicted to drugs may experience malnutrition, retarded growth, hepatitis, and crime in order to obtain the money to keep up their habit.

Families play an important part in the prevention of substance abuse. A stable, loving home environment provides the nurturance and support necessary for adolescents to develop into responsible, self-reliant adults. An examination of the parents' own life-styles is necessary. Setting examples for healthful living helps instill these same habits in their children.

There are many programs available for the rehabilitation of drug abusers. Alcoholics Anonymous has been very helpful for the adolescent who is able to admit a drinking problem. Drug detoxification centers and methadone programs for heroin addicts are also available. In order for any program to be successful, the adolescent must change his or her inadequate self-concept and realize that he or she has the strength and ability to handle day-to-day living without dependence on drugs (Johnson & Klotkowski, 1978).

Nurses can be very instrumental in curbing substance abuse by way of educational programs and role modeling. Programs with a positive emphasis on health can aid in prevention.

Depression is very common among adolescents, often masking serious underlying problems. Adolescent depression is likely to take one of two forms. The first is expressed as a feeling of emptiness and a lack of self-definition. The depressed youths may deny having feelings and complain of not knowing what to do with them or how to evaluate and express them. This kind of depression resembles a state of mourning. A second type of adolescent depression is more difficult to resolve. It has its basis in repeated experiences of defeat over a long period of time. It occurs among adolescents who have tried to find solutions to their problems and to achieve personally meaningful goals, but have been without success, either because of the failure of others to accept or understand, or because of personal inadequacy (Mussen, Conger, & Kagan, 1979).

Adolescents evidence their depression by boredom, restlessness, difficulty in concentration, loss of interest in life, and difficulties in school. Others may act out with drugs, become sexually promiscuous, or withdraw from contact with others. Depression is usually caused by the loss of a meaningful relationship, such as the loss of a parent, friend, or romantic partner.

Nurses dealing with a depressed adolescent need to differentiate between normal periods of depressed moods, which are brief and fade away, and profound or chronic depression, which persists, progresses, and interferes with mastery of developmental tasks. Once the existence and severity of the depression is recognized, appropriate referrals must be sought in order to establish a therapeutic treatment plan. The family of the adolescent will also need support and assistance. They need guidance in identifying any causative factors within family relationships that could have contributed to the adolescent's depression.

There are many opportunities for nurses to use their anticipatory guidance skills in helping to prevent or treat depression. Education of parents concerning developmental norms and behaviors is important. Enhancing parenting skills also helps develop healthy parent–child relationships. Open and honest communication between parent and child contributes significantly to the adolescent's mental health.

Suicide ranks third as a cause of death among 15- to 19-year olds, following accidents and homicides. It occurs more frequently in males than females, although more females attempt suicide. Suicide is often an impulsive plea for help, and shows a direct relationship to the amount of stress placed on the adolescent. The overall rate of attempted suicides to actual suicides is approximately 100 to 1 (Pilliteri, 1981).

The voluntary ending of one's own life, or the attempt to do so, has ramifications not only for the family, but for all of society. Trying to understand what could cause a person to resort to suicide is deeply frustrating. It is particulary incomprehensible that a teenager should feel suicide is the solution to life's problems.

Suicidal methods vary between the sexes. Females are more likely to use passive methods such as the ingestion of pills, while males tend to resort to more quickly lethal methods such as gunshot or hanging.

Causative factors of adolescent suicide are difficult to isolate, but signs of depression usually precede any attempt at suicide. Poor academic function, poor self-image, and feelings of hopelessness have also been identified in adolescents who attempt suicide. Suicidal adolescents are frequently the product of a disrupted family situation (Rohn, Sarles, Kenny, Reynolds & Heald, 1977).

Crisis intervention techniques are successful in averting some suicides, but a real chance for reduction lies in prevention. Adolescents may talk about suicide to others. This is often thought to be an attempt to manipulate others and not taken seriously. Any talk of suicide should not be ignored. Adolescents attempt suicide because they do not see any other solution to their problems. One approach in prevention is education. Therapy should aim to improve adolescents' self-image, identify positive aspects of life, offer alternative solutions to problems, and explore alternative modes of coping.

Two *eating disorders* common in adolescence that have a strong psychological component are anorexia nervosa and obesity. Although there may be a degree of physiological etiology in some cases, emotional difficulties are usually more closely associated.

Anorexia nervosa. Anorexia nervosa is the term given to the disorder characterized by severe weight loss (greater than 25% of total body weight) without an obvious physical cause (Worthington-Roberts, 1985). It is a disorder in which emaciation occurs as a result of self-inflicted starvation. It occurs primarily in adolescent females, rarely in males. Adolescent girls who have this disorder are usually from upper- or middle-class families, well-behaved, academically high achievers, conscientious, conforming, with a high energy level, but lacking a clear sense of identity. They are usually very dependent on their parents, and there is often a history of family strife. The etiology of this disorder, however, is unclear.

Dominating the psychological aspects of this disorder are a relentless pursuit of thinness and a great fear of fatness. The onset is frequently preceded by a year or two of mood swings and behavior changes. The weight loss is usually triggered by some crisis such as the onset of menses, or a traumatic interpersonal incident. Anorexia nervosa consists of three major areas of disordered psychological functioning identified by Bruch (1976). These are a disturbed body image and body concept of delusional proportions, an inaccurate and confused perception and interpretation of inner stimuli, and a paralyzing sense of ineffectiveness that pervades all aspects of daily life.

Girls who are anorectic generally overestimate their size and the size of others. They refuse to eat, have an entire repertoire of excuses not to eat, but are simultaneously markedly preoccupied with food. They frequently cook, talk constantly about food, read books or magazines dealing with food, and exercise incessantly.

The goals of treatment and management of anorexia nervosa are to correct the physiological state of malnutrition and resolve the psychological component. Treatment is difficult and requires long-term management. Intravenous and tube feedings are often necessary to treat the malnutrition. This is done simultaneously with psychotherapy and family therapy to treat the underlying psychological disorganization. Weight gain alone is not considered a cure for anorexia nervosa, as relapses are common.

It is necessary for nurses to be kind and supportive, while firm in managing the care of an anorectic, so as not to cause her to be passive-dependent. A continued behavior modification program is usually the most beneficial mode of therapy. Psychotherapy is aimed at assisting the adolescent to resolve her identity crisis and distorted body image.

A disorder closely related to anorexia nervosa is bulimia or bulimarexia. Bulimia is characterized by an insatiable appetite with eating binges followed by self-purification in the form of self-induced vomiting or diarrhea (purging). Bulimarexia is bulimia accompanied by voluntary starvation (Mahan & Rees, 1984). These symptoms may be a part of anorexia, but also comprise a separate syndrome.

Bulimia usually occurs in women aged 18 to 29, but is also frequently seen in adolescents. Bulimics have many of the same personality traits as anorectics, but are generally not as disordered psychologically. They are usually characterized by depression and guilt. They do, however, tend to realize that their eating behavior is abnormal, which is in contrast to anorectics.

The physiological consequences of bulimia from vomiting, laxative abuse, and overuse of diuretics can be severe, and include cardiac arrhythmias, renal problems, gastrointestinal disorders, and electrolyte disturbances (Worthington-Roberts, 1985). The treatment for bulimia is patterned after the approach used with anorectics.

Obesity. There is probably no disorder so obvious to others, difficult to treat, and with such long-term psychological and physical effects as obesity. It is the most common nutritional disorder of childhood. Approximately 15–30% of adolescents are obese, and 80–85% of obese children become obese adults. The associated increase in mortality and morbidity associated with obesity from both physical and psychological reasons makes this a very serious condition.

Obesity results when one's caloric intake consistently exceeds caloric requirements and expenditure. Heredity plays an important factor, but may be due more to environmental conditions and family habits than genetics. Obesity is distinguished from simply being overweight by an excessive (more than 20% of ideal weight) deposition of adipose tissue or body fat.

Obesity is a serious handicap to the social life of adolescents. It usually results in poor body image, low self-esteem, social isolation, feelings of rejection, and depression. Obese teenagers are frequently passive, feel awkward in social situations, and isolate themselves from social contacts.

Adolescent-onset obesity is closely related to the inability to master the developmental tasks of this period. As a result, adolescents regress to the self-satisfying tactic of overeating to compensate. This only creates a greater obstacle to achieving these tasks. Their obesity serves to ward off pressure impinged by the changes of puberty and the outside world. Obesity becomes their safeguard. They may see their obesity as responsible for all of their disappointments, and thus avoid making the adaptations necessary for growth and maturation. Eating is a means of coping with the normal drives of adolescence. Obese adolescents become increasingly dependent on food as a means of gratification, and this creates a vicious cycle (Whaley & Wong, 1987).

Due to the self-perpetuating nature of adolescent obesity, treatment is frequently disappointing. As stated previously, many obese teenagers become obese adults. Drugs and surgical techniques are not usually used with adolescents. When dealing with adolescents, it is important to remember that weight gain and anabolism are normal and necessary for healthy adolescent development. Strict diets may deprive them of necessary nutrients for healthy development.

Nurses usually play a central role in weight loss programs. Motivation is always the key to any successful weight loss program. Diet, exercise, and behavioral therapy are the most successful modes of therapy. Prevention is, of course, the optimal solution. Healthy dietary habits need to be instilled early in childhood, and role modeling by parents and other significant adults is important.

The causes and consequences of these maladaptive behaviors involve not only adolescents, but their families, schools, and society. Nurses may not always be in a position to provide direct intervention, but are in a position to make important contributions. Nurses must place emphasis on casefinding to identify potentially troubled youth, education for adolescents and their families, and providing nurturance, support, and understanding.

NURSING ASSESSMENT

When making an assessment of a family with an adolescent, it is important for the nurse to have a strong background in growth and development, and knowledge of individual and family developmental tasks. The family must always be incorporated into any plan of care for an adolescent. A family assessment includes a thorough personal and family health history, data concerning health habits and family health perceptions, family strengths and weaknesses, life patterns and life-styles, family structure and functions, family communication patterns and decision-making practices, and growth and developmental data (Friedman, 1981; Jones, Lepley & Baker, 1984).

An example of a format that could be used in assessing the family with an adolescent is shown in Table 8–3.

TABLE 8–3. ASSESSING THE FAMILY WITH AN ADOLESCENT

	Environmental Data
Provisions for care	Who is major catetaker?
	How many and who are living in house together?
	What type of school does adolescent attend?

	Communication Patterns
Adolescent	What is level of language development?
	To whom does adolescent communicate? (peers, family, others)
Between adolescent and caretaker	How do caretaker(s) and adolescent communicate? Do they communicate regularly and openly?
Among family members	What are methods of communication in family? (constructive, nonconstructive, level of participation by each member)
	How do siblings communicate?

	Problem-Solving Skills
Decision-making abilities	How are major decisions made; does caretaker make any decisions independently from other adults in household; roles of family members during decision making/implementing.
Use of health care system	When instituted and for whom, location, accessibility, cost, purposes as perceived by family.
Support from significant other(s)	Viewed as positive or negative by major caretaker and adolescent, areas of strongest support, areas of weakest support (as viewed by caretaker, adolescent, and as viewed by nurse).
Societal interactions	Use of public agencies (welfare, crippled children's school, etc.), ability of caretaker to deal with or circumvent "the system" when appropriate, business communicative skills.

	Life-Style
Role of adolescent in family	What is family structure?
	What are family and personal responsibilities of adolescent?
	Is adolescent employed?
Socioeconomic status (SES)	Estimated yearly income, financial assistance, direction of SES mobility, wage earner's feelings about status.
Family roles	Traditional or nontraditional pattern, level of satisfaction with roles.
Work patterns	Wage earners in family, amount of work hours per day or week, anticipated job change.

TABLE 8–3. ASSESSING THE FAMILY WITH AN ADOLESCENT *(continued)*

	Environmental Data
Recreational patterns	Use of free time, amount of planned activities per month, amount of time spent in recreation/leisure by each family member, amount of group recreation.
Safety	Visible hazards, use of safety features, adults' and adolescent's knowledge of accident prevention, first aid, poison control.
	Potential Stressors
Conflicts in parenting	Parent(s)' perception of parenting role, own recognition of conflicts, potential for unrecognized problems.
Interferences with family tasks	Goals of family members, present health of family members.
Conflict with society	Incorporation of adolescent and involvement with society, societal acceptance of family and adolescent.
Family response patterns	Restructuring or reordering goals, determining priorities, identifying realistic, practical approaches to meeting goals, changing family structure or life-style.

Some specific questions that the nurse could ask to elicit data during an assessment with an adolescent are listed in Table 8–4. Questions should also be asked to assess the occurrence of and the adolescent's coping with menstruation and nocturnal emissions. The nurse should evaluate the need for further teaching or discussion of sexuality and normal adolescent development (Jones, Lepley, & Baker, 1984). If an adolescent is thought to be sexually active, this area of assessment must be treated delicately. Establishing trust and assuring confidentiality are the first step. Questions must not be judgmental. When inquiring about sexual activity, instead of asking if the adolescent has ever had sex, ask open-ended questions. An example is, "Other teens have questions about sex concerning birth control, sexually transmitted diseases, or how to know when you've met the right person. What questions do you have?" After this is discussed, ask if he or she is presently sexually active. Most adolescents will eventually open up and express their concerns if treated as adults in a caring and supportive manner.

Several tests mentioned in Chapter 6 to assess physical and mental development can also be used for adolescents. These include the Slosson Intelligence Test (SIT), Peabody Picture Vocabulary Test (PPVI) and Wide Range Achievement Test (WRAT). The Social Readjustment Rating Scale (SRRS) is a tool useful in assessing stress for adolescents. This tool (Tables 8–5 and 8–6) adapted by Coddington (1972) for use with junior-high and high-school-aged youth is used in the same manner as the ones used for school-aged children and adults. These scales are guides to the assessment of environmental stresses placed on adolescents within a 12-month period. While the total of the life change units (LCUs) is used as a predictor of life crisis, it does not

TABLE 8–4. QUESTIONS A NURSE COULD ASK IN ASSESSING AN ADOLESCENT

Tell me about your family
Does your family get along well together?
What sort of restrictions do you have at home?
How does your family feel about your friends?
What is your family support system, that is, who helps in times of need for assistance, counseling, and support?
Who influences you and gives you feelings and values about growth, development, new experiences, and communicating with others?
How are family decisions made?
Who makes health decisions?
Do members of your family use tobacco, alcohol, or drugs?
What kind of school do you go to?
What do you like best and least about your school?
Are you satisfied with your education up to now?
Have you ever considered dropping out of school?
Why do you think you have been depressed or feeling low lately?
What do you do to relax?
What sort of exercise do you get?
What do you typically eat in one day?

project the outcome of exposure to a particular level of stress. These tools can be useful for nurses in assessing stress levels and the potential for problems in those adolescents with high LCU scores so that supportive and preventive strategies can be implemented. They can also be used as counseling tools to aid adolescents in understanding the stresses they have in their lives, and help them identify coping strategies (Wold, 1981).

ALTERATIONS IN HEALTH

Acute Alterations in Health

As in all developmental stages, temporary and acute health alterations are obvious potential stressors. Many of these alterations in adolescents are a result of the pubertal development, while others are also common in later adult years.

Accidents are the leading cause of death and accidental injury in adolescents. The tragedy of this is that most fatal accidents are preventable. Motor vehicle accidents, drownings, and firearm incidents are common causes of accidents in this age group. Adolescents have feelings of confidence, strength, and indestructibility that they have not had before. They also have a lot of energy and curiosity, which is often spent impulsively and without logical thinking. This makes them especially prone to risk-taking behavior, which frequently leads to accidents.

TABLE 8–5. LIFE CHANGE UNIT VALUES FOR JUNIOR-HIGH-SCHOOL-AGE YOUTH

Rank	Life Event	Life Change Units[a]
1	Unwed pregnancy of child	95
2	Death of a parent	94
3	Divorce of parents	84
4	Acquiring a visible deformity	83
5	Marital separation of parents	77
6	Jail sentence of parent for 1 year or more	76
7	Fathering an unwed pregnancy	76
8	Death of a brother or sister	71
9	Having a visible cogenital deformity	70
10	Discovery of being an adopted child	70
11	Becoming involved with drugs or alcohol	70
12	Change in child's acceptance by peers	68
13	Death of a close friend	65
14	Marriage of parent to stepparent	63
15	Failure of a grade in school	62
16	Pregnancy in unwed teenage sister	60
17	Serious illness requiring hospitalization of child	59
18	Beginning to date	55
19	Suspension from school	54
20	Serious illness requiring hospitalization of parent	54
21	Move to a new school district	52
22	Jail sentence of parent for 30 days or less	50
23	Birth of a brother or sister	50
24	Not making an extracurricular activity he or she wanted	49
25	Loss of job by a parent	48
26	Increase in number of arguments between parents	48
27	Breaking up with a boyfriend or girlfriend	47
28	Increase in number of arguments with parents	46
29	Beginning junior high school	45
30	Outstanding personal achievement	45
31	Serious illness requiring hospitalization of bother or sister	44
32	Change in father's occupation requiring increased absence from home	42
33	Change in parents' financial status	40
34	Mother beginning to work	36
35	Death of a grandparent	35
36	Addition of third adult to family (i.e., grandparent, etc.)	34
37	Brother or sister leaving home	33
38	Decrease in number of arguments between parents	29
39	Decrease in number of arguments with parents	29
40	Becoming a full-fledged member of a church	28

[a]Abbreviations: 0–149 LCU = no life crisis; 150–199 LCU = mild life crisis; 200–299 LCU = moderate life crisis; 300 or more LCU = major life crisis.

From Coddington, R.D. (1972) The significance of life events as etiologic factors in the diseases of children. I. A survey of professional workers. Journal of Psychosomatic Research 16(1), 15–16.

TABLE 8–6. LIFE CHANGE UNIT VALUES FOR SENIOR-HIGH-SCHOOL-AGE YOUTH

Rank	Life Event	Life Change Units[a]
1	Getting married	101
2	Unwed preganancy of child	92
3	Death of a parent	87
4	Acquiring a visible deformity	81
5	Divorce of parents	77
6	Fathering an unwed pregnancy	77
7	Becoming involved with drugs or alcohol	76
8	Jail sentence of parent for 1 year or more	75
9	Marital separation of parents	69
10	Death of a brother or sister	68
11	Change in child's acceptance by peers	67
12	Pregnancy in unwed teenage sister	64
13	Discovery of being an adopted child	64
14	Marriage of parent to stepparent	63
15	Death of a close friend	63
16	Having a visible congenital deformity	62
17	Serious illness requiring hospitalization of child	58
18	Failure of a grade in school	56
19	Move to a new school district	56
20	Not making an extracurricular activity he or she wanted	55
21	Serious illness requiring hospitalization of parent	55
22	Jail sentence of parent for 30 days or less	53
23	Breaking up with a boyfriend or girlfriend	53
24	Beginning to date	51
25	Suspension from school	50
26	Birth of a brother or sister	50
27	Increase in number of arguments with parents	47
28	Increase in number of arguments between parents	46
29	Loss of job by a parent	46
30	Outstanding personal achievement	46
31	Change in parents' financial status	45
32	Being accepted at a college of his or her chcoice	43
33	Beginning senior high school	42
34	Serious illness requiring hospitalization of brother or sister	41
35	Change in father's occupation requiring increased absence from home	38
36	Brother or sister leaving home	37
37	Death of a grandparent	36
38	Addition of third adult to family (i.e., grandparent, etc.)	34
39	Becoming a full-fledged member of a church	31
40	Decrease in number of arguments between parents	27
41	Decrease in number of arguments with parents	26
42	Mother beginning to work	26

[a]Abbreviations: 0–149 LCU = no life crisis; 150–199 LCU = mild life crisis; 200–299 LCU = moderate life crisis; 300 or more LCU = major life crisis.

From Coddington, R.D. (1972) The significance of life events as etiologic factors in the diseases of children. I. A survey of professional workers. Journal of Psychosomatic Research 16(1), 15–16.

Other health alterations commonly occurring during the adolescent years are acne, menstrual disturbances, and infectious diseases such as mononucleosis and influenza.

Acne vulgaris is one of the most common and embarrassing health problems of adolescence. It is an almost universal disorder, and its peak incidence is in 16- to 20-year-olds. It is estimated that 90% of all adolescent males and 80% of all adolescent females suffer from some degree of acne. Although this is a self-limiting disease, it may persist well into adulthood, and its impact on adolescents cannot be underestimated.

Acne is an inflammatory disturbance involving the pilosebaceous follicles (hair follicle and sebaceous gland complex) of the face, neck, back, shoulders, and upper chest. Although usually classified as a sebaceous gland disorder, acne does not result from an abnormal gland, but from the glandular secretion of sebum initiated by androgens. The etiology is not clearly understood, but several aggravating factors are emotional stress, premenstrual hormonal changes, and stimulant and steroidal drugs. There is no evidence that any specific foods cause acne in general, although certain individual may notice outbreaks after ingestion of certain foods. This may be due to an allergic response.

Acne should not be dismissed as an inevitable part of growing up that must simply be lived with and ignored. Treatment seldom shortens the course of the disease or cures it, but management can control it, reduce the inflammatory process, lessen scarring, and improve the adolescent's appearance. Acne occurs at a time when identity development is crucial, and the injury to self-esteem can be as great as the actual physical manifestations of the disease.

Treatment of acne is aimed at removal of the lesions, reducing the formation of lesions, controlling infection, and preventing scar formation. There is no single treatment protocol agreed upon by dermatologists, and treatment for inflamed and noninflamed lesions is different. Some general management measures include adequate rest, sufficient exercise, good personal hygiene, elimination of unnecessary emotional stress, correction of any menstrual irregularities, and elimination of foods if there is a specific food sensitivity.

Menstrual disturbances, particularly irregularities in timing of periods and amount of flow, are very common during adolescence. Irregularities, however, usually resolve themselves by the third year after onset of menarche. The unpredictability of the onset of a period is frustrating and may cause insecurity. Dysmenorrhea, or discomfort during the menstrual flow, is also common. Many females experience cramping, abdominal pain, backache, and legache. The pain may be mildly discomforting or intolerable and incapacitating. Dysmenorrhea is the leading cause of recurrent school absenteeism among adolescent girls in the United States (Klein, 1980). Treatment of dysmenorrhea consists of medications (usually aspirin or a prostaglandin inhibitor), application of heat to the painful area, and exercises such as assuming the knee-chest position and breathing exercises. In severe cases, cyclic estrogen therapy (birth control pills) to prevent ovulation is most helpful. Adolescent females need information regarding the normal physiology of menarche and the expected irregularities they may experience. Anticipatory guidance is vital, as well as continued support and reassurance.

Adolescents are generally resistant to most communicable diseases, but *mono-nucleosis* and *respiratory infections* are common. Infectious mononucleosis is a mildly contagious viral disease also known as the kissing disease. The Epstein-Barr virus (EBV), a herpes-like virus, is thought to be the causative agent. It is believed to be transmitted by direct contact with contaminated saliva of an infected individual. The affected person typically suffers symptoms of fever, malaise, sore throat, and lymphadenopathy. There is no treatment effective in its prevention or cure. Management involves comfort measures to relieve symptoms, such as aspirin and rest. Acute symptoms usually subside within 10 days, and fatigue disappears in about 2 to 4 weeks. Some may need to restrict their activities for 2 to 3 months. Adolescents with mononucleosis need assurance that their confinement is only temporary, and that activity can be gradually resumed after the acute phase of the illness. If care is not taken, relapses back into the acute phase are common.

Influenza is a highly contagious viral infection of the respiratory tract. Adolescents are susceptible because of their inattention to nutrition, rest, and sound sanitary practices. High fever, sore throat, cough, nasal congestion, headache, malaise, and muscular aches are the clinical manifestations. Treatment is aimed at providing comfort measures to control symptoms, preventing secondary infections, and controlling spread. Vaccines are available to aid in preventing influenza.

Ramifications for the Family.   Illness in one family member affects the whole family. Family functions, schedules, finances, and interactions are all disrupted because of an illness. Parents may feel guilt, worry, and fear. They may have to spend more time caring for the sick child at the expense of other family and household responsibilities. This may cause anger, jealousy, or resentment from other children or from a spouse. The ramifications discussed in Chapter 7 can also apply to adolescence. Nurses are in a position to assist families in recognizing potential or actual stresses imposed by illness, and in helping them to make necessary decisions regarding care and treatment.

Ramifications for the Adolescent.   Adolescents with a temporary or acute health alteration are affected in much the same way as a school-age child. School attendance may be necessarily disrupted, interfering with cognitive development as well as peer interaction. Forced dependency on parents or other family members may be difficult to accept, as adolescents are striving to maintain independence and control and establish identity. Confinement and limitation on activities is particularly stressful, as this is a period of much social activity.

Adolescents are generally narcissistic regarding their bodies, and any illness may be a threat to their body image. Any disfigurement, loss of function or mobility, or change in appearance is especially difficult to handle. Nurses must assist adolescents and their families to cope with illness and its accompanying ramifications, and to restore normal family functioning as much as possible.

Response to Hospitalization.   Hospitalization is a stressful experience for anyone. Adolescents have the most well-developed coping mechanisms of any childhood age group and are better able to deal with stress, but they still are vulnerable to the stresses of illness and hospitalization. The main threats of hospitalization for adolescents are: (1) loss of control, especially in terms of loss of independence and identity; (2) fear of altered body image; and (3) separation from peers (Whaley & Wong, 1987; Smith, Goodman & Ramsey, 1987).

Adolescents are particularly threatened by any sense of loss of independence or identity. Hospitalization incurs an enforced dependency and a sense of depersonalization on adolescents. Adolescents have an acute need to control situations affecting them. Hospital restrictions on meals, activity, visiting hours, and bedtime interfere with this need. Nurses should aim to set limits that encourage the adolescent drive toward self-control rather than dependency (Teung, 1982). They should plan nursing care with them, allowing them opportunity for decision making.

Many fears of adolescents during hospitalization center on body image changes. They believe their bodies are a main criteria by which others accept or reject them, and illness and hospitalization cause great insecurity. Adolescents may respond to hospitalization by asking many questions, withdrawing, rejecting others, or conveying a blase attitude. They may also overcompensate for their fears with overconfidence. A careful assessment of how much they know and understand must be made in order to clarify any misconceptions and provide opportunities to ventilate feelings. It is often easy to assume that adolescents know more than they do. Provision of privacy is also important for adolescents, as they are going through sexual and body changes. They are modest and especially sensitive to being displayed in front of strangers, even if the strangers are health care personnel.

Separation anxiety from parental absence is not nearly as acute for adolescents as is separation from peers. They may fear losing their status in a group, missing out on sports events and social activities, and being forgotten. Allowing visitation with friends is as needed for adolescents as is mother's for infants.

Nursing Goals.   The nursing goals in working with an acutely ill adolescent are to resolve the health deviation and minimize its stress on the adolescent and family and to prevent future crises. The nurse should strive to identify and reinforce strengths of the adolescent and family, and to encourage verbalization of feelings and fears. As much control as possible should be given the adolescent in order to help maintain a sense of identity, self-esteem, and control. Illness, hospital routines, and treatment should be explained openly and honestly, and in an adult manner. The adolescent wants to be treated as an adult. Being aware of the adolescent's level of development, coping mechanisms, and support systems will aid the nurse in providing the kind of care necessary for a healthy return to normalcy after the stress of illness and/or hospitalization is over.

Chronic Alterations in Health

Chronic illnesses in adolescents are of major significance. Whether life-threatening or not, they place great strain on healthy physical and emotional development and can be devastating. Among the most common chronic health alterations affecting adolescents are scoliosis, sexually transmitted diseases, obesity (which has already been discussed), as well as many of the chronic health deviations of the school-age child and young adult.

Scoliosis, a lateral deviation of the spinal column from midline, is the most common skeletal deformity of adolescence, and is commonly identified and treated during the adolescent growth spurt. It is seen in approximately 15% of children between ages 10 and 21, and occurs mainly in females (Hill & Romm, 1977). This deformity is usually present before puberty, but the rapid vertebral growth that occurs during adolescence makes the characteristic C- or S-shaped curvature more apparent. Severe spinal deformities can result in cardiopulmonary malfunction or neurological damage as a result of tethered nerves. Damage to self-image can also occur as a result of the visibility of the deformity.

Early identification of scoliosis is stressed because early intervention improves the prognosis and decreases the length of time needed for treatment. Yearly screening for scoliosis for all school-aged children is advocated. Treatment usually involves bracing or spinal fusion, and both are long ordeals that require much cooperation from the child and parents. Bracing places an additional stress on the adolescent's body image, as it is usually necessary to wear the brace 23 hours a day. The psychosocial impact of this requires a great deal of understanding and support, as the adolescent will have many concerns about peer acceptance, normal sexuality development, and body image. Spinal fusion requires surgery and often the insertion of a Harrington rod and a long postoperative period.

Parents are important in the management of scoliosis, as it is long-term and requires cooperation with the therapeutic regime. Parents can help their child feel attractive and in control and lessen the negative impact of this deformity.

Sexually transmitted diseases (STD), commonly known as venereal diseases, are among the most prevalent and dangerous of the communicable diseases in the United States, reaching epidemic proportions. An increasing number of adolescents and young adults are contracting STD, with the peak ages between 15 and 24. Sexually active adolescents are particularly at risk because they often refuse to or do not recognize symptoms, and are late in seeking medical attention. Embarrassment, guilt, and fear also prevent them from admitting they may have a venereal disease.

Gonorrhea ranks first among the reportable diseases, despite the discovery of penicillin. Genital herpes is not a reportable disease, because there is no cure, so its exact incidence is not known; however, it is increasing in prevalence yearly. Chlamydial infections are also becoming more prevalent.

Although AIDS is not commonly seen in adolescents, it should be a major concern. The overall incidence is rising and adolescents should be educated about its transmission. The primary mode of transmission is by direct contact with blood or blood products, and intimate sexual contact in which semen and blood mix. There is no evidence that casual contact can spread the virus (Centers for Disease Control, 1986). There is presently no cure for AIDS, and its course is painful and debilitating.

The effects of STD can be devastating both physiologically and psychologically. The clinical manifestations of STD are varied, ranging from pain and discharge to being asymptomatic. Most can be effectively treated if diagnosed. Many STD have long-term effects and can be transmitted to infants during birth. The psychological trauma of these diseases can be particularly hard on adolescents. Guilt, shame, and fear of rejection are common. The necessity of naming sexual contacts also is difficult. Nurses play a vital role in preventive education regarding STD, and in casefinding and encouraging prompt treatment.

Ramifications for the Family. The family of an adolescent with a chronic illness will be placed under additional stress as it attempts to accept and deal with the problem. The same difficulties discussed for school-age children apply to adolescents. Much long-term support is needed, and nursing care must not only include attention to the physical health of the child and family, but the emotional health as well.

Ramifications for the Adolescent. The presence of a chronic illness has a profound influence on an adolescent's development. The adolescent must incorporate the illness into an already changing self-concept. A child who develops a chronic illness or acquires a disability during adolescence has more difficulty adjusting than one who has been affected since early childhood. It seems that the earlier the onset, the better able the child is to adapt. The adolescent with a newly acquired disorder has the additional task of grieving for loss of perfection, while simultaneously adjusting to the normal changes of puberty (Whaley & Wong, 1987).

Severity, type, and visibility of the illness also influence the adolescent's adjustment. There are obvious limitations imposed by chronic debilitating disorders such as cardiac disease, inflammatory bowel disease, and uncontrolled epilepsy. Health alterations resulting in disfigurement, such as burns, paralysis, or the advent of a colostomy, have dramatic effects on an adolescent's body image, self-esteem, and identity formation. Nonvisible conditions such as diabetes or cardiac disease may cause problems of compliance with therapeutic regimes because of the adolescent's distorted perception of the seriousness of the condition, or because of denial (Whaley & Wong, 1987).

The fear of peer rejection is another problem with adolescents. Whether the condition is visible or nonvisible, the fact that they are different and may require special adjustments in activities of daily living poses a threat to peer acceptance.

The Adolescent's Concept of Death. Adolescents tend to view death as both fearsome and fascinating. They live in a very intense present. Everything important and valuable lies in the immediacy of life or the near future, and death sits off in the distance, as a natural enemy. Adolescents are able to perceive the irreversibility and universality of death, but resent it, as they are acutely aware of losing everything just as they are achieving adult status. The threat of death poses a great obstacle in their quest for an identity and independence. Death causes them to mourn things never experienced or achieved.

Nursing Goals. The ideal nursing plan for a chronically ill adolescent involves managing the disabling condition and facilitating optimal growth and development. The adolescent needs information concerning the condition, the treatment, and expected outcomes. There also needs to be time allowed for the expression of anger, rejection, fear of being rejected, sadness, and loneliness.

Because most adolescents are concerned with physical attractiveness, attention should be focused on the normal aspects of their appearance and capabilities. The subject of sexuality and how it relates to the illness is also a concern for adolescents, but may not be openly voiced. Nurses must be alert to signals indicating concern about sexuality, development, and reproduction.

Peer interaction is especially important during adolescence, and isolation because of exacerbations of an illness deprives them of this. Maintaining peer relationships and participating in activities appropriate to the condition should be encouraged.

It is important to foster independence as much as possible. Allowing adolescents to make decisions concerning their illness and its treatment, encouraging self-management of the disease, and helping them plan for the future will help give them a sense of autonomy. Nurses need to answer their questions honestly and treat them as mature individuals. Nurses must also provide parents the opportunity to ask questions, ventilate feelings, and express concerns.

NURSING RESPONSIBILITIES

Adolescents are generally a healthy group. Disease level is low, but because of hormonal, physiological, and emotional changes, there is much concern about the body and developing sexuality. Health promotion of adolescents is mainly health teaching and guidance.

Adolescents are very vulnerable to practices that are hazardous to their health. They need someone with whom they are free to express fears and feelings and seek guidance. Nurses have the opportunity to provide them with factual information concerning their bodies and the changes taking place, and to clarify misconceptions regarding menses, nocturnal emissions, and other pubertal changes. Nurses are also in a position to educate and counsel about potential health hazards such as substance abuse, STD, and pregnancy. Group discussions are often preferable, because peer support is available.

Mental health problems are substantial during adolescence. Nurses must be alert for clues indicating a problem, such as fatigue, poor school attendance, withdrawal, or acting-out behavior. Nurses are in a position to identify those who are likely to have difficulties and take preventive action.

The overall goals of nursing care for adolescents are:

1. To aid the adolescent in continuing optimal biopsychosocial growth and development
2. To reinforce healthy lifestyle behaviors and discourage negative ones, in order to ensure the development of a mature, responsible, and healthy adult.

Parents also need support and guidance as they try to understand and cope with the changes taking place in their children. They have to prepare to let go and to promote independence.

Health maintenance, promotion, and anticipatory guidance for adolescents is a monumental task, and involves assessment, education, and guidance in the following areas:

1. Physical assessment
2. Accidents
3. Substance abuse
4. Self-concept and body image
5. Sexuality education

Adolescents should be seen by a primary care provider at least every 2 years, even if there are no known problems. Routine health visits should include physical assessment, guidance and counseling on dental hygiene, nutrition, exercise, personal hygiene, and issues of sexuality. Adolescence is a peak time for dental caries, and professional dental hygiene care should, therefore, occur every 6 months. Nutritional needs are high. The rapid increase in height, weight, and muscle mass that occurs during the growth spurt is accompanied by an increased need for calories, protein, calcium, and iron. Eating behaviors are often erratic, and nutrition is neglected. Failure to develop habits of good dental hygiene and nutrition at an early age results in the perpetuation of problems. Relating these issues to the body and appearance often makes adolescents more receptive to health education.

As stated previously, accidents are the leading cause of death among adolescents. Safety education should include driver education, water safety, sports safety, and emergency care measures. Many deaths could be prevented if adolescents were better able to handle their new freedom, independence, and energy.

Self-concept and body image are of primary concern to adolescents. They are not always comfortable asking questions about their body changes, so it is often necessary to anticipate their questions and educate them accordingly. They will notice variations in one another's development and compare themselves to others. These differences produce anxiety in those who may develop earlier or later than their peers, and they must realize that these variations are not abnormal.

Adolescents desperately need information and education about their sexuality. This is a complex area in which much knowledge, understanding, and objectivity are needed. Adolescents need to recognize how their sexuality can help or harm them, and that they must learn to make mature and responsible decisions concerning their sexual behavior. Education for adolescents on sexuality should include anatomy and physiology, information regarding AIDS, STDs, and other sexual functioning, intimacy, contraception, pregnancy, abortion, marriage, parenting, and discussions of value systems. It cannot be overemphasized that the respecting of confidentiality is one of the most important elements in obtaining the trust of adolescents, which is necessary for effective counseling.

An important issue in sex education is sexual experimentation. It is simply not true that sexual urges cannot be controlled. The best guard against teenagers' participating in promiscuous sexual experimentation at a time when their sex drive is high and peer pressure heavy is for their family to promote self-esteem. When adolescents believe in and like themselves and have a strong self-concept, they are better able to take a stand on moral issues. Parents can help their children to think through situations in advance and consider the consequences of their actions. This anticipatory guidance helps them to be able to handle difficult situations and not become caught up in a situation or the intensity of emotion (Tackett & Hunsberger, 1981).

With the increasing number of young people who are engaging in sexual intercourse, it seems it is never too early to begin teaching about contraception. Options must be made known so those who are sexually active can make informed decisions regarding birth control.

Nurses can make significant contributions in the area of sexuality and promoting healthy behaviors, because they are knowledgeable, respected health care providers in a position to provide information and identify problems. Healthy life-style habits must be emphasized. Adolescents should be given facts, made aware of consequences, and offered alternatives.

CARE PLAN FOR THE ADOLESCENT WITH ANOREXIA NERVOSA

Situation

J. S. is a 16-year-old white female. She is 5 feet 5 inches tall and weights 92 pounds. She was brought to her pediatrician by her mother because of recent weight loss and amenorrhea. J. makes straight As in school, is very active physically, and exercises at least 2 hours a day. She loves to talk about food and cook, and frequently bakes cookies and cakes. Her daily intake of food usually consists of a lettuce salad with oil and vinegar dressing and several diet drinks and glasses of unsweetened iced tea. J. has one older sister who is in college away from home. Her sister was a high school homecoming queen, very popular, and very intelligent. J. has a younger brother who is 14 years old. He is very athletic. J.'s father is a prominent attorney who works long hours. Her mother does not work outside the home, but is very active in local social activities and charities. J. states that "my mother tries to control my life and make me perfect like my sister." She does not have many close friends. J. does not think she is too thin and frequently argues with her mother about this. J. says that she thinks her weight is right for her and appears angry when anyone suggests she is too thin.

Nursing Diagnosis

The medical diagnosis for J. S. is Anorexia Nervosa. The primary nursing diagnoses for J. S. and her family are:

1. Alteration in nutrition related to an alteration in body image.
2. Ineffective family coping

The following care plan addresses the primary diagnosis of alteration in nutrition.

SAMPLE CARE PLAN

Nursing Diagnosis	Goals	Interventions	Evaluations
Alteration in nutrition related to an alteration in body image.	J. S. will no longer make statements that she does not think she is too thin J. S. and her family will begin family therapy J. S. will begin to eat a balanced diet, gain weight, and maintain a healthy, normal weight for her age and height range	Obtain a psychiatric referral for J. S. to begin psychotherapy Encourage J. S.'s family to begin therapy Implement a high-calorie diet Give J. S. positive reinforcement for any progress made Help J. S. find other and more appropriate modes of maintaining control and having a positive sense of self Monitor J. S.'s physical activity to decrease the amount of her exercising Support measures for resolving malfunctioning family processes	J. S. will begin to see her body size realistically and develop a healthy body image J. S. will achieve a weight of 112 pounds J. S. and her family will attend family therapy regularly

REVIEW QUESTIONS

1. What are the major developmental tasks of the adolescent and his or her family? How can the nurse promote healthy accomplishment of these tasks?

2. How does physical sexual maturation affect the emotional development of the adolescent?

3. What are some potential problems an adolescent with a poor sense of identity might encounter?

4. What is the major cause of stress in adolescence?

5. How can parents help their adolescent children adapt to the stressors of this period in a healthy manner in order that they emerge as mature and independent adults?

References

Bengston, V. L. (1975). Generation and family effects in value socialization. *American Sociological Review 40*(3), 358–471.

Bruch, H. (1978). *The golden cage: The enigma of anorexia nervosa.* Cambridge, MA: Harvard University Press.

Centers for Disease Control (1986). *Morbidity & Morality Weekly Report 35*(5), 76–79.

Coddington, R. D. (1972). The significance of life events as etiologic factors in the diseases of children. I. A survey of professional workers. *Journal of Psychosomatic Research 16*(1), 15–16.

Duvall, E. M. (1977). *Marriage and family development* (5th ed.). Philadelphia: Lippincott.

Erikson, E. H. (1963). *Childhood and society* (2nd ed.). New York: Norton.

Erikson, E. H. (1963). *Childhood and society* (2nd ed.). New York: Norton.

Fredlund, D. (1970). Juvenile delinquency and school nursing. *Nursing Outlook, 18*(5), 57–59.

Friedman, M. M. (1981). *Family nursing, theory and assessment.* Norwalk, CT: Appleton-Century-Crofts.

Hall, G. S. (1905). *Adolescence: Its psychology and its relations to physiology, anthropology, sociology, sex, crime, religion, and education* (Vol. I). Englewood Cliffs, NJ: Prentice-Hall.

Havighurst, R. (1972). *Developmental tasks and education.* New York: McKay.

Hill, P., & Romm, L. (1977, May/June). Screening for scoliosis in adolescents. *American Journal of Maternal-Child Nursing,* 156.

Jarvis, V. (1983). Runaway kids. *Imprint, 30*(2), 31.

Johnson, E., & Klotkowski, D. (1978, May). Turning an addicted patient onto turning drugs off. *RN,* 91.

Jones, D. A., Lepley, M.K., & Baker, B. A. (1984). *Health assessment across the life span.* New York: McGraw-Hill.

Josselyn, I. (1975). The adolescent today. In W. Sze (Ed.), *Human life cycle.* New York: Aaronson.

Kappelman, M. (1977, August). When your teenager needs you the most. *Family Health,* p. 44.

Klein, J. R. (1980). Update: Adolescent gynecology. *Pediatric Clinics of North America, 27,* 141–152.

Kohlberg, L. (1969). *Stages in development of moral thought and action.* New York: Holt, Rinehart, & Winston.

Lempp, R. (1978, April). Psychological damage to children as a result of sexual offenses. *Child Abuse and Neglect,* 1478.

Mahan, L. K. & Rees, J. M. (1984). *Nutrition in adolescence.* St. Louis: Mosby.

Murray, R. B., & Zentner, J. P. (1985). *Nursing assessment and health promotion through the life span* (2nd ed.). Englewood Cliffs, NJ: Prentice-Hall.

Mussen, P. H., Conger, J. J., & Kagan, J. (1979). *Child development and personality* (5th ed.). New York: Harper & Row.

National Institute on Drug Abuse (1980). National Survey on Drug Abuse. U.S. Department of Health and Human Services, Rockville, MD.

Piaget, J. (1961). *The growth of logical thinking from childhood to adolescence.* New York: Basic Books.

Pilliteri, A. (1981). *Child health nursing, care of the growing family* (2nd ed.). Boston: Little, Brown.

Remsberg, C., & Remsberg, B. (1977, May). An American scandal: Why some parents abuse teens. *Seventeen,* 154.

Rohn, R. D., Sarles, R. M., Kenny, T. J., Reynolds, B. J., & Heald, F. P. (1977). Adolescents who attempt suicide. *Journal of Pediatrics, 90*(4), 636–638.

Rowe, C. J. (1975). *An outline of psychiatry.* Dubuque, IA: Brown.

Satir, V. (1972). *Peoplemaking.* New York: Science and Behavior Books.

Smith, M. J., Goodman, J. A., & Ramsey, N. L., (1987). *Child and family: Concepts of nursing practice* (2nd ed.). New York: McGraw-Hill.

Tackett, J. J. M., & Hunsberger, M. (1981). *Family-centered care of children and adolescents.* Philadelphia: Saunders.

Teung, A. G. (1982). *Growth and development, a self-mastery approach.* Norwalk, CT: Appleton-Century-Crofts.

Upsurge in violent crime by youngsters: Results of a story (1978, July 17). *U.S. News and World Report,* p. 55.

Wahlroos, S. (1974). *Family communication.* New York: Macmillan.

Whaley, L. F., & Wong, D. L. (1987). *Nursing care of infants and children* (2nd ed.). St. Louis: Mosby.

Whitehurst, G., & Vasta, R. (1977). *Child behavior.* Boston: Houghton Mifflin.

Wold, S. J. (1981). *School nursing, a framework for practice.* St. Louis: Mosby.

Wold, S., & Brandon, J. (1977, Summer). Runaway adolescents' perceptions of parents and self. *Adolescence,* p. 175.

Worthington-Roberts, B. (1985). Eating disorders in women. *Focus, 12*(4), 32–41.

The youth crime plague. (1977, July 11). *Time,* p. 18.

9

The Family and the Development of the Young Adult Aged 20–44

Mary Ann S. Rogers

OBJECTIVES

Upon completion of this chapter, the student should be able to:

1. Identify developmental tasks of the young adult and beginning family member
2. Summarize societal expectations of the young adult
3. Outline common life-style patterns and relationships
4. Recognize stressors that may affect life during this period of maturity
5. Create an intervention plan for the young adult that will promote health
6. Contrast tasks for the family of origin with tasks for the family for procreation
7. Give examples of needs for the young adult

CONCEPTS

Young adult: Person aged 20 to 44

Family of origin: One's mother/father/siblings

Peers: Friends in the workplace

Family of procreation: Young family that bears children

Status symbols: Cars, money, clothes, education, houses, jewelry, and position titles

Goals: What one wants to achieve

Priorities: Deciding what is most important for continuation of health or life's goals

Family relationships: Dealings with all members of a family

Need response patterns: Ways of getting one's needs met that are learned and are used over and over

Young adults comprise a very large group in today's society: 42.8% of the population of the United States is aged 20–44 years. Never before in history has the young adult had so many opportunities, privileges, choices, responsibilities, and liabilities as in today's affluent American society. The meaning of adulthood has changed as people have been propelled toward more education, money, and leisure time, and longer life expectancy. Schell (1975) states that the roles of the young adult have become more complex as he or she moves quickly into changing roles of fundamental importance. With these changes come demands and pressures that some individuals handle more readily than others. It is in these areas that the nurse has an opportunity to use his or her skills to assess, plan, implement, teach, evaluate, and help the client and family toward a more productive life.

This chapter will address the individual's orientation to the family of origin. The changes in this family's structure during the young adult period are many and occur at different phases as the young adult matures and embarks on a separate life pattern. Marriage, parenthood, subsequent childbearing, child rearing, divorce, and remarriage are transition points that make heavy demands on the individual family.

FAMILY TASKS

The tasks listed under "Tasks of the Family of Origin of a Young Adult" (Table 9–1) represent the needs of the family group. The family strives to maintain continuity while simultaneously adjusting to changes as the young adult establishes a separate identity.

Continuance of Physical Care

With maturity and inclination to increased independence, the young adult becomes more responsible for physical care. Physical growth and development are completed by the mid-twenties. These years represent the height of attractiveness, physical agility, speed, and strength. An occasional gray hair may signal that one is getting older, but young adults do not seem to be bothered by small changes in their physical appearance. As the young adult moves toward complete independence in matters of dental care, eye care, grooming, hygiene, nutrition, rest, exercise, and shelter the family of origin continues to be supportive of these physical care needs until this independence is attained. Example: The young adult breaks a pair of glasses. The family of origin helps pay for the unexpected expense of new glasses.

TABLE 9–1. TASKS OF FAMILY OF ORIGIN OF A YOUNG ADULT

1. Continuance of physical care
2. Redefining need-response pattern
3. Support for maturation of the individual
4. Allocation of resources
5. Maintaining family relationships
6. Establishing priorities and maintaining goals

Redefining Need-Response Pattern

The young adult no longer gets all emotional needs met through family and peers but moves into a marital relationship, parenthood, and job requirements that necessitate major adjustments in orientation (Schell, 1975). The family expands to accept these new relationships and sees as one of its tasks the incorporation of these additional people into its system.

Relationships in families are sometimes incomplete and imperfect, but avoiding them is an even more devastating choice (Blank, 1982). As the young adult begins to break away and become independent, relationships change. Bad feelings may surface over breaking away. The easy way to solve this dilemma would be to pull away completely. However, dealing with family members, though difficult, will give members an opportunity to build a relationship based on mutual respect and avoid the loss of relationships that can never be salvaged. Healthy families redefine their need-response patterns. Parents let young adults become independent and meet their own needs through new arrangements that support personal needs. Families that are unafraid of change construct reality rather than fighting it, and continue to relate to one another and work toward stronger relationships within the family.

Support for Maturation of the Individual

A healthy family continues to support the maturation of the individual. The family loosens its hold on the young adult but continues to be supportive in successes and defeats. Many families continue to allocate monies for the young adult for education, until a secure job is found, or in some instances, until the young couple is stable financially.

According to Schell (1975), early adulthood lasts longer for young adults in the upper middle class than for a member of the working class. The upper class sees this as a time for exploration. Lower-class young adults use this time to choose a job, marry, become parents, and accept responsibilities. Consequently, their choices are made without having a chance to explore all options before making decisions that will change their lives.

Not all people get married, settle into careers, or become parents at exactly the same age. As the young adult matures, he or she has expectations of behaviors appropriate for various ages that are derived from society, family, and one's own experiences. The family of origin continues to allow for maturity but at the same time continues its interest in the life of the young adult. Example: Parents usually insist on some continued contact through phone calls, letters, family dinners and birthdays, and holiday events.

Allocation of Resources

The allocation of resources is an important issue for the young adult's family of origin. The family at this time may still be the primary source of income if the young adult is still in college and has not started becoming established in a career. Some families earn more than others. The occupation of the head of the family helps or hinders the median-income young adult with choices he or she can make about education, travel, and job opportunities. Young adults of the middle and upper classes have various differential advantages. There may be early planning for the young adult's leaving home to go to college or start a career. Educational or technical opportunities during childhood, along with financial planning, contribute to the young adult's establishment in a career.

As the young adult matures and physically departs from the family of origin, resources for monetary support are lessened. The family then reallocates its money. Still, the family continues to support the young adult when he or she needs money. Financial planning continues as the family begins to think about the inheritance it will leave its members.

The single-parent family will feel the same pressures as two-parent families to meet the needs of the young adult. This will place upon these families the burden of being even more creative in meeting the financial needs of the young adult. Many children from these homes feel a responsibility for meeting their needs earlier than their peers and accept the challenge of being on their own earlier in life.

Maintaining Family Relationships

The young adult who is venturing forth into the adult world sometimes feels the need to break away from old family traditions such as family dinners, birthday parties, and outings, and holiday celebrations. The family usually adjusts its expectations to allow for more freedom, but will not allow a complete break. Members continue to seek the presence of the individual at family gatherings. As the young adult becomes more able to meet his or her own needs, the response pattern of the family adapts. They will give the person a chance to form family relationships for himself or herself. These family relationships change but remain a source of comfort, strength, or, in some cases, aggravation and despair.

Through compromise, family traditions may become a source of great happiness for the young adult. Much depends on the degree to which the young adult seeks to preserve an internal or external relationship that he or she needs or thinks is needed. Some relationships may become strained beyond repair. The family of origin will allow the young adult to begin family traditions of his or her own (Tinkham & Voorhies, 1977).

Establishing Priorities and Maintaining Goals

During this time priorities for the family change. Once a new car, a house, a membership in the country club, clothes, books, a new television set, video games, and needs of the young adult's siblings may have been high on the priority list. Now the focus shifts to education for the young adults in the family, their beginning career, or starting new relationships. Parents and siblings find themselves caught up in this embarking period. The family priorities revolve around the young adult and his or her needs. Parents put children's needs ahead of their own for many years. Siblings are also a priority. The young adult's needs will sometimes be secondary to problems of other family members.

Duvall (1977) states that rearranging physical facilities becomes a priority. The young adult's room remains empty while he or she is away at college, only to become alive during return trips home. The family car becomes a source of struggle with all siblings, and parents have to vie for a time to use it.

As young adulthood closes, the family readjusts its priorities to accommodate the changes that have taken place through the years. Many families of procreation find this a time of new affluence and prosperity. Father's career is usually at its peak, and mother is beginning to enjoy a new freedom. To contrast the early young adult period where one was seeking independence from the family of origin, the late thirties bring a need for family stability. There is a reassessment of priorities. Some men and women use this time to have a second career. They begin to see life moving very fast and see this as their last chance for self-actualization.

INDIVIDUAL TASKS

As one begins to look at individual tasks, one can see that there is no single best model for reaching maturity. Although men and women have an equal opportunity in the workplace, there still remains differences. Some of these differences depend on beliefs about sex-role behavior, social class, education, and one's own unique developmental history (Schell, 1975).

Physical Tasks

During this time, most people's bodies are the best they will ever be; therefore, the young adult is very conscious of physical fitness. Healthy young adults stand erect and walk with a firm step. Their bodies are at the peak of attractiveness, physical agility, speed, and strength. Gradually physical changes begin to appear, weight is gained, and muscle tone begins to slacken.

Shelter.   The young adult begins to look after his individual physical needs. As he or she begins a college career, a new job, marriage, or any number of activities that help the individual embark on a new beginning, he or she begins to look toward a new place of shelter. It may be a room, an apartment, or a house. Nevertheless, this is usually the first time the young adult has had total control over furnishings, decoration, cleaning, and many daily responsibilities. Also for the first time, he or she becomes responsible for personal safety. Example: Parents no longer see to it that the car has brakes, or that the door is locked.

Nutrition.   Nutrition becomes a big factor. As they break ties with home, young adults tend to eat what they like or what is convenient. After a year of eating out, junk food, or freezer meals, young adults usually begin to see the need for balanced meals. This sometimes happens because they realize that they have a decreased energy level or rapid weight gain.

TABLE 9–2. NUTRITIONAL NEEDS OF THE YOUNG ADULT[a]

30% fat (low saturated)
55% carbohydrates (complex starch rather than refined sugar)
15% protein
Fiber

[a]If pregnancy occurs, nutritional needs should be adjusted.
Adapted from Sorensen, K., and Luckman, J. (1979). Basic nursing: *Philadelphia: Saunders.*

According to Sorensen and Luckman (1979), age influences the types of food and amounts one eats. The number of calories needed depends directly on the level of physical activity and daily routine. Young adults have little difficulty meeting both calorie and nutrient needs unless the budget is too tight to include good nutrition or they do not know about a balanced diet. Table 9–2 displays items the diet for an average young adult should include.

Sleep. Sleep needs vary among young adults. According to Crips and Stonehill (1976), age, sex, and personality affect the sleep needs of adults. The average adult person needs from 6 to 9 hours of sleep in 24 hours. The young adult may enjoy staying up all night when he or she begins independence. However, the old patterns of rest will be hard to break, and the individual will return to previous sleep habits.

Dental Care. Dental care was once parents' total responsibility. "Brush your teeth!" was a common phrase. By young adulthood, teeth are a source of either pride or shame. Braces will have come off for those able to have such appliances. A pattern of "good" teeth or "bad" teeth, with many cavities, will be set. Dental checkups every 6 months may no longer be feasible. Still, need for dental care continues. Sometimes the cost can be a shock to a young person. Here again the person may not feel the need for care, but eventually it will return.

Exercise. Exercise serves several functions. It helps depress appetite, releases tension, aids sleeping, keeps body muscles firm, and promotes cardiovascular and respiratory health (Phipps, Long, & Woods, 1983). It should be regular and appropriate to one's physical condition. There has been an increased interest in exercise, especially aerobics. Aerobic exercises are activities that require oxygen for prolonged periods of time and improve the body's capacity to handle oxygen.

Young adults participate in a variety of physical activities. Walking, jogging, running, and aerobic dancing seem to be the exercises most used by the young adult (Cooper, 1982). Other popular forms of exercise are skiing, swimming, cycling, handball, racquetball, squash, basketball and tennis.

A program of exercise with a gradual increase in intensity of exertion allows the body to adapt to physical demands. If the young adult chooses a pattern of inactivity, he or she may experience having less energy and more physical complaints, and may become obese.

Personality Tasks

Personality is defined by Clayton (1985) as the unique organization of traits, characteristics, and modes of behavior of an individual. It determines how others react to a person. Personality is the mental aspects of the individual rather than physique. It includes attitudes, interests, and the sum total of a person's life adjustment.

Erikson (1968) defines the task of the individual in adulthood as intimacy versus isolation. Intimacy is characterized by a deep and true psychosocial relationship with another person. It will be found in friendships and erotic encounters. Intimacy is achieved through commitment, sacrifice, compromise, work productivity, and satisfactory sexual relationships. Isolation exists when the young adult is self-absorbed, distances himself or herself from others, and has problems interacting with others.

Self-Concept. Because young adulthood is relatively free of physical changes, the individual can concentrate on developing a strong self-concept and interacting with others. Self-concept development begins at an early age and continues to develop and change throughout life as the individual moves toward maturity and fulfillment. A young adult who has a positive self-concept can move forward, hoping to achieve his or her highest potential. If the young adult has a low self-concept, he or she will spend time trying to find out what is wrong, defending thoughts, actions, and perceptions. It is during this period that one realizes that being able to love oneself frees one to love others (Fromm, 1956). Until this happens, young adults spend their time trying to figure out what is wrong with them. Such questions as: "Why didn't I get the best job?" "Why doesn't Sally want to marry me?" can become preoccupations, and the young adult does not move forward to maturity because confidence in the self is stymied. The self-concept is made up of many parts. These include body image, self-ideal, self-esteem, and roles (Stuart & Sundeen, 1979).

Body Image. Today's society, with its overwhelming focus on youth and beauty, puts a great deal of pressure on the young adult (Murray & Zentner, 1979). One's *body image* (how one looks) is a very important concept of self. If one can look in the mirror and like what one sees, it can help the self-confidence needed to pursue other tasks. The young adult begins to see some stability of body change as the traumas of adolescence are passed. When the individual values the body and acts to preserve and protect it, the body image becomes a basis for more secure feelings about the self. Comparison with others is an important issue during this time. A good body image strengthens the self-concept. Men generally rate taller and bigger as desirable. Women have traditionally been conditioned to seek the approval of men for their appearance (Murray & Zentner, 1979).

Self-Ideal. The *self-ideal* is the part of the self concept that puts together the individual's perception of how he or she should behave given a set of personal standards (Stuart & Sundeen, 1983). The self-ideal is the person one wishes at one's best. It is not only what one wishes to be, but also one's perception of what others wish one to be. The self-ideal is based on norms of society, age group, culture, educations, and one's own standards. One's self-ideal may be realistic, based on goal expectations and abilities, or unrealistic, which leads to anxiety and feelings of failure. The young adult comes to terms with individual abilities and goals and directs life toward a specific outcome. By maintaining a realistic self-ideal, the young adult sets goals neither too high nor too low and thus nourishes the self-concept.

Self-Esteem.   The part of the self-concept that deals with how one feels about the self is *self-esteem.* The self-esteem of the young adult is high. One is at the peak of life. One can do what one wants, when one wants to, for the first time in one's life. The decisions are one's alone. If a young adult has had successes in earlier life, he or she faces this period of life with optimism. High self-esteem is the result of believing in one's self. It increases with age but begins to stabilize as one reaches maturity.

When a person sets a goal and reaches that goal, this increases self-esteem. Making the team, passing an examination, getting a date, landing that first job, getting a driver's license are examples of events that increase one's self-esteem. It is also increased when a seemingly insurmountable obstacle is conquered and one does not give in to defeat. Self-esteem comes from within the person.

Role Assumption.   *Roles* are socially accepted behaviors associated with a job or title. The young adult tries many different jobs, recreational activities, community activities, and social functions during the beginning of early adulthood.

One of the roles of the family is to prepare the next generation for its role in society (Tinkham & Voorhies, 1977). The roles must be congruent with the roles of society if this purpose is to be fulfilled. The values of the community are inherent guidelines that families use in role assignment.

Decisions about roles made in early life can be changed. This is not an easy concept for a young adult to comprehend. All things seem possible in the twenties. As the person moves into the thirties, commitments are made, broken, or renewed, and this becomes the age of changes and expansions in life's horizons (Sheehy, 1976). As the thirties come to a close, one finds a mature adult ready to face the challenge of tomorrow knowing that the roles he or she has chosen are the ones that will help him or her fulfill life goals. Some of the roles common to this age period are listed in Table 9–3. One holds many roles at one time, so it is highly possible that roles can become confused.

Sexuality.   Sexuality of the individual encompasses more than physical intimacy. The psychosocial development in human sexuality is concerned with sexual identity, which includes awareness of gender identity and gender roles. In American society sex-role stereotyping has led to conflicts that are being addressed in today's social movements. Sex roles have become less rigid since the 1970s (Woods, 1984).

Calhoun and Acocella (1978) describe young adulthood as a period of maximum sexual self-consciousness. It is during this phase, according to Sigmund Freud (Freedman, Kaplan, & Sadock, 1976), that the individual strives to achieve the first phase of sexual genital maturity. Physiological maturation of systems of genital

TABLE 9–3. ROLES OF THE YOUNG ADULT

1. Worker	10. Student
2. Boyfriend or girlfriend	11. Peer group participant
3. Mate (husband/wife)	12. Friend
4. Offspring (son/daughter)	13. Peer
5. Sibling (sister/brother)	14. Teacher
6. Grandchild	15. Mentor
7. Aunt/uncle	16. Religious group member
8. Cousin	17. Civic club member
9. Father/mother	18. Team member

functioning and attendant hormonal systems leads to intensification of drives (Freedman, Kaplan, & Sadock, 1976). Erikson (1968) states that the body and mind must be masters of the organ, which means that even though one is physically capable of sexual relationships, one must stop and think before acting.

During the young adult years premarital intercourse is prevalent (Woods, 1984). The effects of premarital intercourse differs with the individual. More people now judge the acceptability of sexual behavior on the basis of the amount of affection in the relationship.

Evidence points to a heightened freedom of expression and pleasure in married people's sexual relationship not present in sexual relationships without commitment (Delora, Warren, & Ellison, 1981). There is still some question as to the contribution of a good sexual relationship to the overall success of a marriage. Some women do not want to risk losing their sexual inhibition because they worry about what their husbands will think of them (Delora et al., 1981).

Assuming the role of parent can affect a person's attitude about sexuality. Generally people become less permissive after the birth of a child (Schell, 1975). Women oftentimes do not feel sexual after childbirth. For many women the baby becomes the love object and replaces the husband (Still, 1986). There are different ways to express sexuality during pregnancy and after childbirth. There are different levels of desire, all of which are normal and acceptable. Communication of these desires will bring a couple closer together (Colman, 1977).

A young adult's sexuality depends on many factors. They include: early conditioning, attitudes of family, significant others, friends, level of maturity, and hormones. Feelings about oneself as a sexual being, body image, and self-concept also affect sexuality. Changes occur with the passage of time and can cause changes in sexuality. Sexuality is intangible. It encompasses many modes of sexual expression that are left to the individual's preference.

Interpersonal Relationships

Interpersonal relationships are primarily a result of experiences with others as one grows. Sometimes the young adult finds he or she is propelled into a world of social activity because of college, career, chosen life-style, or locale.

There is a tendency for young adults to postpone marriage in favor of career or education. According to Dion (1984) in the Bureau of the Census Report, the number of young adults living in nonfamily households (persons living alone or sharing homes with someone who was not a relative) was 21.2 million. This is an increase from 11.9 million reported in 1970.

Significant Others.   While the striving for intimacy is profound for the young adult (Erikson, 1968), sexual intimacy is only part of what the young adult seeks. Interpersonal relationships with peers and significant others (parents, sexual partners, marriage partners) encompass many relationships vital to the young adult. These people have a profound importance in one's life. Significant others are loved, hated, feared, wanted, and depended on in time of need. There is as much concern with the other's feelings and needs as with one's own.

Harry Stack Sullivan (Freedman et al., 1976) points out that significant others change through the years. The interpersonal relationships formed through the years are the basis of security. The young adult will continue to develop or delete relationships as they fill a need in life.

The first sense of stagnation and discontent occurs around age 28–33 (Sheehy, 1976). Relationships are reassessed, and earlier decisions and commitments to such entities as work, play, society, oneself, and family relationships are changed or intensified.

Parents.   Parents and the young adult continue to try to maintain good relationships. It is a challenge when family tasks conflict with individual tasks. Often parents use their financial resources to control their children. Sometimes parents find it difficult to accept the young adult's need for emotional independence. During this time, young adults may seem uncaring about parental relationships. They seem to be insensitive to parents' needs to maintain contact. While developing their own intimate relationships, they do not "need" parents. This is part of the maturing process. A balance between the two families will be reached through patience, caring, and consistency of the openness of the parents to accept the young adult. The parent may have to be the one to initiate the contacts for a while. A mature relationship is possible, but parents must be willing to support the separation (Schenk & Schenk, 1978).

Sexual Relationships.   Erik Fromm (1956) states that a sexual relationship is the major self-actualizing function that mitigates the feelings of aloneness that accompanies being human. Young adults have a biological need to be sexually intimate. It relieves loneliness. The sexual interaction of two close, caring people is highly symbolic and expressive. Sexual relationships and sexual performance continue to be important concerns during adulthood.

The opportunity for meeting other young adults and selecting a sexual partner varies with the individual's sex, occupation, area of residence, and personal attractiveness.

Availability according to marital status is exemplified by Table 9–4. Thus one

TABLE 9–4. MARITAL STATUS, U.S. ADULTS AGES 20–40

	Age (yr)	Percent				Total
		Single	*Married*	*Widowed*	*Divorced*	
Males	(20–24)	74.8	23.5	—	1.6	100.0
	(25–29)	37.8	56.8	.1	5.3	100.0
	(30–34)	20.9	69.8	.1	9.1	100.0
	(35–40)	9.5	80.1	.3	10.0	100.0
Females	(20–24)	56.9	39.4	.1	3.6	100.0
	(25–29)	25.9	65.6	.6	7.9	100.0
	(30–34)	13.3	74.2	.8	11.6	100.0
	(35–40)	6.6	77.5	21.0	13.8	100.0

From U.S. Department of Commerce, Bureau of Census (1986). Statistical abstract of U.S. (106th ed.). Washington, DC: Bureau of Census.

can see that as age increases for a female, the availability of eligible males decreases. Females tend to be widowed at an earlier age. More females are divorced in the 20–40 age group.

An upper-middle-class male who lives in an apartment house in a large urban area is most likely to find many opportunities for either casual or committed sexual relationships. The person with the least chance to have a meaningful sexual relationship is an older female with a low income living in a small town or rural area (Delora et al., 1981).

A type of sexual relationship that has been thrust into the public eye in the past 10 years is that of homosexuality. Although the "gay movement" has been popularized, it is estimated that only 10% of the population lead homosexual life-styles. Of this estimated 10%, about 6% are male and 4% female. Only 1% of the 10% make no conscious effort to hide their homosexuality. Two percent to three percent are exclusively homosexual (Fromer, 1983). One homosexual relationship does not make a person homosexual. Some young adults classify themselves as bisexual (enjoying sex with both male and female partners.)

The young adult involved in sexual activity should consider the possibility of pregnancy. Although mechanisms for preventing reproduction have been known for centuries, it is only recently that technologies to separate the recreative from the procreative aspects of sex have been available in the American society (Woods, 1984). They include the following, listed in Table 9–5.

When selecting a contraceptive, individuals and couples will want to consider these factors: cost, effectiveness, ease of use, risks or disadvantages. Oral contraceptives (birth control pills) are one of the most widely used and effective methods available. When taken correctly, oral contraceptives are 98–99% effective (Cupit, 1984). Other methods (see Table 9–5) range between 70 and 80% in effectiveness. The newest forms of contraceptives, the cervical cap and the sponge, have been available in the United States market for only a few years, and their complete effectiveness has

TABLE 9–5. COMMON FORMS OF CONTRACEPTION

Mechanical	Chemical	Behavioral	Sterilization
Condom	Spermicidal foam,	Abstinence	Vasectomy
Diaphragm	cream, or gel	Rhythm	Tubal ligation
Sponge	Hormonal-oral (pill)	Coitus interruptus	
	Spermicidal	Celibacy	
	suppository		

not yet been determined. Sexual relationships and sexual performance continue to be important concerns during adulthood.

Marriage and Mate Selection.   Rubin (1973), in his study of young adults and the people they marry, found that men fall in love more quickly than women, tend to be more satisfied with the woman's qualities, and to be more romantic. Rubin (1973) found young adult women to be more selective. They tend to be more practical about whom they marry.

In the Census Report of 1986, 45% of those 18–34 years old were married and had their own households. The census found that a male was 24.1 years old before his first marriage, while the median age was 22.3 for women. This represents a rise from 1970 when the median for males was 22.5 and females was 20.6. This rise in the age of both sexes is attributed to a stronger desire to pursue advanced education and to be higher on the corporate ladder before marriage.

Marriage is being recognized as a close, loving partnership between two people rather than as a social institution where the man is the head of the house and the wife is a childbearer (Murray & Zentner, 1979). Marriage provides opportunities in four areas: sexuality, birth and rearing children, domestic and economic services, and property. It is recognized as the socially accepted way for two people to live together and be intimate. However, marriage is not required for today's young adults to have the same opportunities.

Marriage is not a state but a process (Willi, 1982). It demands the courage to allow real growth and change that may put one's freedom at risk. Marriage can last an entire lifetime. Marriage passes through different stages, over a period of time, as human beings live together.

During this time, couples encounter the inevitable hurdles and face the complexities of true human need. No two people can correlate all of their developmental needs, but must be willing through communication, mutual respect, and desire to work through problems and let each partner grow according to his or her own developmental time line.

The first years of married life are generally the most active in the relationship. During this period the couple establishes an identity as a couple, establishes their place in society, and makes many decisions that will give their marriage definite form (Willi, 1982).

When children become part of the family, the couple's relationship undergoes a major transformation. The couple no longer has much time alone to direct their attention only to themselves. The period of exclusive intimacy comes to an end. Sometimes jealousies develop between partners as attention is turned toward children.

During the next 20 years, marriage partners may grow apart. Because the children have grown up, there is no urgent necessity for prolonging the marriage. The partners may need to decide whether or not it is worthwhile to continue.

Establishing a Home.   No matter what kind of living arrangement is made, there are a number of factors that go into starting a home. In today's society young adults have many choices about the people with whom they share their home. Choices of young adult living partners are included in Table 9–6.

Management of resources is of top priority. Many problems stem from inherited attitudes about money. They are: who handles the money; do they have a joint bank account or is it separate; who pays the bills; who makes major purchases; and plans for the future. Discussion before marriage will help allay some of the frustration.

Division of labor is another important area. Decisions are made about sharing home responsibilities. Who will make the beds, buy groceries, cook, clean, and do the laundry needs to be discussed. If the wife does not work outside the home, she will probably do these chores. If she does have a career, the couple will divide these tasks. Another choice is an outside-of-family person (housekeeper) to help with these necessary jobs. If another living arrangement is made (see Table 9–6), these decisions will still have to be made.

Couples also need to make a decision about birth control and number of children. Control of family size permits women to enter the work world with its greater opportunity for new relationships and self-actualization.

As a home is established, marriage partners will find there is a need to establish themselves as a pair, become better communicators with each other, decide how their life will be lived (goals and priorities), share problems, give mutual support, and encourage each other's self-actualization. All living arrangements will have an element of the tasks necessary for establishing a home.

Starting a family is usually a high priority. According to Duvall (1977), in American society most couples have a year or two before the child arrives. Becoming a mother or father has an important effect on both partners and demands major

TABLE 9–6. CHOICES OF LIVING PARTNERS OF YOUNG ADULTS

1. Traditional marriage
2. Cohabitation with male or female friend
3. Living together without marriage
4. Housemate
5. Commune living
6. Living alone

readjustments in the marital relationship (Schell, 1975). Before parenthood, there is but one relationship—husband and wife. After the first child arrives and with all subsequent children, there is an increase in family relationships and responsibilities. It does not seem to be the number of children a couple has or the spacing that is crucial to marital happiness, but that the couple have the number they want (Schell, 1975).

In 1984, the number of family households with children was 50.1%; the number of married couples was 48.6%, male householder was 39.4% and female householder was 59.8% (Statistical Abstract, 1986). This shows that there are parents who raise children virtually alone. This also means that the single parent has a heavy role assumption. These single parents must assume economic functioning, household responsibilities, authority, psychological support, and social interaction for the remaining members. Since the mother usually, but not always, is awarded custody of the children, she will usually be the one to have this responsibility (Duvall, 1977). A more in-depth discussion of family tasks is reflected in the chapters for age groups of children.

Extended Family and Support Systems. The family of the young adult continues to expand to include in-laws and new babies. Friends seem to multiply as one moves about more freely. Neighbors become a source of support because of commonalities shared. Sometimes an older neighbor becomes a surrogate parent. Young adults expand their world as they meet new people through the workplace. As adults begin to establish a self-concept and interface with society, this frees them to care about others.

Competency and Achievement

As the young adult progresses toward achievement, he or she will incorporate an inherited belief about education. If education is important to a job or seen as a way to become socially mobile, it will be an important aspect of life, and the young adult will pursue it through higher degrees or continuing education programs. There are many opportunities for young adults in the workplace. They are not restricted to certain jobs because of gender or stereotyping. Many young adults find themselves pursuing careers that a few years ago did not exist. (Examples: female lumberjills and increased number of men in nursing.) Some seem to know exactly what they want, while others try many options before they decide. Whatever the choice, the chances are that with motivation, intelligence, perseverance, and a little luck, one can achieve desired goals.

Intellectual Skills. Learning, memory, and performance of motor skills are usually at their peak. This is a time of maximum flexibility to form new concepts, shift the way one thinks, and solve problems. Creativity (finding unique and original solutions to problems) is heightened during this period (Schell, 1975).

Parenting Skills. Most young adults are not prepared either emotionally or intellectually for the responsibility of children. Parenting is a challenging experience. It involves facing the unknown with hope, because no one can predict the outcomes of human relationships. Parents grow by taking each day at a time and realizing the joy that can be a part of the years. Parenting skills are learned from a variety of sources. The family of origin, childbirth classes, and books on parenting are only a few ways the young adult learns about parenting. Generally, there is no formal continual educative process that will aid adults as they parent. Parenting is mostly through experience and belief in one's own judgment.

Society and Culture

The young adult begins to take an active interest in civic responsibility. He or she becomes a member of civic groups, i.e., Lions Club, Rotary Club, Jaycees, or takes on the responsibility of volunteer fireman, police or civil defense, or Red Cross. He or she may become a leader of Girl Scouts or Boy Scouts, Campfire Girls, Little League baseball, football, or other groups. Many adults look upon these activities as a way to return to the community some of the nurturing experiences that helped him or her to grow.

Young adults have a renewed sense of pride in differences. It is no longer mandatory to be like everyone else, as it once was in the teenage years. A pride in ethnic, religious, and class differences emerges.

POTENTIAL STRESSORS

There are many potential stressors in the life of a young adult. Much of this is due to the great number of changes the young adult encounters. Change is a complex phenomenon and brings with it new desires, goals, and responsibilities. Changes at this time include deciding on a career, independence, where to live, new relationships, money, food, clothing, getting married, becoming parents, and many more. Most young adults manage these stresses fairly well. Some see them as a part of growing up and are willing to take the bad with the good. Many view these changes as an exciting challenge.

Physical Stressors

This group of stressors includes acute and chronic illnesses. Young adults are susceptible to many physical diseases. They will have their share of accidents that will significantly change their lives. It is during this age period that surgery will be a major stressor in many lives. Each group of physical stressors will have an impact on body image, work responsibilities, interpersonal relationships, and self-esteem. Physical stress may accelerate the young adult's worrying about the future because of the responsibilities of raising a family. Most young adults, however, are relatively healthy and lead productive lives.

Some physical stressors are from deprivation of normal health needs such as rest, nutrition, and exercise. As young adults' activities accelerate, their need for sleep also increases. One can adjust to short periods of interrupted rest and sleep, but prolonged periods can contribute to physical problems such as fatigue, malaise, or lethargy. Lack of sleep can also slow a person down on the job, which may cause accidents and psychological stress.

Nutritional problems in young adults frequently stem from their life-styles. Because of increased activity they forget to eat or do not take the time to eat a meal of the basic four food groups. Poor nutrition can lead to a lessening of physical stamina, which may lead to illness.

Exercise serves several purposes in the young adult's life. It helps control appetite, release tension, and aid sleep. A sedentary life-style can lead to problems of elimination, weakened muscles, and fatigue.

Pregnancy.   Due to the growth of the fetus, the woman's body undergoes many physical changes. As her body enlarges, she may have backaches, varicose veins, hemorrhoids, edema, and cramps (Quilligan, 1983). These conditions may make her uncomfortable. She also experiences an increase in blood volume and cardiac output, change in respiratory pattern, and a lengthening of the ureters and urethra (which contributes to the development of cystitis).

Accidents.   Motor vehicle accidents can cause serious injury or death. Accidents such as falling down the steps, breaking an arm, or tripping over a rug will incapacitate the young adult. This leads to further frustration due to loss of time on the job and money. Industrial accidents and drowning also rank high as major causes of accidents (Murray & Zentner, 1979). Other injuries such as dislocations, abrasions, fractures, and lacerations put stress on the young adult's performance.

Diseases.   For the young adult this is a period of maximum health. Their bodies are healthy, and the contagious diseases of childhood (chicken pox, mumps, measles) are behind them. However, there are some diseases that may be present when younger and continue to need care into the young adult years. There are also some diseases that will appear during this time and cause physical stress. This category includes diabetes, heart disease, Addison's disease, bacterial infections, mononucleosis, and asthma. These are only a few of the diseases found in the young adult. Some of these are discussed further in the section on alterations in health.

Smoking.   Smoking is a habit that most young adults have begun earlier in life. Smoking can become a physical stressor when it causes problems in the respiratory system. Since the Surgeon General's warning that cigarette smoking can be dangerous to a person's health, there has been a concerted effort to help people stop smoking. This habit can be costly. It is becoming socially unacceptable to smoke in public in today's society.

Work. This is a period of heightened excitement about work. The young adult is responsible for his or her economic welfare and that of others. In an effort to get ahead, the young adult becomes a workaholic (concentrating on or spending time at work in excess of requirements for employment). Young adults are sometimes blocked in their need to achieve, and frustrations may be manifested by headaches, stomachaches, fatigue, and restlessness. If the job is not satisfactory, a quest for a different one will cause the young adult a period of uncertainty. This may heighten the physical signs of frustration.

Social-Emotional Stressors

A completely safe society is one in which no choice is possible (Schenk & Schenk, 1978). Today one finds himself or herself in the midst of choices and change. Change is a major stressor. The risks are tremendous, but so are the chances for self-actualization. Societal changes occur when the rules of conduct break down, social controls become meaningless, and relationships become confused or unacceptable. These changes cause confusion and need to be understood by the young adult. Emotional stressors are those caused by the inner needs of the young adult. They include passions, love, anger, hate, fear, and anxiety. Biological changes such as rapid heart beat, increased respiratory activity, vasomotor reactions, and changes in muscle tone may result from emotional stress.

Careers. Society has accepted a woman's right to enter the work force. Fifty-one percent of married women were in the labor force in 1982 (FYI/Reports, 1984), up from 14% in 1940. Wives have boosted their family's incomes, and 49% of mothers of preschool children were working in 1982 (FYI/Reports, 1984). The U.S. Dept. of Commerce Bureau of Census (1986) report shows that women accounted for 59% of the increase in the labor force. It also reported that college enrollment for women 25 to 34 tripled between 1970 and 1984.

Divorce. The divorce rate is very high in the American society. In the U.S. Department of Commerce *Statistical Abstract of U.S.* (1986), the divorce rate is 4.9% per 1000 people. This is a decrease from the 1979 and 1981 reports, in which divorce was at its highest—5.3% per 1000 people. The median age at divorce after first marriage was 33.6 years of age for males and 31.1 years of age for females. The median duration for a first marriage was 7.0 years. This shows that young adults may wonder about the permanance of relationships because of the high divorce rate in today's society.

The divorce rate seems to be falling. The decrease in divorce rate is probably due to many factors. According to Leo (1984), a gradual shift toward conservatism is underway. During the early 1970s, marriage, motherhood, and the family were not popular with counterculture feminists and radicals. By the late 1970s marriage became more attractive to the women of that generation. Women came to see that job, family, and freedom could be combined and the trend began to shift toward marriage and family. Seventy percent of young divorcees remarry within 5 years after divorce (Delora et al., 1981).

An uncertain economy may have played a part in the new conservatism. No cause-and-effect relationship has been demonstrated, but sex therapists say that sexual permissiveness seems to follow the stock market (Leo, 1984). Another factor may have been the "de-establishment of a person's belief system" (Leo, 1984) brought about by the Vietnam war. The end of the war and the onset of a recession brought the system back to more stability.

Remarriage.   In the United States, 60–70% of younger divorced women remarry within 5 years (FYI/Reports, 1984). Remarriage, adapting to change, is a challenge. The acquisition of a new mate brings with it new step relatives and ready-made ("blended") families. Divorce rates after the second marriage are as high or higher than after first marriages (FYI/Reports, 1984). Fears about marrying the same kind of man or woman, marrying for security, not love; marrying because one is lonely and someone finally asked you to marry—all these put tremendous stress in the form of worry, guilt, and unworthiness on the individual.

Abortion.   The term *therapeutic abortion* was coined during the Supreme Court decision in 1973 (Quilligan, 1983), which made abortions legal in the United States. Abortion may be spontaneous or induced expulsion of the product of conception before the fetus is legally viable. Therapeutic abortion is now one of the safest procedures done in the United States (Quilligan, 1983). The dilemma for the young adult is termination of pregnancy versus an unwanted child. A new societal dimension, legality and acceptance of abortion, has been added to the decision problem.

The psychological stress placed on an individual or a couple deciding to terminate a pregnancy is immeasurable. According to the CDC Report (Atrash, Rhodenhiser, Hogue, & Smith, 1986) in 1983, the national abortion rate was 24 legal abortions per 1000 women. The women tended to be young, white, and unmarried, with no history of live births.

External Crises.   Gerald Caplan defines situational crises as chance events that are viewed by the person as unpredictable (Burgess, 1981). An example of a situational crisis is unexpected loss.

Loss of a part of the body can affect body image. Loss of a job, a partner, family unit, or possessions, or loss by death can deal a blow to the individual that causes major stress. Every loss takes time to get over, and according to Kübler-Ross (1969), the person must take certain steps before grief can be resolved. Loss is individualized. What may seem insignificant to one person may constitute a major loss to another. Sometimes with a loss comes a strength the individual did not know he or she possessed. Loss is definitely a challenge for the individual and family.

Boredom. As the young adult begins to settle into a routine, life may become boring. Young adults may feel goals have been accomplished and that life is passing them by. After a year or two of marriage, boredom in the relationship may become a problem. It can be a major cause of communication breakdown, especially as children grow and become the focus of attention. A certain amount of monotony is inevitable as one settles into habits and routines. Boredom can also occur with other aspects of life.

Adaptation to Family Structure. A husband and wife and other people living together have distinct personalities. Building a life together can be challenging. It can also lead to intense stress. Communication may be blocked, and values, beliefs, goals, and desires will have to be defined. Living together will have its rewards, but it will also demand that changes take place.

Changes in Family Structure. Changes in family structure can be caused by either the addition or deletion of members. The nuclear family (father, mother, and their children) are sometimes alienated from their kin because a parent's job moves them to a distant destination. They may feel isolated from the extended family, who can give material and social support. When a young parent needs help with children, he or she can feel very stressed. If relatives are close by and can help, it is very rewarding for the young parent.

Addition of in-laws in a common adjustment for the young adult. The classic rivalry pattern is seen as being between the mother-in-law and son-in-law. However, the most destructive rivalry is between the mother-in-law and the daughter-in-law. These women vie for the affection of the son from the first day the son's relationship becomes serious. If they realize that there are two kinds of love at work here, the relationship may be salvaged. The mother wants her son to marry and be happy. She cannot, however, relinquish her caring for her son overnight just because another woman has entered his life. The daughter-in-law may see the mother as her enemy. Mother has no interest in the eros type of love her son has for his new wife. Mother is proud he is married and looks forward to grandchildren. If the two women involved are educated about the dynamics of this love-hate relationship, a stronger bond can be built in the family, and the potentially stressful situation can be avoided.

Some young adults find themselves living with their parents. Because of the economic stressors of today's society, a job with enough money to pay for an apartment or house may not be feasible. Clear lines of responsibility need to be established with the young adult having as much freedom over his or her activities as possible. The need to establish an independent household remains important.

Conflicts with Family Tasks

Each family will have different areas of strengths and weaknesses. They will also have differences in their ability to function and coping mechanisms.

Conflicts arise when the family cannot get its needs met or when priorities conflict. The basic needs of maintaining adequate shelter, nutrition, and health can be a struggle depending upon the economic resources of the family. Budgets, cleaning, cooking, yard work, and all tasks of daily living are potential conflict for families (Burgess, 1981).

Teaching children the skills of daily living and helping them grow in their abilities to meet the demands and stresses of society requires support and compromise. Other areas of conflict may be with helping children form friendships, playing sports, taking music lessons, and traveling. As the child grows, readjusting space and resources take on a new dimension. Family-of-origin tasks (see Table 9–1) can cause conflicts for the family that has a young adult who is embarking on a life of his or her own.

As marriage partners struggle to have open communication and continue sexual intimacy, conflicts can arise as pressures mount. One partner may be absorbed by work, and the other may be preoccupied by family responsibilities. The family's ability to resolve conflicts while at the same time meeting the needs of its members is a never-ending task and responsibility for all family members.

COPING MECHANISMS

Coping mechanisms, according to Stuart and Sundeen (1983), can be either constructive or destructive. They can be constructive when a stressor is treated as a warning signal and the person accepts it as a challenge (Hagerty, 1984). Destructive coping mechanisms are used to protect oneself from positive resolution. The coping mechanism that helps the person successfully deal with a stressor is the one usually chosen over and over.

Health Beliefs and Behaviors

Health beliefs and behaviors are learned from experience, family, and culture. Swanson and Hurley (1983) believe that individuals and families need to pay more attention to the context of cultural values. They state that the individual is oriented to values, acquires particular values, and applies them to life situations from his or her cultural group. These values are brought to all relationships and behaviors.

Some of the health beliefs that are associated with relief of a stress include masturbation, exercise, vitamins, and diet. Values concerning sexual activities change with transforming social conditions (Woods, 1984). Several values that have remained constant in American culture are the incest taboo (sex between family members) and forbidden sex between adults and children. In American culture romantic love and sexual expressions are intertwined. Beliefs about contraception, abortion, and size of family add other dimensions to the health care of young adults.

These are but a few of the values and beliefs that shape the beliefs of the young adult. Each one must deal with his or her own set of beliefs. How the young adult deals with these beliefs will shape the life-style he or she will live. Each young adult will have to define for himself or herself what optimum health means and how to accomplish it. The young adult will find access to the health care system when the need arises. The system used will be the one that has always been used by the family of origin (clinic, private physician, i.e., family doctor, emergency room, or medical centers). Eventually young adults will choose the medical system that services them best.

Responses to Stressors

Adaptive Responses.   There are many successful ways to cope with stressors. The young adult can respond in an adaptive way by making a realistic appraisal of the stress.

An adaptive coping mechanism will include: (1) appraisal of the stressor, (2) naming the actual threat, (3) seeing it as a challenge and making a plan to overcome the stress, (4) mastery of the stress. One must be capable of insight and be able to accept reality. Acknowledging the stress may be the most difficult part of all. Some strategies for coping are shown in Table 9–7. It is important to note that each person will have his or her own unique way of coping.

Maladaptive Responses.   There are many maladaptive coping responses used by the young adult. Maladaptive coping responses are listed in Table 9–8.

Maladaptive coping strategies are manifested in individual ways, and a young adult may use a combination of strategies to deal with the stress.

Abuse. A maladaptive response that is commanding much attention in today's society is child abuse (Thorman, 1980). An abusive episode has three stages: (1) building of tension, (2) outburst of physical or emotional assault, and (3) a period when the abuser demonstrates remorse and loving behavior toward the victim (Schultz & Dark, 1986). Child abuse seems to be a product of psychological tension and external stress, which affects all families at all social levels (Newberger, 1977). The abuser is characterized as having low self-esteem, being dependent and socially isolated, lacking trust, and having dysfunctional personal relationships (Schultz, 1986).

TABLE 9–7. STRATEGIES OF COPING

1. Talking it out with partner, friend, or family
2. Emotional response: crying, laughing
3. Physical activity (exercise)
4. Reappraising and reordering priorities in work and private life
5. Confronting the stress
6. Working it off by doing tasks
7. Seeking professional guidance
8. Spending money
9. Enhancing problem-solving skills
10. Using biofeedback
11. Using defense mechanisms
12. Being flexible

TABLE 9–8. MALADAPTIVE RESPONSES

1. Psychiatric disorders (depression, anxiety, stress)
2. Withdrawing from the problem
3. Somatizing (complaints about the body)
4. Suicide (attempted)
5. Over- or under-eating
6. Taking illegal drugs
7. Rebelling against authority
8. Losing control of one's temper
9. Isolating oneself from family and friends
10. Chemical abuse (alcohol and cigarettes)
11. Abuse of wife, husband, or child and elderly

The number of victims is difficult to determine. It is estimated that there are over 1.5 million cases in a year. Approximately 1000 children die each year from physical abuse (Thorman, 1980).

Wife abuse is also prevalent in the American society. Each year over a million women are slapped, kicked, shoved, or brutally beaten by the men in their lives (Weingourt, 1979). A recent Harris poll shows that 20% of all Americans approve of hitting a spouse on appropriate occasions (Weingourt, 1979). An example of the cycle of abuse is that the husband accuses the wife of not being faithful; he brutally beats her; he begs her not to leave him and promises never to hit her again. She returns home and waits for it to start all over again.

Gelles (1979) states that women do not break off these relationships because: (1) they have negative self-concepts, (2) they believe their husbands will reform, (3) economic hardship, (4) they have children who need a father's support, (5) they doubt they can live without him, (6) they do not believe in divorce, and (7) it is difficult for a woman with children to get a job. For whatever reason, wife abuse is on the rise in the American society (Schultz & Dark, 1986).

NURSING ASSESSMENT

The use of a structured framework for assessing the young adult will enable the nurse to consider the myriad of activities and stressors which impinge upon task accomplishment. Table 9–9 indicates priority areas of assessment.

TABLE 9–9. ASSESSING THE FAMILY OF A YOUNG ADULT

Environmental Data
Living conditions: type of dwelling, maintenance, availability of necessities, hazardous conditions, number of occupants, type of neighborhood
Family size: relationship of member(s) to individual, roles/contributions to family

Communication Patterns
Within family: verbal and nonverbal patterns, maladaptive/inappropriate responses, member that young adult perceives as most responsive
With society: family member that interacts most with society, business communicative skills

TABLE 9–9. ASSESSING THE FAMILY OF A YOUNG ADULT *(continued)*

Problem-Solving Skills

Decision making: use of systematic approach, major decision maker(s), responses by other members
Use of health care system: recognition of need, access to system, frequency of use, cost, compliance to health regimen
Support from significant others: viewed as positive or negative, areas of strongest/weakest support (as viewed by young adult and as viewed by nurse)
Societal interaction: use of agencies, ability to deal with or circumvent the system as appropriate

Life-Style

Role within family: young adults view of self within family, view of own roles, view of roles of other member(s)
Socioeconomic status: estimated yearly income, young adult's estimation of adequacy, use of other financial assistance, direction of SES mobility
Work patterns: number of wage earners in family, amount of work hours per day, anticipated job change, amount of job satisfaction
Recreational activities: use of free time, amount of planned activities per month, amount of time spent in recreation/leisure by each family member, amount of group recreation
Personal health care: usual eating habits, usual amount of sleep, use of tobacco, alcohol, drugs, over-the-counter medications, exercise regimen
Safety: use of safety features at home and work, young adult's knowledge of accident prevention, first aid, poison control, visible hazards around home

Potential Stressors

Interferences with developmental tasks: role conflict, individual and family goals, current health status, potential for unrecognized problems
Conflicts with society: individual involvement with society, perception of social support system, societal influence on personal/family goals
Response patterns: ability to cope, problem solve, and prioritize, communication patterns within family and with society, approaches to meeting goals, use of professional health services, presence of maladaptive responses

Excellent assessment skills are essential because a missed point may be the key to the problem. One needs a quiet place, free from interruption, to do an assessment. Sometimes nurses leave an assessment for an aide or nursing assistant to do. This should be a priority of the nurse, since he or she is educated to do the assessment.

ALTERATIONS IN HEALTH

There are many physical health problems that can cause an alteration in the health of the young adult. The acute problems are those that require immediate attention. They are, according to Thomas (1985), sharp, severe, having a rapid onset, severe symptoms and short course.

Chronic illnesses are confirmed, habitual, deep-rooted, persistent, of long duration, and require continuing care (Clayton, 1985). They tend to show little change or be of slow progress. They make major changes in the young adult. The person may require constant care for the rest of his or her life. These illnesses can cause major alterations in life-style.

Acute Alterations in Health

Accidents and Injuries.   Motor vehicle accidents are the most prevalent accidents in the 20–24-year-old age group. Because motor vehicle accidents affect the young disproportionately, injuries from these accidents are the third leading cause of death (*Mortality & Morbidity Weekly Reports* [MMWR], 1986).

Young adults are people on the go. They are traveling to and from work, home, school, and social events much of the time. With the increase in travel time comes an increased chance of car accidents. Swimming, motorcycle accidents, and work accidents are traumas that may alter a life-style. Sports injuries are a problem because the young adult is very active physically at this point in life, and is at the peak of physical condition. These injuries cause much pain and suffering for the young adult. Many hours of lost work time are attributed to accidents. Recurring problems from accidents lead to stress for the young adult (Luckman & Sorensen, 1980). The return to health from these accidents depends on the extent of the injury, successful treatment, the will to live, and family support.

Respiratory Conditions.   Acute conditions of the upper respiratory tract, infection, and influenza occur more frequently in the young adult than do other acute illnesses (Luckman & Sorensen, 1980). The MMWR (1986) show respiratory illnesses to be the tenth largest cause of deaths in the United States. The cause could be related to poor health practices, which include inadequate rest, sleep, exercise, and nutrition. They could also be contracted through excessive smoking, unnecessary chills, and environmental pollutants. These infections include the common cold, influenza, pneumonia, and acute bronchitis.

The young adult should be encouraged to see a health care provider when any of these illnesses arise. They can be treated with medication and proper nutrition, rest, and hydration.

Infertility.   Infertility is an acute condition that demands attention during the childbearing years. According to Woods (1984), 10–14% of American couples of childbearing age are infertile. Most couples presume they can conceive. When they find they cannot, this can become a major loss. Infertility directly involves sexuality. Being infertile affects the way people feel about themselves. Infertility can become a major stressor for the couple. Many women experience the loss of sexual desire when they are infertile, and this can cause a change in the couple's sexual relationship. Today there are many ways to help the infertile couple (Table 9–10).

TABLE 9–10. INTERVENTIONS FOR INFERTILITY[a]

Surgically correcting blockage in the reproduction system
Pharmacological interventions
  Changing present medications that influence sexual potency
  Beginning a series of fertility drugs
Dietary: heavy women sometimes are infertile
Immunological: through condom therapy, the female is shielded from sperm that reduces the antibodies
Endometriosis: this causes the alteration of tubal and ovarian physiology. It accounts for 25–30% of all infertility problems. It is the most common cause of infertility in women over 25 years of age

From: Kistner, R. (1983).

If the interventions listed are unsuccessful, there are other options that can be considered. They include:

1. *In vitro fertilization (IVF):* A woman's egg is surgically removed from her ovary, then fertilized with her husband's sperm under laboratory conditions. Once the egg is successfully fertilized (cell division begins), it is returned to her womb
2. *Artificial insemination by donor (AID):* This has been widely practiced since 1960 (Friedrich, 1984)
3. *Surrogate mothers:* Women who contract to bear babies for other couples, have become more common since the late 1970s.

These practices have many legal and ethical complexities. Although their use has risen sharply since the 1960s, society has yet to define and solve all the problems that belong to the birth revolution. Experts differ on just how optimistic couples should be about having a baby, but much more help for the problem of infertility is now available.

Sexually Transmitted Diseases.   It is estimated that 10 million people in the United States contract one of the sexually transmitted diseases each year (Luckman & Sorensen, 1980). The three diseases most commonly seen are gonorrhea, syphilis, and genital herpes.

Gential herpes has increased in incidence. It is caused by a virus and is treated with Acyclovir in ointment or capsule form to relieve the symptoms. Treatment is begun either with onset of symptoms or continuous as a prophylaxis against outbreaks. Currently there is no cure.

Gonorrhea is one of the oldest known diseases. It is easily transmitted; it has a variable incubation time (usually 3–8 days). Bacteria are the causative agent. In women the most common site is the cervix. The MMWR (1986) shows that it is the number one sexually transmitted disease. Penicillin has been used effectively for 30 years as a cure. However, a strain resistant to penicillin has been discovered (Quilligan, 1983). It is diagnosed by taking material from the cervix of a woman and from the urethra of a man.

Syphilis is the eighth most common notifiable communicable disease in the United States (MMWR, 1986). Its incidence has increased in the past few years. All genital sores (chancres) should be considered syphilitic until proven otherwise. Syphilis is treated with penicillin. If primary syphilis is not treated, it will continue into the secondary stage, when the chancre heals, the person then has no outward symptoms but can still infect others (Delora, et al., 1981). Diagnosis can be made through microscopic examination of fluid of the chancre or a blood test.

The newest sexually transmitted disease is acquired immunodeficiency syndrome (AIDS). The number of people infected in the United States is estimated to be between 1 and 1.5 million. Difficulty with estimation of infected persons is a cause of concern among health care givers. Ninety percent of the victims are 20 to 49 years old; 93% are men, 60% white, 25% black, and 14% Hispanic (MMWR, 1986). Acquired immunodeficiency syndrome is spread through transmission of body fluids (blood, plasma, semen). It can be spread through sexual intercourse, intravenous drug use (dirty needles), blood transfusions, and possibly in other ways not yet documented. There is no evidence, at present, that saliva can transmit the virus so kissing is not a vector.

Homosexual men or bisexuals have the highest risk of acquiring the disease. Consequently, heterosexuals can acquire the disease through sexual contact with an affected person. The risk of AIDS can be lessened through the use of condoms during sex, not using intravenous drugs or sharing needles, knowing your sex partner and reducing the number of sex partners (American College Health Association, 1987). At the time of this writing there is no known cure.

Emotional Adjustment Problems.   This set of acute problems encompasses those problems associated with adjustments to life. They are suicide, depression, and drug abuse. They become life-threatening when clients cannot take care of themselves and forget to eat or drink.

Depression may become a problem for the young adult, particularly between the ages of 25 and 40. It is most common in high achievers, persons who have had recent physical disorders, people exposed to overuse of alcohol and drugs, and people living in crowded conditions. Adults suffering from depression are overwhelmed by feelings of helplessness, hopelessness, and sadness. Theories about depression are many. Depression occurs in all social groups, but is more prevalent in lower socioeconomic groups. It occurs twice as often in women as in men (Lobel & Hirschfeld, 1985).

According to Burgess (1981), men between the ages of 35 and 40 are at the greatest risk for suicide. Women make more attempts, but more successful suicides are done by men. Suicide is the fourth leading cause of death in the United States (MMWR, 1986).

The most common form of attempted suicide is the ingestion of a sedative or hypnotic drug for women and the use of a gun or jumping from high places for men (Aguilera & Messick, 1986). Suicide warning symptoms include depression, loss of appetite, weight loss, inability to sleep, loss of interest, social withdrawal, apathy, and despondency. These people feel so helpless and hopeless they can see no other solution to their problem.

Chemical abuse is an acute problem when it interferes with the ability to perform the tasks of everyday living. The person on drugs begins to forget things. Sometimes people forget when they ate last and become anemic. An overdose of pills or alcohol can cause death. Young adults continue to believe that mind-altering drugs and alcohol are a social aid to relieving stress, therefore allowing them to forget problems. They rarely see drug use as a problem. There is little desire to stop (Rakel & Coon, 1978). Drugs vary widely in their use. Alcohol including beer seems to be the most prevalent followed by cigarettes and marijuana and cocaine (Kandel & Logan, 1984). The age for first-time use of each drug is shown in Table 9–11 (Kandel & Logan, 1984). Although first-time use usually begins before young adulthood, these drugs continue to be used for many years. The use of marijuana and alcohol declines sharply after age 20. Withdrawal from many of these drugs can be dangerous and therefore becomes an acute illness. Substance abuse can become a chronic illness if not caught early.

TABLE 9–11. AGE FOR FIRST-TIME USE OF A DRUG

Drug	Age
Alcohol	15
Cigarettes	19
Marijuana	20
Psychedelics	21
Cocaine	24

From Kandel, D., and Logan, J. (1984). Patterns of drug use from adolescence to young adulthood: Periods of risk for initiation, continued use and discontinuation. American Journal of Public Health, 74(7), 660–665.

Chronic Alterations in Health

Diabetes.   Diabetes is a physical illness which requires the affected person to be careful about diet, exercise, and rest (Phipps, 1983). It can be controlled through diet, oral hypoglycemic agents, or insulin injections. It can produce major permanent disabilities, such as loss of eyesight and impotence in untreated cases.

Diabetes may develop at any age. Many 20–40-year-olds have had diabetes since childhood. Diabetes is a major illness that must be monitored all of a person's life.

Diabetes is usually found in persons over 40 but can be found in young adults (Phipps et al., 1983). It is the thirteenth leading cause of death in all age groups (MMWR, 1986). Diabetes is a complex metabolic disease involving disorders in protein, carbohydrate, and fat metabolism. It causes a change in the body's production of insulin. It is more common in females (Phipps et al., 1983). Diabetes can be a major problem for young adults.

Cancer.   The factors that cause cancer are many and are not fully understood. According to the MMWR (1986), there are over 2,308,000 Americans who died of cancer in 1984. It is the second highest cause of death in the United States.

According to Lewis and Collier (1987) breast cancer is the second most common malignancy in American women. The mortality rate of 27 per 100,000 women has changed only slightly in the last 45 years. Lung cancer is the leading cause of cancer death for men. However, lung cancer is rising sharply among both sexes. Colon–rectal cancer is prevalent in both sexes with leukemia/lymphona following closely behind.

When cancer strikes, it affects everyone within the family system. The individual, with support from the family and physician, will have to make the decision about treatment and how it will effect the rest of life. Cancer is no respector of race, color, or station in life; it is a very feared disease hitting across all age groups and both sexes.

Survival rates have significantly increased due to: (1) better diagnostic techniques, (2) diagnosis at earlier stages before metastasis (spreading) occurs, (3) earlier treatment, (4) new and more sophisticated treatments (chemotherapy, immunotherapy, radiotherapy, and surgery), (5) the public has more knowledge about carcinogens within the environment, (6) education of the public has led them to seek help earlier, and (7) an emphasis on cancer research (Phipps et al., 1983).

Cancer is not just another chronic disease. It evokes many of the deepest fears of mankind. Despite excellent treatment, it can spread throughout the body. It can affect the social and emotional domains, drastically disrupting families. The family with a young adult who has cancer will find each member will be challenged to cope with the havoc cancer can cause (Weisman, 1979).

Sterility. Sterility is a permanent or incurable infertility. There is some hope today for sterile couples, such as in vitro fertilization. Many couples adopt children (Dedonder, 1986). No one knows for certain how many children are adopted in the United States. There is no central government agency that regularly tabulates this information (Feigelman & Silverman, 1983). The individual of the couple who is sterile has a heavy burden placed upon him or her. It requires much understanding, commitment, and communication to keep the marriage strong when sterility is the problem.

Cardiovascular Disease. Heart disease is the leading cause of death throughout the world (Luckman & Sorensen, 1980). Diseases of the heart are the third largest cause of death in the United States (MMWR, 1986). More than 1 million people a year die from cardiovascular ailments (Luckman & Sorenson, 1980). Because of greater understanding of cardiovascular disease and its causes and risks, this area of medicine is one of the most progressive.

Individuals in their 20s and 30s have been known to suffer from coronary heart disease in the form of anginal attacks and myocardial infarctions. Men below the age of 40 are eight times more likely to be stricken than young women. White males die more frequently from cardiovascular heart disease than do nonwhites (Luckman & Sorensen, 1980).

Prognosis for patients with cardiovascular disease is good, but successful rehabilitation will require months and sometimes years of treatment following discharge from the hospital. The overall goal is to help the patient live a full, vital, and productive life within the limits of his or her physical condition.

Hypertension. Hypertension is diagnosed by persons having a persistent blood pressure of over 140/90 (Luckman & Sorensen, 1980). It affects both males and females. It can cause serious health problems if untreated. Hypertension can be aggravated by stress. Consequently, the life-style of the young adult can contribute to the development of hypertension.

Chronic Developmental Diseases. As with other stages of life, the young adult encounters disabling conditions that include mental retardation, cerebral palsy, and motor dysfunction. Employment depends on the level of skills. Epilepsy (abnormal discharge of brain cells) causes seizures in 1 of 50 persons in the United States (Wilgerink, 1979). Eight percent of all seizures are controlled. These problems cause the biggest employment and living problems for the young adult. Many innovative and creative employment opportunities for this group have come to the forefront in recent years. These young adults once were thought only to be burdens. Now with the new opportunities available to them, they lead productive and independent lives (Reichert, 1976).

Alcoholism. Chronic alcoholism is a family disease in the sense that every individual who has the disease has family and friends who suffer along with him or her (Fisk, 1986). Habitual drunkenness has a high cost in terms of human misery. In recent years the concept of alcoholism as a disease has been accepted by society (Minshull, 1985).

According to Clark and Midanik (1981), the percentage of women who drink is highest in the 21–34-year-old age range. Evidence points to the fact that their drinking may be related to reproductive cycles. Heavy drinking by women is more often in response to a buildup of emotional stress and more often precipitated by a crisis (Rakel & Coon, 1978).

Male alcoholics outnumber females. Men usually begin drinking at an early age to relieve inhibitions. It is easy for the young adult male to drift into heavy drinking. Habitual heavy consumption to relieve tensions and anxiety generates more tension and guilt. This is then followed by more drinking. It becomes a vicious cycle. The onset of drinking begins at home with family members, extends to away from home settings with peers and then, in later years, returns to the home setting (Hartford, 1984). Few other drugs have such a variety of harmful effects on nearly all the organ systems of the human body.

Chronic Mental Illness. A population of young adult chronically mentally ill patients who have spent relatively little time in hospitals are now living on the streets in America's cities. The reduction of residents from state hospitals nationwide has contributed to this problem. These young adults carry many labels—schizophrenia, other psychoses, and personality disorders. A reluctance to accept help and acknowledge an ongoing need for medication is the major concern. The work of developing more effective ways of dealing with the young adult chronic patients will be a challenge for the coming decade (Pepper, Kirshner, & Ryglewicz, 1981).

NURSING RESPONSIBILITIES

Health Promotion

Young adults face a variety of situations dealing with themselves and their families each day. These situations cause different reactions in each person, such as fear, anxiety, anger, and frustration. The young adult can be helped to face these emotional arousals by the nurse who is empathetic and concerned with helping him or her maintain wellness.

The nurse can offer continuing education courses that deal with nutrition, emotions, communication, safety, contraception, exercise, and other areas of interest to the young adult. She or he helps the young adult maintain optimum health by teaching skills, disease processes, and recognition of psychological and physical components of stress.

The nurse teaches the young adult ways to cope with problems of the work world, parenting, and maintaining healthy family relationships.

The nurse, by his or her own life, can set an example for others to follow. A nurse who takes care of himself or herself through weight control, regular exercise, working, continuing education, having fun, laughing, being supportive, and religious practice sets a good example. The female nurse can be a role model for peers by showing the way to be a wife, mother, and professional. The increased number of men in nursing helps demonstrate that men are also excellent caregivers and health providers. This brings to nursing a dimension much needed by the profession.

In a professional relationship with the young adult, the nurse needs to be approachable and an active listener. Active listening consists of paying attention to what the person is saying verbally and nonverbally. This encourages the person to believe that one values him or her as a person and encourages disclosure.

The nurse can be a counselor of young adults. Because young adults are involved in achieving independence from their families, many have trouble accepting suggestions from their parents. People outside the home can be very helpful in solving problems by letting young adults have an opportunity to express their ideas and ask questions about the things that interest them. Counseling in health matters such as birth control, losing weight, and interpersonal relationships are examples of problems that can be brought to the nurse. Confidentiality is of prime importance in the nurse–client relationship.

The nurse should be an advocate for the young adult. The nurse can help protect the rights of young adults and ensure that they get the best care possible as clients. The nurse can promote a positive self-concept through self-appraisal, interpersonal relationships, and individual therapy.

When the physical body has matured, one can concentrate on the other areas of maturation for young adults. A regimen of productive measures to maintain optimum health is essential.

Preventive Measures

The goal of primary intervention is general health promotion. Secondary or preventive nursing action is aimed at early recognition and treatment of disease. Through these levels of intervention, the nurse can use expertise and competence to prevent illness (Clayton, 1985). Some of the nurse's actions may include:

- Helping the patient reduce stress by teaching the art of relaxation
- Helping prevent health problems by developing with the patient a regimen to control hypertension. This will be a program of nutrition, exercise, rest, and blood pressure monitoring
- Teaching classes about cessation of smoking, taking drugs, and alcohol consumption
- Teaching women to do breast self-examinations
- Encouraging patients to have regular checkups
- Helping the patient talk positively about himself or herself
- Teaching the patient to be future-oriented by setting goals that are individualized and of interest to a young adult

- Helping the patient avoid or deal with guilt. Guilt about choices made can cause a young adult stress
- Teaching the patient how to give himself or herself permission to have fun and enjoy life. Sometimes the young adult concentrates too much on earning a living
- Letting a patient express feelings about dying at a young age
- Giving support to the young adult's family members as the grief process unfolds

The nurse can be a primary source of referral. With the insight that she or he has into the professional arena, the nurse can refer patients to the most appropriate person to help clients when it is no longer feasible for the nurse to continue treatment. Nurses recognize that not every problem can be solved through nursing. It is at that point that referral takes place. Example: A young divorcee needs to see social services about welfare support.

Acute Caregiver

The nurse acts as an acute caregiver in clinics, hospitals, and doctors' offices. When the young adult is in need of direct care, the nurse provides what is needed. Through this approach the nurse becomes involved as a primary caregiver by: (1) assessment of the problem, (2) development of a plan of care with the patient, (3) putting the plan into action, (4) evaluating its effectiveness. The circadian rhythm (biological clock) of the young adult may be different from the hospital schedule. Tailoring care to the individual would help the young adult adjust to the hospital routine. Example: The patient likes to take a bath in the afternoon rather than in the morning. This can be arranged. Give as much control over activities of daily living as possible.

The young adult will probably not like to ask for medication for pain. Offering medications as necessary and reassuring that the medication is for relief of pain after a procedure or necessary for maintenance of health will alleviate fears about drugs and feeling of inadequacy because he or she takes medication. The young adult will be independent about the activities of daily living (bath, mouth, hair, nail, and eye care). Seeing to it that they have the necessary items to perform these functions will be the nurse's task.

The young adult nurse will have to deal with his or her feelings about taking care of someone the same age. This can be particularly stressful if the young adult has a terminal illness. Getting a young adult to follow the doctor's orders can be challenging, especially if one is of the same age.

Along with taking care of a young adult with acute problems, the nurse does health teaching, plans care, and gives emotional support and hope.

SUMMARY

This chapter has focused on the young adult as an individual, family-of-origin member, and family-of-procreation member. The tasks of the individual include physical tasks, enhancing intimacy versus isolation, developing interpersonal relationships, establishing a home, determining support systems, building competency and achievement, and doing what society expects from the group aged 20–40. Potential stressors such as illnesses, motor vehicle accidents, poor nutrition, pregnancy, physical attributes, diseases (diabetes, cardiovascular, hypertension, heart), work, divorce, remarriage, and careers are addressed. Alterations in the health of the young adult are explored. Finally, the section on nursing responsibilities looks at the way nurses can help the young adult achieve a life of optimum health.

Care Plan for the Young Adult with Job-Related Anxiety and a Problem-Solving Technique Deficit

Situation

Sandra is a 23-year-old white female who lives with a female roommate. She is a police officer for a small college town. She moved away from home a year and a half ago and has maintained her own home, living expenses, and health needs. She comes to the clinic with complaints of headache, tiredness, difficulty sleeping, and loss of appetite, and states: "I have not been feeling like myself for several months. It is beginning to interfere with my job."

Nursing Diagnosis

1. Anxiety related to job stress.
2. Problem-solving technique deficit.

SAMPLE CARE PLAN

Nursing Diagnosis	Goals	Nursing Intervention	Evaluation
Anxiety related to job stress	Reduce level of anxiety	The nurse will: Teach how to reduce anxiety	The patient will: Have relief of anxiety
		Assess coping techniques	List own coping techniques
		Teach new coping techniques	Explore ways to deal with anxiety
		Assess positive and negative feelings about job	List positive and negative feelings about job
		Plan one-to-one therapy	Discuss feelings of anxiety, fear, stress, relationships, self-confidence about job
	Promote development of rest, sleep, activity, and appetite	Assess rest and sleep pattern	Practice relaxation techniques each day
		Assess nutritional status	Maintain nutritious eating patterns

SAMPLE CARE PLAN *(continued)*

Nursing Diagnosis	Goals	Intervention	Evaluation
		Teach basic four food groups	Plan interesting meals
	To have insight about personal stress	Teach relationship between anxiety and psychological stress	Participate in one-to-one therapy
Learn problem-solving techniques		Teach problem-solving techniques	Demonstrate new problem-solving techniques
			Role play

Review Questions

1. Identify and discuss tasks of the young adult.
2. Identify and discuss tasks of the young adult as a member of a beginning family.
3. Discuss how the young adult can maintain self-identity, grow, and at the same time establish an intimate relationship with a partner.
4. Discuss the tasks of the family of origin during the embarking period for the young adult.
5. Discuss the societal and cultural expectations of the young adult.
6. Discuss life-style patterns and relationships of the young adult.
7. Analyze stressors of the young adult.
8. Analyze adaptive and maladaptive coping behaviors of the young adult.
9. Write a care plan for a young adult.

REFERENCES

Aguilera, D., & Messick, J. (1986). *Crisis intervention* (5th ed.). St. Louis: Mosby.

American College Health Association, Task Force on AIDS (1987). AIDS . . . what everyone should know. Rockville, Maryland.

Atrash, H., Rhodenhiser, E., Hogue, C., & Smith, J. (1986, August). Abortion surveillance: Preliminary analysis 1982–1983. *MMWR Surveillance Summaries, 35*(255).

Blank, T. (1982). *A social psychology of developing adults.* New York: Wiley.

Burgess, A. (1981). *Psychiatric nursing in the hospital and the community* (3rd ed.). Englewood Cliffs, NJ: Prentice-Hall.

Calhoun, J., & Acocella, J. (1978). *Psychology of adjustment and human relationships.* New York: Random.

Clark, W., & Midanik, L. (1981). Alcohol use and alcohol problems among U.S. adults. In *Alcohol consumption and related problems* (NIAAA Alcohol and Health Monograph No. 1). Rockville, MD: National Institute of Alcohol Abuse and Alcoholism.

Clayton, R. (Ed.) (1985). *Taber's cyclopedic medical dictionary*. Philadelphia: Davis.

Colman, B. (1977). *Making love during pregnancy*. New York: Bantam.

Cooper, K. (1982). *The aerobics program for total well-being*. New York: Bantam.

Crips, A., & Stonehill, E. (1976). *Sleep, nutrition and mood*. London: Wiley.

Cupit, L. (1984). Contraception: Helping patients choose. *Journal of Gynecological Nursing, 13*(2, Suppl.), 23–29.

Dedonder, J. (1986, May/June). Adoption as a positive option. *Pediatric Nursing, 12*(3), 202–204.

Delora, J., Warren, C., & Ellison, C. (1981). *Understanding sexual interaction*. Boston: Houghton Mifflin.

Dion, M. (1984). We, the American women. U.S. Department of Commerce, Washington D.C.

Duvall, E. (1977). *Marriage and family development* (5th ed.). New York: Harper & Row.

Erikson, C. (1968). *Youth identity and crisis*. New York: Norton.

Feigelman, W., & Silverman, A. (1983). *Chosen children*. New York: Praeger.

Fisk, N. (1986). Alcoholism: Ineffective family coping, *American Journal of Nursing* (May): 586–587.

Freedman, A., Kaplan, H., & Sadock, B. (1976). Harry Stack Sullivan. In *Modern synopsis of psychiatry II*. Baltimore: Williams & Wilkins.

Friedrich, O. (1984). A legal, moral, social nightmare. *Time*, pp. 54–56.

Fromm, E. (1956). *The art of loving*. New York: Harper & Row.

Fromer, M. (1983). *Ethical issues in sexuality and reproduction*. St. Louis: Mosby.

FYI/Reports. (1984, March/April). *Children Today*, pp. 15–17.

Gelles, R. (1979). *Family violence* (pp. 95–119). Beverly Hills, CA: Sage.

Hagerty, B. (1984). *Psychiatric mental health assessment*. Princeton: Mosby.

Hartford, T. (1984). Situational factors in drinking. In Miller, P., & Nurenberg, T. (Eds.), *Prevention of alcohol abuse*. New York: Plenum.

Kandel, D., & Logan, J. (1984). Patterns of drug use from adolescence to young adulthood: Periods of risk for initiation, continued use and discontinuation. *American Journal of Public Health, 74*(7), 660–665.

Kistner, R. (1983). Endometriosis. In E. Quilligan (Ed.), *Current therapy in obstetics and gynecology*. Philadelphia: Saunders.

Kübler-Ross, E. (1969). *On death and dying*. New York: Macmillan.

Leo J. (1984, April). The revolution is over. *Time*, pp. 74–83.

Lewis, S. & Colliec, I. (1987). *Medical-Surgical Nursing* 2nd ed. New York: McGraw-Hill.

Lobel, B., & Hirschfield (1985). Depression—What we know.

Luckman, J., & Sorensen, K. (1980). *Medical-surgical nursing*. Philadelphia: Saunders.

Minshull, D. (1985, July 3). Sick or self indulgent. *Nursing Mirror, 161*(1), 15–18.

Morbidity and mortality weekly report. (1986, May 16). Center for Disease Control (Vol. 35, No. 19). Washington, DC: U.S. Department of Human Health Services.

Murray, R., & Zentner, J. (1979). *Nursing assessment and health promotion through the life span*. Englewood Cliffs, NJ: Prentice-Hall.

Newberger, E. (1977). Pediatric social illness: Toward an etiologic classification. *Pediatrics, 60,* 178–185.

Pepper, B., Kirshner, M., Ryglewicz, H. (1981, July). The young adult chronic patient: Overview of a population. *Hospital and Community Psychiatry, 2*(7).

Phipps, W., Long, B., & Woods, N. (1983). *Medical-surgical nursing* (2nd ed.). St. Louis: Mosby.

Quilligan, E. (1983). *Current therapy in obstetrics and gynecology.* Philadelphia: Saunders.

Rakel, R., & Coon, H. (1978). *Family practice.* Philadelphia: Saunders.

Reichert, K. (1976). *Primary care of young adults.* Flushing, NY: Medical Examination Publishing.

Rubin, Z. (1973). *Liking and loving.* New York: Holt, Rinehart & Winston.

Schell, R. (Ed.) (1975). Early adulthood: selecting the options. In *Developmental psychology today* (2nd ed.) (pp. 387–425). New York: Random House.

Schenk, Q., & Schenk, E. (1978). *Pulling up roots.* Englewood Cliffs, NJ: Prentice-Hall.

Schultz, J., & Dark, S. (1986). *Manual of psychiatric nursing care plans* (2nd ed.). Boston: Little, Brown.

Sheehy, G. (1974). *Passages.* New York: E. P. Dutton & Co., Inc., Morrow.

Sorensen, K., & Luckman, J. (1979). *Basic nursing.* Philadelphia: Saunders.

Still, H. (1986). Sexuality during and after pregnancy. *Canadian Family Physician, 32,* 2177–2179.

Stuart, G., & Sundeen, S. (1979). *Principles and practices of psychiatric nursing.* St. Louis: Mosby.

Swanson, A., & Hurley, P. (1983). Family systems: Values and value conflicts. *Journal of Psychosocial Nursing, 21,* 24–30.

Tinkham, C., & Voorhies, E. (1977). *Community Health Nursing: Evolution and Process.* New York: Appleton-Century-Crofts.

Thomas, C. (Ed.) (1985). *Taber's cyclopedic medical dictionary.* Philadelphia: Davis.

Thorman, G. (1980). *Family violence* (pp. 18–55). Springfield, IL: Thomas.

U.S. Department of Commerce, Bureau of Census. (1986). *Statistical abstract of U.S.* (106th ed.). Washington, DC: Bureau of Census.

Weingourt, R. (1979, April). Battered women: The grieving process. *Journal of Psychiatric Nursing, 17*(4) 40–47.

Weisman, A. (1979). *Coping with cancer.* St. Louis: McGraw-Hill.

Wilgerink, R. (1979). *Developmental disorders.* Baltimore: Paul Brooks.

Willi, J. (1982). *Couples in collusion.* New York: Hunter House.

Woods, N. (1984). *Human sexuality.* St. Louis: Mosby

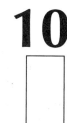

The Family with the Middlescent 45–65 Years

Vickie A. Lambert and Clinton E. Lambert Jr.

OBJECTIVES

Upon completion of this chapter, the student will be able to:

1. Describe family and individual tasks as they relate to the middlescent
2. Identify potential stressors for the middlescent
3. Explain the coping mechanisms utilized by the middlescent
4. Describe the salient components of a nursing assessment for the middlescent and his or her family
5. Identify common acute and chronic health alterations experienced by the middlescent
6. Plan nursing care for the middlescent in regard to health maintenance, health promotion, and preventive measures

---

CONCEPTS

Generativity: the act of establishing and guiding future generations

Stagnation: to become dull and without interest in taking part in life's activities

Empty-nest syndrome: a sense of loss due to the departure of children from the home

Multigenerational communicator: one who can effectively impart information to individuals of all age groups

Grandparenting: the act of caring for the children of one's children

Adaptation: the appropriate use of coping mechanisms to deal with stressors

Maladaptation: the inappropriate use of coping mechanisms to deal with stressors

Illness: an alteration in physiological function and/or psychosocial integrity that impedes an individual's ability to achieve an optimal level of performance

Stressors: demands that tax or exceed the resources of the individual

Conflict resolution: the successful termination of an event that has been perceived to hold opposing impulses or desires

Anticipatory guidance: the act of helping someone to plan for forthcoming events

---

Middlescence, the time frame between the ages of 45 and 65 years, is when evaluation of personal achievements and attempts to successfully guide the next generation via the family or through community activities is accomplished (Streff, 1981). This time frame of one's life encompasses the launching-center stage and the middle-aged-parent stage of the family life cycle (Duvall, 1977), and involves the psychosocial tasks of generativity versus stagnation (Erikson, 1963). Within the context of these developmental and psychosocial aspects, this chapter will address family and individual tasks, personal stressors and coping mechanisms, and health care problems relevant to the middlescent. How the nurse can intervene and appropriately deal with each of the aforementioned components will be presented.

FAMILY TASKS

There are three major family tasks facing the middlescent. These tasks include: (1) evaluation and maintenance of socioeconomic security for the future, (2) evaluation and maintenance of family accomplishments, and (3) change and maintenance of family relationships. Successful attainment of each of these tasks requires the family to function as a unit, while recognizing that each family member is a unique being.

Socioeconomic Security

Assessment of financial resources and expenditures in order to identify present socioeconomic status and to determine future needs is the first major family task facing the middlescent. To assess financial resources, the middlescent family needs to examine total annual household income, as well as supplemental incomes such as investment returns, part-time employment income, alimony, and/or child support payments. In addition to monetary assets, the family should take into account such acquisitions as real estate, stocks and bonds, cars, valuable art objects, and jewelry.

Major expenditures for the middlescent family are derived from such expenses as house and car payments, medical costs, food, clothing, and educational support. Due to the exodus of the children from the home during this time, educational expenses for professional or vocational school increase. Financial support from the family also may go toward the cost of a wedding, the establishment of a business, or the setting up of a home or apartment for a departing child. In addition, due to the aging process, medical expenses for the middlescent tend to increase, because chronic physical illnesses, such as diabetes mellitus, cardiovascular disease, and arthritis are more prevalent (Strauss et al., 1984).

In order to determine the family's socioeconomic status, a comparison between financial assets and financial expenditures must be made. Families who evaluate their assets as adequately outweighing their expenditures will, no doubt, determine their socioeconomic status to be satisfactory. If, however, assets do not sufficiently outweigh expenditures, the perception of an unsatisfactory status may be determined.

The family that determines its socioeconomic status as satisfactory most likely will believe that continuing its present financial practices is sufficient. However, the family that does not perceive its socioeconomic status as satisfactory will need to determine what financial practices to alter. For example, does the family need to reduce certain expenditures? If so, which ones? Do family members need to obtain supplemental employment? If so, how and where? What the middlescent family needs to consider are which resources and which expenditures are important to the economic functioning of the family unit so that financial security can be maintained. In some circumstances financial counseling may be advisable.

Family Accomplishments

The second task confronting the middlescent family is the evaluation and maintenance of family accomplishments. In other words, has the family achieved its perceived goals? These goals will vary among families, and are based upon culture, socioeconomic status, religious affiliation, geographical location, and family size. For some, family goals may include the successful departure of children from the home, the provision of higher education for children, the completion of financial debts and mortgages, the achievement of desired occupational endeavors, and/or societal recognition as a successful family.

The family that believes it has achieved perceived goals will manifest a sense of accomplishment and satisfaction. Such a family will have the capability to look toward the future, to formulate new goals, and to move ahead. However, should the family believe it has not adequately achieved its perceived goals, a sense of disappointment and, possibly, a sense of failure will prevail. This will impede goal planning and implementation for the future. As a result, the family unit is likely to find it difficult to progress as a unit, because the component of middlescent family accomplishments has not been resolved.

Family Relationships

Change and maintenance of family relationships comprises the third family task of middlescence. It is during middlescence that children leave home, new members are added to the family unit by way of marriage and through the birth of grandchildren, and elderly relatives often become residents in the home. These changes in the family structure require alterations in the relationships that exist among family members.

Parents who have invested a great deal of energy in childrearing early in their marriage may have failed to develop a sound and close relationship with each other. Now that their children have departed the home and they finally are alone, they may find they have nothing in common (Streff, 1981) and truly feel that their nest is empty. According to Knafl and Grace (1978), when dealing with the *empty-nest syndrome*, women report experiencing more dramatic changes in their daily activities than do men. Women, however, who are engaged in gainful employment outside the home or have established activities outside the home view the empty-nest syndrome as a natural, essentially problem-free issue. Parents who have progressively developed their relationship as a couple throughout the parenting experience are less likely to view each other as strangers when children depart the home and are more inclined to progress as a creative unit. Such couples are likely to view life without children as simpler, more relaxed, and allowing more available time together. Couples, however, who have failed to develop a sound relationship may find their marriage ending in divorce now that their one common bond, their offspring, is gone (Lambert & Lambert, 1977).

As children leave home, new positions within the family structure are created for the remaining siblings, thereby altering the existing relationships within the family. Younger children, often informally, are promoted to the rank of oldest (Karpel & Strauss, 1983) with a prized room or other "perks" accompanying the promotion. The new positions created for and by the remaining siblings involve certain family responsibilities. As the second oldest child moves into the oldest child position, he or she is expected to fulfill that role. The child may be expected to provide supervision for younger siblings, to serve as parental confidant, and/or to contribute to the household income. If the child does not live up to the family expectations in regards to the new role, he or she may feel inadequate and further disrupt the maintenance of family relationships.

The departing child also is faced with a new position within the middlescent family structure. He or she may assume a removed role in the family unit due to the creation of his or her own family unit. Or the child may continue to assume a contributing role, but in a peripheral sense. An example is the college student who is financially supported by the parents, but is leading a life separate from the family unit. This child may continue open communication with the family and come home on holidays, but not be involved in the day-to-day family decision-making process. The development of such a child may be a painful experience, if he or she is leading a life-style the parents consider unacceptable or if he or she prolongs the act of dependency upon the parents.

Relationships in many middlescent families are altered due to the addition of new members through marriage and or the birth or adoption of grandchildren. Due to the marriage of their children, the middlescent couple is required to take on the role of in-laws and its accompanying responsibilities. These responsibilities may involve providing financial support, serving as a confidant, and furnishing social outlets to the new adult family member. When parents are in support of the marriage of their children, assumption of the role of in-law is made with ease. If, however, the parents are in opposition to the marriage of their children, in-law role assumption is likely to be perceived as being difficult. The establishment of healthy relationships between the middlescent parents and their new in-law is dependent upon all parties being in agreement regarding the responsibilities and expectations of the in-law role.

Like the in-law role, the grandparent role forces relationship alterations among family members. Grandparents today are more likely to be middle-aged, to be working, and to perceive themselves as youthful (Troll, 1975). Therefore, they are less likely to be actively involved in rearing activities and more likely to be involved in leisure activities with their grandchildren on holidays and/or special occasions.

The assumption of the role of grandparent tends to be a positive experience for most middle-aged adults. However, if the new grandparent perceives the label "grandparent" as indicating "oldness," the role may not be assumed with ease. To avoid using the label "grandparent," some middlescents have insisted that their grandchildren address them on a first-name basis and relate to them as buddies rather than as mature adults. Such behavior necessitates relationship alterations within the family unit, particularly if the parents of the child see the grandparenting role from a different perspective.

Elderly relatives becoming residents in the home is the third form of altered family relationships that can occur during middlescence. These relatives may include parents, grandparents, aunts, uncles, and even cousins. Such family additions tend to expand the generational dimensions within the family structure and place additional responsibility upon the middlescent because the middlescent generation tends to serve as the communicator and interpreter between generations (Anderson & Polk, 1983). Having multigenerations within the family unit can provide a rich network for interactions and/or the division of labor. On the other hand, difficulties can arise in the maintenance of relationships within the family unit if misunderstandings occur across generations in regards to each generation's need. For example, the elderly relative may become irate about the adolescent children's extended usage of the bathroom and attempt to place unacceptable demands upon the middlescent parents to resolve the issue. To maintain relationships within the family unit, it becomes necessary for all involved members to openly identify, discuss, and negotiate perceived rights and privileges.

INDIVIDUAL TASKS

Along with family tasks, the adult in middlescence is faced with five specific individual tasks. These tasks can be categorized as physical changes in the body, personality development, interpersonal relationships, competencies and achievements, and societal and cultural endeavors. These tasks may or may not occur simultaneously; however, they all exist and must be dealt with at some point during the middlescent years.

Physical Changes

Physical changes that occur in the body during middlescence involve major hormonal changes, decreased activity level, weight gain, changes in physical appearance, and alterations in sensory function. Generally all of these physical changes occur rather insidiously.

The major hormonal changes that occur during middlescence are associated with menopause, which tends to occur in women between the ages of 40 and 55 years. Ovarian function gradually diminishes, and thus decreased amounts of estrogen and progesterone are produced. The decrease in production of these hormones leads to the cessation of the menstrual cycle, which may abruptly stop or may gradually cease. Symptoms that tend to be associated with menopause are hot flashes, the cause of which is unknown; atrophic vaginitis, in which the vaginal mucosa becomes thin and dry; and osteoporosis, which is not necessarily a product of menopause but often accompanies or follows it as bone demineralization is accelerated in the absence of estrogens (Rankoff, 1980).

In most cases, menopause is unlikely to create serious health problems for the middlescent woman. In fact many women state that the nice thing about menopause is "not having to bother with menstruation." At present there tends to be considerable disagreement among researchers and practitioners about the effectiveness of compensatory hormone treatment for menopause. The consensus seems to be that little, if any, generalized therapeutic value results except for specific lessening of symptoms, such as hot flashes (Rankoff, 1980). Estrogen replacement therapy seems to postpone, not avert, hot flashes. Once compensatory hormonal treatment is discontinued, the hot flashes usually reappear (Seaman & Seaman, 1977).

Psychological changes, such as mood swings, nervousness, insomnia, and mild transitory depression, often accompany menopause. However, most of these symptoms are experienced by women throughout their lives and, indeed, are even experienced by men. These symptoms may not be precipitated by the hormonal deficiency but may be more appropriately related to the adjustments and adaptations of middlescence.

There are no physical changes in men comparable to the menopausal changes in women. Androgen levels tend to decline, but do so at a very slow rate (Keele, Neil, & Joels, 1982). A decreased sex drive may occur in the middlescent male; however, his reproductive capabilities tend to continue. The sexual changes that the male may begin to notice in the late middle years include: a longer time needed to achieve full erection and to reach a climax, fewer genital spasms with a reduction in both the force and amount of ejaculate, and a longer refractory period (intervals between erections) (Hatcher & Stewart, 1978).

The level of physical activity tends to decrease during middlescence due to degenerative changes in the joints, a decrease in pulmonary vital capacity, reduction in cardiac muscle strength, a decrease in cardiac output, and a steady loss of skeletal muscle strength, particularly in the back and leg muscles (Chinn, 1971). These physiological changes are normal and can affect the individual's tolerance for physical activity. Individuals, however, who have been physically active throughout life tend to remain the quickest in their peer group (Haan & Day, 1974). For the middlescent to maintain appropriate physical strength and functionability, a regular exercise program that is interspersed with rest periods and done at a slower pace is advisable. Exercise not only strengthens and improves the circulation in cardiac muscles, but it also reduces the severity of arteriosclerosis (Cantu, 1982). Exercising the leg muscles, as through jogging and cycling, facilitates the flow of blood to the heart and thus, indirectly, maintains body function in all areas, including the brain.

As a result of decreased physical activity, along with a slowed metabolic rate, weight gain in the middlescent is common. In adolescents only 10% of body weight is fat, while fat comprises at least 20 to 25% of body weight in the middlescent, with most of it settling about the waist (Troll, 1975). The weight gain that results may have detrimental effects on other body systems. For example, research has shown that individuals who are overweight are more prone to diabetes mellitus, cardiovascular disorders, and renal disease (Cavallo-Perin et al., 1981; Kannel & Gordon, 1979; Tobian, 1978). Undoubtedly, weight gain in the middlescent is the result of the affluence of Western society. Food is abundant and accessible; the standard of living is high, with large amounts of time being available for recreational activities; and most forms of entertainment involve the consumption of food and drink.

Along with changes in weight, perhaps the most obvious changes in physical appearance involve the hair and skin. During the forties, particularly in men, the hairline recedes, the hair becomes thinner, and baldness increases. At the same time, grayness increases, so that by the fifties most men and women have a noticeable amount of gray hair, with some being white-haired. Another less noticeable hair change includes the appearance of stiff hair in the nose, ears, and eyelashes of men and on the upper lip and chin of women. Men find they need to shave less often, while women need to shave more often. Skin changes involve the loss of elasticity, an increase in coarseness and darkness on the face, neck, arms, and hands, the appearance of wrinkles, and the formation of bags and dark circles under the eyes (Malasanos, 1981). Therefore, it is most understandable why middlescent men and women become increasingly preoccupied with their physical appearance.

Alterations in sensory function during middlescence involve changes in vision, hearing, taste, smell, and touch. An increased tendency to farsightedness is prevalent due to the loss of lens elasticity, causing inability to focus accurately. This change is evidenced by decreased near vision and can occur in individuals who have never before had vision problems. Some middlescents find they may need reading glasses for close work, while others find bifocals necessary (Cadogan, 1984).

Thickening of the lens also occurs, causing a decrease in visual acuity, a lengthening of time for visual adjustment from light to dark environments, and a decrease in peripheral vision. Because the diameter of the pupil also tends to decrease around 50 years of age, less light enters the eye, thus requiring the presence of greater light intensity to appropriately discern the environment. Dim lighting in restaurants and theatres can make the middlescent functionally blind, even though he or she is able to read without glasses while sitting on a sunlit porch.

Yellowing of the lens makes it difficult for the middlescent to distinguish certain color intensities, especially cool colors like blue, green, and violet. Warm colors such as yellow, red, and orange tend to be seen more easily (Corso, 1981).

During middlescence most hearing alterations are not noticed because they involve the loss of sound receptions that are not required for daily function (Timiras, 1972). Alterations in hearing that do occur involve a gradual loss of high-pitched frequencies (above speech frequencies). This is due to progressive degeneration of the sensory hair cells, supporting cells, and the stria vascularis of the cochlea (Cadogan, 1984). After age 55 this loss is more prevalent in men than in women (Timiras, 1972).

No blatant changes in either taste or smell sensitivity occurs during middlescence. There may be, however, a slight loss in the ability to distinguish the finer nuances of certain tastes, due to atrophy of the papillae on the lateral edges of the tongue (Malasanos, 1981). Food that seems bland to the middlescent may be perceived as highly flavorful to a child.

Touch sensitivity begins to decline around age 45. Sensitivity to pain remains steady until 50 years of age, at which time it begins to decline. In light of a decreased sensitivity to pain, pain tolerance may increase, so that the individual reacts to more pain with less distress. Woodrow, Friedman, Siegelaub, and Collen (1972) found that reported tolerance of superficial pain tends to increase with age. In support of this finding, Bellville, Forrest, Miller, and Brown (1971) noted that young patients reported more pain initially after surgery and less pain relief following the administration of an analgesic than did their older cohorts.

Personality Development

Personality development during middlescence involves the utilization of intellectual functioning and certain desired personality traits in relationship to the task of generativity (the need to help younger persons become integrated human beings). Traditionally it has been believed that intellectual functioning declines after 30 years of age. Recent longitudinal studies, however, show a gradual improvement in general intelligence until approximately age 50, and stabilization until shortly before death (Kimmel, 1974). The patterns of change in adult intelligence vary, depending upon the specific mental ability being measured. Fluid intelligence consists of those abilities related to neurological development and involves associative power, memory, figural relationships, and visual-motor flexibility. Due to degenerative neurological changes, fluid intelligence may decline during middlescence. Crystalline intelligence involves abilities that arise out of experiences and the accumulation of learning, and includes verbal comprehension, formal reasoning, and general information. Crystalline intelligence improves with age (Schaie, 1975). Generally, individuals who have maintained a high level of intellectual functioning throughout the young adulthood years will continue to do so during middlescence. One must keep in mind, however, that such factors as education, social class, motivation, illness, and personality traits will influence maintenance of intellectual functioning.

The presence of desired middlescent personality traits is dependent upon successful achievement of each developmental task of childhood and early adulthood. Such tasks include the development of trust, autonomy, initiative, industry, role identity, and intimacy. By the time one reaches middlescence, personality already has been well established, because it is the result of many years of development. However, there may be some changes in attitude toward such activities as childrearing, marriage, and religion. Desired personality traits that have been noted to exist in

TABLE 10–1. THEORISTS AND THE FAMILY WITH THE MIDDLESCENT

Name	Source	Age Group	Concepts	Remarks
Erik Erikson	*Childhood and society,* 1963	Middlescent: 45–65 years of age	Generativity versus stagnation	This time frame in one's life encompasses the launching-center stage and the middle parent stage of the family life cycle. During this time frame a vital interest outside the home occurs with a major focus on establishing and guiding future generations with an optimistic hope of bettering society.

the middlescent include: being able to invest meaningful emotion in new activities, new relationships, and new experiences; being satisfied with self; being open-minded; feeling whole, worthwhile, and happy; having a genuine concern for others' well-being; feeling satisfied with his or her body; and being able to mesh sexual desires with other aspects of life (Peck & Berkowitz, 1964).

The middlescent who is capable of demonstrating generativity through the utilization of his or her intellectual functioning and desired personality traits has some central perspective and direction in life that provides a meaningful sense of unity and purpose (see Table 10–1). This purpose integrates past experiences with expectations and hopes for the future. In other words, the generative middlescent has come to see himself or herself in comparison with what others expect and now is faced with the psychosocial task of being concerned for others versus being preoccupied with self (Erikson, 1963).

By comparison, the middlescent who fails to manifest sufficient generative personality traits will, most likely, portray a sense of stagnation. As a result, the individual will become engulfed in satisfying personal needs and acquiring self-comforts because he or she believes that there is only one chance left for succeeding in life. The outcome will be a sense of interpersonal improverishment resulting from a state of self-absorption.

Interpersonal Relationships

Renewal and development of friendships and reaffirmation of family ties are the two types of interpersonal relationships that are of significance during middlescence. Middlescence provides a time when the adult finds it necessary to re-examine relationships with others due to changes in family structure (brought about by deaths, children leaving home, and the adding of family members).

Renewal and development of friendships is important for expanding one's horizons, for increasing self-esteem, and for combating loneliness, which can occur when activities that existed previously have decreased or ceased. Now that family and career demands have changed, the middlescent tends to focus on renewing and developing a few significant friendships. These relationships provide personal contact with others, intellectual stimulation, and opportunities for self-actualization. The middlescent is most likely to renew and develop relationships with individuals who have similar interests and needs. For example, it is not uncommon for the middlescent to seek out old cronies and high school and college classmates via reunions and parties. A common interest develops in learning and sharing what others have accomplished over the years. In attempting to make new friends, the middlescent often finds the religious groups, social clubs, and adult-only housing areas to be appropriate avenues to meet others.

The activities of young adulthood (active childrearing and career development and advancement) tend to slow down in the middle years, leading to a reaffirmation of family ties. The middlescent recognizes the need to redirect energy toward relationships with the spouse, significant others, or family members. Over the years, relationships with these individuals may have been neglected or taken for granted and, as a result, a chasm may have developed. Although there is an increasing awareness of the need to share the joys and apprehensions of a new life stage with another, the middlescent may find that he or she has nothing in common with those deemed to be significant (Streff, 1981). A less subtle message focuses on the realization that advancing years are approaching and one must renew significant relationships before it is too late.

Competencies and Achievements

It is during middlescence that one takes the time to evaluate his or her competencies and achievements. The two aspects of life that are most extensively evaluated are attainment of personal accomplishments and achievement of career goals (Lidz, 1980).

The middlescent tends to assess the attainment of personal accomplishments in relationship to what he or she perceives as significant and/or important. What is of significance and/or importance will vary in regard to socioeconomic status, educational experience, and perceived family expectations. For example, an individual from a high socioeconomic level may find importance in possessing valuable material objects, such as cars, homes, and jewelry, while a middlescent from a low-income family may find significance in having supported a child through college. What one's family deems as meaningful can influence the middlescent's determination of successful acquisition of personal goals. Families who believe that appointment to community positions of importance are essential by middlescence may not acknowledge achievement of the middlescent who has not been so appointed.

Evaluation of achievement of career goals in light of one's personal value system comprises the second individual competency examined by the middlescent. Goals and ideals toward which the individual strove in earlier years are reassessed in a more realistic manner. Because limited time is left until retirement, occupational goals may need to be revised toward more reasonable expectations. Questions frequently asked are: Have I accomplished what I intended to accomplish by this time in my life? Are my career expectations realistic for this stage in my life? Do I wish to continue aspiring to the career goals I set earlier in my life?

The awareness of middlescence causes the individual to question his or her purpose in life and often is accompanied by the decision to get out of the rat race and to start to enjoy life. Individuals who find their jobs mundane and unfulfilling or determine that their jobs are at risk due to the expertise of younger employees may believe that a change in career focus is necessary. Therefore, alterations in career goals are not uncommon during middlescence and may involve returning to school for additional training and/or credentials. Education, however, may be pursued as an end in itself for self-development or achievement of previously denied aspirations unrelated to one's career. For example, it is not uncommon for the middle-aged woman to return to school now that the children are "out from underfoot."

Societal and Cultural Endeavors

With the decreased or completed responsibilities of childrearing and/or career endeavors, the middle-aged individual finds that more attention can be focused toward involvement in other arenas. As a result, the concluding individual task of middlescence encompasses participation in societal and cultural endeavors. The two components comprising this participation are expanded involvement in community activities and increased participation in leisure endeavors.

Being involved as decision maker for society is common during middlescence. Earlier life stages have prepared the individual for expanded involvement in community activities. This is readily noted by the middlescent's assumption of responsible positions in social and civic activities, organizations, and community functions. The emphasis changes from striving to obtain positions of responsibility to attaining and maintaining positions of importance. The middlescent tends to be selected as the leader of civic endeavors and is identified as the individual who has the potential to better the world for future generations.

Along with an increased involvement in community activities an increased participation in leisure endeavors occurs. During the early middle years the individual may intentionally make time in his or her schedule for leisure activities. With advancing years, however, the emphasis changes to dealing with an increased availability of time. For the middlescent who previously had not cultivated leisure activities, the increased availability of leisure time may be perceived as a negative experience. Using leisure time in a satisfying and creative way can prove to be fulfilling. It is not uncommon to hear the middlescent comment, "Now that I have the time, I finally have begun to enjoy life." However, researchers who sampled a population of middlescents on their attitudes toward leisure time found that 90% of the men and 80% of the women desired to continue working, even if they did not need work, because they gained more satisfaction from work than from leisure activities (Pfeiffer & Davis, 1971).

The general types of leisure activities in which the middlescent engage tend to be less home-centered, less physically demanding, absent of the need for quick reflexes, and oriented toward health maintenance activities such as swimming or exercising (Abbick, 1983). These activities are selected because the individual has greater freedom and more available money to spend on leisure, is more easily fatigued, does not have as quick reflexes as when younger, and has a concern for maintaining an adequate state of health.

POTENTIAL STRESSORS

Three major categories of potential stressors exist for the adult facing middlescence. These include: physical stressors, social and emotional stressors, and stressors related to conflict with family tasks. Understanding what role each potential stressor plays during middlescence aids in preparing one for action to deal with each stressor.

Physical Stressors

Physical stressors facing the middlescent involve dealing with bodily changes due to the aging process and adjusting to the development of chronic illnesses. Bodily changes, or more specifically, changes in bodily appearance are the most apparent signs of aging (Weiner, Brok, & Snadowsky, 1978). Although we are unsure of the precise cause of aging, we can describe a number of changes that seem to occur. The body's ability to regulate levels of blood pH, blood sugar, and pulse rate under various and changing conditions tends to decline with age. Research has shown that there is almost a linear decline of approximately 1% a year in most integrated body functions in adult life (Bierman & Hazzard, 1973). In spite of this fact, it has been shown that older people maintain basic homeostatic balance as efficiently as younger individuals under resting conditions. What tends to be problematic is that with advancing age one's ability to favorably readjust body functioning after a stressful circumstance is greatly impaired (Kimmel, 1974), explaining why the middlescent is forced to deal with a decreased physical activity level.

Until recently it was widely accepted that aging involved the progressive loss of cells. Cell loss was thought to be responsible for symptoms of aging such as impairment of cerebral functioning and decreased muscle strength. Although still of some importance, the theory of cell loss currently is not considered the primary factor in the aging process (Weiner et al., 1978).

Scientists who are in disagreement with the decreasing importance of cell loss as a factor in aging believe that human cells have a finite life span. Hayflick (1970) and Bierman and Hazzard (1973) found that human cells grown in tissue cultures do not divide indefinitely, but show a decreasing capacity for cellular division as aging occurs. Other scientists believe that the aging process is the result of the accumulation of "errors" in "the genetic matrix which generates the many physiochemical systems supporting cell biosynthesis and homeostatic regulation" (Jarvik & Cohen, 1973, p. 234). It appears that problems arise over time in the genetically programmed DNA-RNA enzyme protein synthesis required for normal cellular functioning.

Several other untested theories explaining the aging process have been proposed (Kimmel, 1974). One involves the belief that aging occurs due to cellular poisoning over time by metabolic waste products that have accumulated. Another theory proposes that the body builds up immunity to its own tissues over time through the production of autoimmune antibodies, which leads to cellular dysfunction and death.

A difficulty encountered in regards to the aging process from a biological perspective is that many of the physical changes observed during middlescence may be the result of chronic illness related to age rather than to the aging process itself. As previously pointed out, individuals experience a decline in integrated body functions as age progresses. Many scientist believe that no one really dies from the aging process, but rather death is the result of illnesses that are in some way correlated with aging. Aging may be a process that increases the probability of illness (Bierman & Hazzard, 1973). The middlescent is faced with the inevitable fate of having to deal with bodily changes brought about by the aging process in concert with the increased incidence of chronic illness.

Social-Emotional Stressors

The two major social and emotional stressors facing the middlescent include occupation-related stressors and the increasing prevalence of a diminishing social support system. Particular attention tends to be paid to occupation-related stressors such as job security, workload, threat of unemployment, constant need to remain current in one's field, and mandatory retirement. The results of these concerns leads to disengagement from work as a source of personal fulfillment.

Even though there tends to be an increase in power, prestige, and satisfaction with work during middlescence, research (Tamir, 1982) shows that in comparison, especially to young adults, a male's job satisfaction fails to contribute to a sense of well-being. Less educated men experience a decrease in self-esteem regardless of the satisfaction they say they derive from work. More educated men tend to lack zest in spite of satisfying jobs. It appears that the rationale for these findings is that by middlescence one's occupation recedes in importance for self-fulfillment.

Although work may not be as fulfilling as it once was, the middlescent is aware that there is a need for definitive action to ensure economic stability for the later years. The individual may have made appropriate economic plans for changes in job status; however, never before have the realities of the economic situation been so evident. The fear of having to resort to some type of financial assistance, such as welfare, becomes increasingly prevalent. These concerns contribute to the female middlescent's re-entry or initial entry into the work force to supplement the family income or to serve as primary breadwinner. Re-establishing career credibility or learning a new occupational skill certainly incites additional stressors.

Due to the departure of children, divorce, and the death of spouses, parents, and significant others, middlescents are forced to deal with a diminishing social support system. The individuals upon whom they can rely for assistance become increasingly fewer, forcing establishment of new relationships. For the extrovert, such an activity may be perceived as an exciting adventure, while the introvert may find making new acquaintances stressful.

Stressors Related to Conflict with Family Tasks

Children leaving home, the marriage of children, the arrival of grandchildren, and the increased dependency of aging parents are the major stressors related to conflict with family tasks. All of these situations create alterations in existing family relationships and force the middlescent to evaluate and potentially establish new and/or different role relationships.

Children leaving home forces the middlescent to examine his or her marital relationship and determine the nature of its stability. Research has shown that during middlescence, awareness tends to increase concerning one's marital relationship and its problems, both past and present (Tamir, 1982). Those couples who have remained together for the sake of the children may now realize that they have little in common and may decide to separate or divorce. On the other hand, now that there is freedom from parenting responsibilities, the middlescent couple may become involved in developing new areas of interest, either individually or together.

Marriage of children and the arrival of grandchildren forces the establishment of the new role relationships of in-law and grandparent. Both roles place demands upon the individual that may be perceived as highly stressful. Both roles may be welcomed and revered by some middlescents, while for others the roles may be disliked and approached with great trepidation.

The increased dependency of aging parents can produce not only increased financial responsibilities but also a change in role. The middlescent may find that he or she now is serving in the parent and decision maker role while the aging parent is assuming the dependent, childlike role. It is not uncommon for the middlescent who is encountering extreme difficulty in dealing with the increased dependency of aging parents to engage in parental abuse. To deal with such a situation, the family requires professional intervention by a psychiatric clinical nurse specialist, a clinical psychologist, or a psychiatrist. On the other hand, being accountable and responsible for aging parents may be viewed as paying one's dues so that he or she will be guaranteed similar care during later years.

Regardless of which of the aforementioned family situations occur, all can be stress-provoking. For a more detailed discussion of this content, refer to the section in this chapter entitled "Family Relationships."

COPING MECHANISMS

Health Beliefs and Behaviors

Examination of the health status of the middlescent generally reveals a variety of health beliefs and behaviors. Each individual's values and beliefs related to health directly influence the way he or she responds in carrying out health care practices. Health may be perceived as a valued commodity or viewed as something that is taken for granted. If he or she believes that health can be maintained or improved by self-care measures, the individual is more likely to take action when an illness arises. On the other hand, if the person believes that his or her actions do not influence health status, then preventive and action-oriented measures either will be negated or simply not explored.

Three related health behaviors tend to emerge during middlescence: delay in obtaining health care, appropriate initiation of health practices, and overinvolvement in health improvement activities.

Delay in obtaining health care often is noted when the middlescent experiences chest pain and wants to see if the symptoms being experienced will subside or worsen before taking action. This delay can range from less than an hour to as long as several days. No doubt delays in seeking health care are due to the fear of potential life-threatening diagnoses. Research has shown that in the case of an individual experiencing a heart attack, approximately 50–70% die within 1 hour after the onset of acute symptoms and prior to obtaining medical attention (Gentry, 1979).

Appropriate initiation of health practices is observed when the middlescent obtains periodic physical examinations, complies with medically directed regimens, and contacts health care providers when the signs and symptoms of illness first appear. In an extensive research study conducted in California over a 10-year period (Walker, 1974), seven health habits emerged as promoting longevity for the middlescent. These habits included: meals at regular times, regular breakfast, exercise, adequate sleep, no cigarette smoking, normal weight, and the consumption of alcohol in moderation. It was shown that a 45-year-old man practicing six of these habits can live 11 years longer than a man the same age who complies with fewer than three of these behaviors. A 7-year gain was noted when data were analyzed on women of the same age.

In conjunction with appropriate health practices, the middlescent's cultural health care practices must be taken into account. To deal with the disequilibrium of illness, practices may include the ingestion of hot and cold foods, the drinking of specific teas, the wearing of pungent herbs or mixtures enclosed in a small cloth bag, and/or the application of mustard plasters (Bullough & Bullough, 1982). Although these practices may be considered foreign to others, their importance to the middlescent must not be negated.

To maintain or regain youthfulness, the middlescent may become overinvolved in health improvement activities such as excess consumption of vitamins, participation in fad diets and rapid weight-reduction programs, and impulsive involvement in physical exercise. While these activities may be the in thing, the end result can cause deleterious effects, since fad diets may not contain adequate nutrients, and impulsive exercising will not allow the cardiovascular system sufficient time to adapt.

Responses to Stressors

The aging process, adhering to health care regimens for the treatment of illnesses, retirement, seeking out new social support systems, and incorporating new members into the nuclear and extended family unit are examples of potential stressors for the middlescent. In dealing with these stressors, the middlescent may respond in an adaptive or in a maladaptive manner. Whether behavior is adaptive or maladaptive will depend on the stressor, the strength of the individual's ego, and the person's ability to effectively use coping mechanisms.

Adaptive Responses. Individuals who manifest adaptive behavior make appropriate use of their coping mechanisms and do not resort to symptoms for relief of anxiety. An adaptive response to stress occurs when the middlescent appropriately confronts the stressor in a constructive, logical, and systematic manner and is capable of continuing to function at an optimal level.

Adaptation is expedited when the middlescent identifies the stressor, collects information about the stressor, examines how this stressor and other stressors have been effectively dealt with in the past, plans and carries out actions related to the stressor, and evaluates the effectiveness of his or her actions regarding the situation. The individual who has successfully adapted to stressors throughout life is likely to continue to do so during middlescence. The middlescent who has a well-integrated personality, has learned to live in harmony with the environment, and has effectively been able to utilize available resources in dealing with stressors in the past is better able to adapt.

Maladaptive Responses. Maladaptive responses to stressors are noted when the individual uses physical and emotional symptoms to relieve anxiety. Diarrhea, migraine headaches, skin eruptions, and irritability are but a few examples of stress-related symptoms. Obsession with being younger than one's age, refusal to comply with recommended health care regimens, frequently returning to the worksite after retirement, denial of the need for new social support systems, and ostracizing new family members are maladaptive responses to stressors that may be observed in the middlescent. The individual who has not appropriately dealt with stress throughout life will undoubtedly continue to have problems adjusting to stressors throughout middlescence.

NURSING ASSESSMENT

Significant changes occur in an individual's life during middlescence. In order to determine the impact that each of these changes impose, a comprehensive assessment of the middlescent and his or her family needs to be conducted. See Table 10–2 for considerations that must be addressed when assessing the middlescent and his or her family.

TABLE 10–2. ASSESSING THE FAMILY WITH A MIDDLESCENT

	Environmental Data
Living conditions	Is the house clean? Is there adequate temperature control? Does the house provide adequate space for the occupants? How many people reside in the home? Are hazardous conditions present in and around the home?
Family size	Is a spouse present? How many children are in the family? Are aged relatives residing with the occupants?
	Communication Patterns
Within the family	What types of verbal and nonverbal communications are used? Who speaks to whom and about what?
With members of society	What types of verbal and nonverbal communications are used? Who speaks to whom and about what?
	Problem-solving Skills
Decision-making abilities	Is a systematic approach used to make decisions? How much time is taken in making a decision? What resources are used to help in decisions? What is the individual and family response to the decisions made?
Use of the health care system	Is there recognition of the need for use of the health care system? Do the individual and the family know how to access the system? How frequently do they use the health care system? For what reasons do they use the health care system? Do they adhere to prescribed health care regimens?
	Life-style
Role within the family	How does the family view the middlescent's role within the family structure? How does the middlescent view his or her role in the family? What are the roles of the middlescent in the family?
Socioeconomic status	Who is head of the household? Who contributes to the family income? What role does the middlescent play in the socioeconomic status of the family? What is the socioeconomic status of the middlescent? What is the income level of the family?
Recreational patterns	What forms of recreation are used by the middlescent and by the family? Do the family members and the middlescent engage in recreational activities on a regular basis? With whom does the middlescent engage in recreational activities?
	Potential Stressors
Income level	Is the income level sufficient to meet the needs of the middlescent and/or the family? What financial considerations are used in making a decision? Who makes the decisions? Is there recogni-

TABLE 10–2. ASSESSING THE FAMILY WITH A MIDDLESCENT *(continued)*

	tion of the consequences of the financial decisions made and of the resources available to the middlescent and/or the family?
Health status	What is the health status of the family and of the middlescent? Has there been a recent change in the status of health in the family and/or the middlescent? Is the middlescent on a pre- scribed health care regimen? Is there anyone with an acute and/or chronic illness in the family?
Family structure changes	Are the children leaving home? Have any of the children recently been married? Have any new grandchildren recently arrived? Have aged relatives recently moved into the home?
Family Response Patterns	
Goal evaluation	How have the goals of the family and of the middlescent changed? If they have changed, how have the family and the middlescent adapted to the changes?
Counseling	Has the middlescent or the family ever sought counseling? If so, for what reasons and where?

ALTERATIONS IN HEALTH

During middlescence there is a slowing of recuperative power so that injuries and acute conditions, which rapidly resolve during young adulthood, may require a prolonged recovery and may result in a chronic condition. An increased prevalence of chronic illness has been noted during middlescence (Strauss et al., 1984), with the most prevalent being cardiovascular disease, cancer, rheumatoid arthritis, diabetes mellitus, obesity, renal calculi, alcoholism, chronic obstructive pulmonary disease, and sleep pattern disturbances. Although acute conditions, such as upper respiratory infections, gastric and intestinal upsets, back pains, and headaches are not uncom- mon, the primary health care focus during middlescence is on dealing with chronic diseases.

The presence of chronic illness during middlescence can have devastating effects. Chronic conditions can interfere with the individual's sense of generativity, can lead to career or occupational changes, can impose undue economic strain, can alter family roles, and ultimately can lead to anxiety and/or depression. For a defini- tion of each of the aforementioned health alterations, please refer to Table 10–3.

TABLE 10–3. HEALTH ALTERATIONS DURING MIDDLESCENCE

Type	Definition
Acute	
Anxiety	A feeling of uneasiness, apprehension, or dread about the unknown.
Depression	A mental state characterized by dejection, lack of hope, and absence of cheerfulness.

TABLE 10–3. HEALTH ALTERATIONS DURING MIDDLESCENCE *(continued)*

Type	Definition
Chronic	
Cardiovascular disease	A pathological condition of the heart and/or blood vessels resulting in inadequate perfusion to the body's tissues.
Cancer	A neoplastic disease in which there is new growth of abnormal cells.
Rheumatoid arthritis	A chronic, systemic, connective tissue disorder of unknown cause that involves inflammatory changes primarily in the small peripheral joints in the hands and feet.
Diabetes mellitus	A disorder of carbohydrate metabolism characterized by an elevated blood sugar and an increased sugar content in the urine, resulting from inadequate production or utilization of insulin.
Obesity	An increase in weight beyond what is considered desirable with regard to age, height, sex, and bone structure.
Renal calculi	A stone formation consisting of a crystallization of minerals found in the urinary system.
Alcoholism	A disorder manifested by loss of control over the consumption of alcohol, resulting in impairment in social or occupational functioning.
Chronic obstructive pulmonary disease	A disease process where obstruction of the small airways occurs, leading to a decreased ability of the lungs to perform their function of ventilation.
Sleep pattern disturbances	An alteration in sleep patterns whereby total sleep time decreases, the number of sleep arousals increase, the percentage of time spent awake in bed increases, and the amount of stage 4 sleep decreases (the time when the heart rate and blood pressure reach their lowest points).

NURSING RESPONSIBILITIES

The responsibility of the nurse is to assist the middlescent in identifying and dealing with the positive and negative aspects of health and in becoming more actively involved in the maintenance and promotion of present and future health needs. The nurse, following a comprehensive assessment of the middlescent and his or her family, can plan nursing interventions under three major categories. These categories include health maintenance, health promotion, and preventive measures.

Health Maintenance

To facilitate the middlescent's maintenance of a high level of wellness, the nurse needs to assist the individual and his or her family in an overall assessment of the accomplishments of individual tasks and of family tasks. The accomplishments achieved should be delineated, as well as determining if the achievements are realistic. For example, has the middlescent family and/or the middlescent achieved the desired socioeconomic security, accepted the family accomplishments, established appropriate family relationships, dealt with physical changes, achieved age-related personality development, established appropriate interpersonal relationships, been successful in personal competencies and achievements, and established societal and cultural endeavors? If the aforementioned are true, the nurse should foster the manner in which these tasks have been achieved by providing positive feedback regarding accomplishments, providing information concerning pertinent community resources related to family and individual tasks, and encouraging continued recognition of and adaptation to stressors. On the other hand, if these tasks have not been accomplished, health promotion and health prevention modalities should be provided by the nurse.

Health Promotion

The purpose of health promotion is to facilitate the middlescent's optimal level of functioning, which can be accomplished through role modeling and by means of health education. Role modeling and health education can be achieved through involvement in support groups, through one-to-one teaching sessions, and through family and middlescent health care planning.

Health-related support groups that may be beneficial to the middlescent include cardiac and arthritic clubs, exercise classes, Overeaters Anonymous, and Alcoholics Anonymous. These groups not only provide exposure to individuals with similar health-related issues, but also provide a medium where health-related information is disseminated and evaluated.

Health care issues that need to be addressed with the middlescent include bodily changes brought about by the aging process, the development of chronic illnesses, the presence of occupation-related stressors, the decrease of social support systems, and the alterations in family relationships. These issues can be addressed through the use of a one-to-one teaching session during any encounter with the middlescent. Printed materials regarding health care issues, whether written by the nurse or obtained from health care organizations, prove beneficial in augmenting verbal instructions.

Family and middlescent health care planning is an ongoing process that requires active participation on the part of the nurse. The nurse may need to assist the family and the middlescent in identifying desired health outcomes. Specific means of accomplishing the outcomes need to be delineated. The middlescent who identifies a need for weight reduction will require a diet with the appropriate calorie count in addition to a regulated exercise program. If enhancing family relationships is the desired health outcome, reviewing and practicing appropriate communication skills are in order. Should coping with a chronic illness be the desired health care outcome, a thorough review of prescribed health care regimens, an examination of the impacts that the physical illness has upon the individual's and the family's life-style, and a delineation of the alternatives for dealing with the impacts created by the chronic illness are necessary (Lambert & Lambert, 1985).

Preventive Measures

Sound health behavior can be accomplished through a variety of measures including anticipatory guidance, stress management, and safety practices. The underlying purpose of each of these measures is to prevent the occurrence or reoccurrence of illness.

Anticipatory Guidance. This is a helpful modality for assisting the middlescent in dealing with family and individual tasks. In providing guidance, it is necessary to point out that hormonal changes will occur, activity tolerance will decrease, weight gain is likely, changes in physical appearance will occur, alterations in sensory function will occur, the likelihood of chronic illness will increase, changes in career endeavors can occur, and interpersonal relations with family and friends tend to undergo change.

   The nurse must work with the individual in planning the most appropriate strategy for dealing with each of these issues. The middlescent female, anticipating hot flashes as a result of hormonal changes, should be encouraged to wear fabrics that provide air flow, to remove layers of clothing, to open a window, and to sip a cool drink when hot flashes are experienced (Woods, 1982).

   When an increase in activity expenditure is expected, the middlescent undergoing a decrease in activity tolerance should be encouraged to space the activity expenditure, to engage in rest periods during the activity, and to carry out warming-up and cooling-down periods before and after the activity. Regular daily exercise should be encouraged, while sporadic weekend exercise should be discouraged, because it can lead to injury. In conjunction with a regular exercise program, a monitoring of caloric intake should occur. A balance between caloric consumption and caloric expenditure will assist the middlescent in weight control. There also should be encouragement to reduce the intake of cholesterol and saturated fats, sugar, salt, and food additives. Fiber and fluid intake may need to be increased to deal with diminished gastrointestinal motility brought on by the aging process and by a reduction in physical activity.

   In providing guidance regarding anticipated changes in physical appearance, the nurse should focus on the realities of potential changes while emphasizing viable means for dealing with these changes. The middlescent may find it desirable to place tints and rinses on the hair when color changes are experienced. In dealing with changes in skin integrity, the middlescent will find it beneficial to use moisturizing creams and lotions to keep the skin supple.

   The primary sensory changes experienced during middlescence involve a decrease in visual acuity, a lengthening of time for visual adjustment from light to dark environments, a need for greater light intensity to appropriately discern the environment, and a decrease in peripheral vision. Yearly eye exams should be encouraged so that appropriate eye correction may be acquired for visual acuity deficits. The middlescent should be encouraged to wait a few moments after entering a dark room to allow the eyes time to adjust to the light changes. In addition, use of adequate lighting should be emphasized so the environment can be easily seen. Moving too quickly after entering a dark room or using inadequate lighting can lead to injury due to falls or to bumping into objects. When crossing the street or engaging in any activity involving moving objects, the middlescent should be instructed to turn the head to correctly assess the presence of objects, because peripheral vision has decreased. Lack of adequate environmental assessment also can lead to injury.

Because the likelihood of chronic illness increases during middlescence, the middlescent should be encouraged to watch for changes in bowel and urinary function, chest pain, increase in thirst, faintness, headaches, bloody noses, difficulty breathing, alterations in sensations, the presence of any palable mass, joint stiffness and pain, weight fluctuations, and changes in sleep patterns. Appropriate health care intervention should be initiated if any of these symptoms are noted. It is advisable for the middlescent to receive periodic health examinations to monitor his or her health status as well as to detect the development of illness.

As career achievements are being assessed, the nurse needs to alert the middlescent that it is not uncommon to make changes in career goals during this time in one's life. The middlescent should be provided information regarding possible job placement and retraining opportunities.

As a result of changes in family structure, the middlescent is faced with alterations in interpersonal relationships with family members and friends. Assuming the role of grandparent, in-law, close friend, and/or intimate spouse are part of the developmental process of the middle years. The nurse needs to assist the middlescent in preparing for these changes by encouraging verbalization of concerns about the new roles and about the interactive process. The intervention should focus on what the middlescent perceives to constitute the new role, what the role means, what activities are inherent in the new role, and how the individual will assimilate the new role responsibilities.

Stress Management.   This provides a second major modality for fostering sound health behavior. By middlescence an individual has experienced numerous stressors; however, the most frequent stressors facing the middlescent include physical changes, societal and emotional changes, and conflicts with family tasks. The nurse needs to encourage the middlescent, to determine how he or she has effectively dealt with stress, and to be prepared to mobilize these coping mechanisms. Generalized aids that may prove beneficial in reducing stress include:

1. Recognizing stress by identifying one's physical and emotional responses (i.e., increased heart rate; cool, pale skin; increased perspiration; diarrhea; urinary frequency; decreased appetite; headaches; difficulty swallowing; decreased ability to follow directions; decreased attention span; and constant need for reassur-

ance). Analyzing what precipitates the reaction, and accepting responsibility for own behavior
2. Reducing pace by doing one thing at a time
3. Providing a period of relaxation daily. Yoga, deep-breathing exercises, meditation, progressive muscle relaxation, biofeedback, and/or guided imagery are suggested techniques
4. Seeking objectivity about concerns by conversing about feelings with friends, family, and/or a counselor/therapist
5. Engaging in physical exercise and/or recreation to increase endorphin levels and to reduce physical tension
6. Developing a fulfilling hobby
7. Establishing realistic expectations of self and others

Safety Practices. These constitute the third modality for fostering sound health behavior. The nurse's role involves assisting the middlescent in a comprehensive assessment and institution of safety factors in the home, neighborhood, and workplace. The need for ready access to emergency phone numbers, smoke detectors, fire extinguishers, appropriate evacuation procedures, cleanliness, control of pollutants, presence of potable water, adequate traffic control, adequate police and emergency health care assistance, and protection from hazardous wastes are essential in each of these environments. Assistance and direction may need to be provided to appropriate individuals, organizations, and community services to assure the presence of a healthy environment.

To further enhance a healthy environment, the middlescent needs to be encouraged to destroy outdated medications, to check the expiration date on food and drug items, to avoid placing objects in pathways inside and outside the home, to keep windows and doors in the home locked, to paint rooms light colors so that visual brightness is enhanced, to avoid self-medication for health care problems, to check all machinery such as lawnmowers and carpentry equipment for compliance with safety regulations, and to inform family and friends of usual daily routines. Such preventive and safety tactics are easy to carry out and may prevent injury and/or illness.

Acute Caregiver

Middlescence is a time when productivity, achievement, and responsibility are major concerns in an individual's life. When an acute illness occurs, goals and expectations are often thwarted for both the middlescent and the family. The nurse needs to be sensitive to the concerns and anxieties brought about by the illness. For example, the woman undergoing a mastectomy may be concerned about her abilities to be sexually desirable to her mate. The individual who has been hospitalized for long periods of time may be concerned about financially supporting the family or providing child care.

The nurse in the acute care situation can be most helpful by assisting the individual and the family in making decisions by offering a variety of options and resources that may help in meeting their specific needs. At the same time, the nurse must be careful not to foster dependence. To be successful in meeting the needs of the middlescent dealing with an acute health alteration, the nurse needs to be knowledgeable about all aspects of growth and development related to the middle years and incorporate this knowledge into nursing care plans and interventions.

SUMMARY

Middlescence, the time frame between 45 and 65 years of age, is when the individual deals with socioeconomic security for the future, achievement of family goals, changing family and friend relationships, bodily changes, generativity, personal and career accomplishments, increased involvement in community and leisure activities, and an increased likelihood of chronic illness. To facilitate the middlescent's optimal level of health, the nurse needs to thoroughly assess the developmental and psychosocial aspects of the individual and his or her family, provide needed acute care, and initiate and foster appropriate health maintenance, health promotion, and preventive measures.

CARE PLAN FOR THE MIDDLESCENT WITH DIABETES MELLITUS

Situation

Mr. Levy, a 55-year-old, married, furniture upholsterer, has had diabetes mellitus, type II, for 10 years. Over the past 9 months he has encountered increasing difficulties with control of his diabetes while being maintained on a regulated diet and oral hypoglycemic agents. Therefore, a month ago Mr. Levy's physician placed him on insulin and a regulated diet. Mrs. Levy has taken the responsibility of administering Mr. Levy's insulin because Mr. Levy is reticent to administer his own insulin. Mr. Levy is resting in the furniture company's dispensary after being treated for a state of hypoglycemia experienced during work. While in the dispensary, Mr. Levy tells the occupational health nurse that he cannot keep his diabetes under control and that he does not understand the reason for his prescribed diet. While conversing with Mr. Levy, the nurse compiles the following nursing diagnoses. Following the diagnoses is a care plan developed by the nurse that addresses Mr. Levy's most prominent diagnosis, knowledge deficit related to proper control of diabetes mellitus.

Nursing Diagnoses

1. Knowledge deficit related to proper control of diabetes mellitus.
2. Alteration in health maintenance related to failure to meet specific dietary health status needs.

SAMPLE CARE PLAN

Nursing Diagnosis	Goals	Nursing Intervention	Evaluation
Knowledge deficit related to proper control of diabetes mellitus.	Mr. Levy will describe three measures to control diabetes mellitus and prevent complications and one measure to monitor control of his illness.	The nurse will review with Mr. Levy, what constitutes an appropriate diet for him, how to correctly administer his insulin, what constitutes an appropriate amount of exercise for him, and how to monitor his blood glucose level.	Mr. Levy will describe three measures to control diabetes mellitus and prevent complications and one measure to monitor control of his illness.

Review Questions

1. Discuss the major areas of concern for the middlescent in regards to the accomplishments of family developmental tasks.

2. Discuss the major areas of concern for the middlescent in regards to the accomplishment of individual developmental tasks.

3. Discuss the role that the nurse plays in assisting the middlescent in accomplishing his or her family and individual developmental tasks.

4. Identify major stressors confronting the middlescent, and describe how the nurse can facilitate the individual's coping process.

5. Define five major chronic illnesses that can occur during middlescence.

6. Identify and discuss four means of anticipatory guidance that the nurse can use to foster sound health behavior.

REFERENCES

Anderson, L., & Polk, G. (1983). The family with an elderly member. In I. Clements & F. Roberts (Eds.), *Family health: A theoretical approach to nursing care*. New York: Wiley.

Abbick, C. (1983). Adult development and the impact of disruption. In S. Lewis & I. Collier (Eds.), *Medical-surgical nursing: Assessment and management of clinical problems*. New York: McGraw-Hill.

Bellville, J., Forrest, W., Miller, E., & Brown, B. (1971). Influence of age on pain relief from analgesics: A study of postoperative patients. *Journal of the American Medical Association, 217*, 1835–1841.

Bierman, E., & Hazzard, W. (1973). Biology of aging. In D. Smith & E. Bierman (Eds.), *Biologic ages of man, from conception through old age*. Philadelphia: Saunders.

Bullough, V., & Bullough, B. (1982). *Health care for the other Americans*. New York: Appleton-Century-Crofts.

Cadogan, M. (1984). The middle adult. In D. Jones, M. Lepley, & B. Baker (Eds.), *Health assessment across the life span.* New York: McGraw-Hill.

Cantu, R. (1982). *Sports medicine in primary care.* Lexington: Collamore.

Cavallo-Perin, P., Sorbo, R., Morra, G., Pagani, A., Tagliaferro, V., & Lenti, G. (1981). Correlation between obesity and other risk factors for coronary heart disease in a group of 4124 volunteers. In G. Enzi, C. Crepaldi, G. Pozza, & A. Renold (Eds.), *Obesity: Pathogenesis and treatment.* New York: Academic Press.

Chinn, A. (Ed.) (1971, July). *Working with older people: A guide to practice.*(U.S. Department of Health, Education, and Welfare Publication, No. 1459) Washington, DC: U.S. Department of Health, Education, and Welfare.

Corso, J. (1981). *Aging sensory systems and perceptions.* New York: Praeger.

Duvall, E. (1977). *Marriage and family development.* Philadelphia: Lippincott.

Erikson, E. (1963). *Childhood and society.* New York: Norton.

Gentry, W. (1979). Preadmission behavior. In W. Gentry & R. Williams, Jr. (Eds.), *Psychological aspects of myocardial infarction and coronary care.* St. Louis: Mosby.

Haan, N., & Day, D. (1974). A longitudinal study of change and sameness in personality development, adolescence to later adulthood. *Aging and human development, 5*(1), 11–39.

Hatcher, R., & Stewart, G. (1982). *Contraceptive technology: Nineteen eighty two to eighty three.* New York: Hatchford.

Hayflick, L. (1970). Aging under glass. *Experimental Gerontology, 1970, 5,* 291–304.

Jarvik, L., & Cohen, D. (1973). A biobehavioral approach to intellectual changes with aging. In C. Eisdorfer & M. Lawton (Eds.), *The psychology of adult development and aging.* Washington, DC: American Psychological Association.

Kannel, W., & Gordon, T. (1979). Psychological and medical concomitants of obesity: The Framingham study. In G. Ray (Ed.), *Obesity in America* (NIH Publication No. 79-359). Washington, DC: U.S. Government Printing Office.

Karpel, M., & Strauss, E. (1983). *Family evaluation.* New York: Gardner.

Keele, C., Neil, E., & Joels, N. (1982). *Samson Wright's applied physiology.* Oxford: Oxford University Press.

Kimmel, D. (1974). *Adulthood and aging.* New York: Wiley.

Knafl, K., & Grace, H. (1978). *Families across the life cycle.* Boston: Little, Brown.

Lambert, C., & Lambert, V. (1977). Divorce: A psycho-dynamic development involving grief. *Journal of Psychiatric Nursing and Mental Health Services, 15* (1), 37–42.

Lambert, V., & Lambert, C. (1985). *Psychosocial care of the physically ill: What every nurse should know.* Englewood Cliffs, NJ: Prentice-Hall.

Lidz, T. (1980). *Phases of adult life: An overview.* In W. Norman & T. Scaramella (Eds.), *Mid-life: Development and clinical issues.* New York: Brunner/Mazel.

Malasanos, L. (1981). *Health assessment.* St. Louis: Mosby.

Peck, R., & Berkowitz, H. (1964). Personality and adjustment in middle age. In B. Neugarten (Ed.), *Personality in middle and late life.* New York: Atherton.

Pfeiffer, E., & Davis, G. (1971). The use of leisure time in middle age. *Gerontologist, 11,* 187–195.

Rankoff, A. (1980). The female climacteric and the pros and cons of estrogen therapy. In J. Gold & J. Josimovich (Eds.), *Gynecologic endocrinology.* Hagerstown, MD: Harper & Row.

Schaie, K. (1975). Age changes in adult intelligence. In D. Woodruf & J. Birren (Eds.), *Aging: Scientific perspectives and social issues.* New York: Van Nostrand.

Seaman, B., & Seaman, G. (1977). *Women and the crises in sex hormones.* New York: Ramson.

Strauss, A., Corbin, J., Fagerhaugh, S., Glaser, B., Maines, D., Suczek, B., & Weiner, C. (1984). *Chronic illness and the quality of life.* St. Louis: Mosby.

Streff, M. (1981). Examining family growth and development: A theoretical model. *Advances in Nursing Science, 3*(4), 61–69.

Tamir, L. (1982). *Men in their forties: The transition to middle age.* New York: Springer.

Timiras, P. (1972). *Developmental physiology and aging.* New York: Macmillan.

Tobian, L. (1978). Hypertension and obesity. *New England Journal of Medicine, 298,* 46–48.

Troll, L. (1975). *Early and middle adulthood.* Monterey, CA: Brooks/Cole.

Walker, A. R. (1974). Survival rate at middle age in developing and western populations. *Postgraduate Medical Journal, 50,* 29–32.

Weiner, M., Brok, A., & Snadowsky, A. (1978). *Working with the aged: Practical approaches in the institution and community.* Englewood Cliffs, NJ: Prentice-Hall.

Woodrow, K., Friedman, G., Siegelaub, A., & Collen, M. (1972). Pain tolerance: Differences according to age, sex, and race. *Psychosomatic Medicine, 34*(6), 548–556.

Woods, N. (1982). Menopause. In G. Hongladarom, R. McCorkle, and N. Woods (Eds.), *The complete book of women's health.* Englewood Cliffs, NJ: Prentice-Hall.

11

The Family with the Senescent Over 65 Years

*Vickie A. Lambert and
Clinton E. Lambert Jr.*

Objectives

Upon completion of this chapter, the student will be able to:

1. Describe family and individual tasks as they relate to the senescent
2. Identify potential stressors for the senescent
3. Explain the coping mechanisms utilized by the senescent
4. Describe the salient components of a nursing assessment for the senescent and his or her family
5. Identify common acute and chronic health alterations experienced by the senescent
6. Plan nursing care for the senescent in regards to health maintenance, health promotion, and preventive measures

Concepts

Aging: a normal developmental process in which certain anatomical and physiological changes take place that are universal, intrinsic, progressive, and eventually deleterious to the organism

Retire: to withdraw from one's mode of gainful employment

Ego integrity: one's sense of acceptance of past triumphs and disappointments

Despair: a sense of hopelessness

Poverty: the serious lack of means for proper existence

Grandparenting: the act of caring for the children of one's children

Isolation: to detach or separate one's self from others

Powerlessness: the perception that one's own actions will not effect change in self or the environment

Dependence: the act of relying upon another individual for assistance, aid, or support

Loss: a condition whereby an individual experiences deprivation of, or complete lack of, something that was previously present

Illness: an alteration in physiological function and/or psychosocial integrity that impedes an individual's ability to achieve an optimal level of performance

Adaptation: the appropriate use of coping mechanisms to deal with stressors

Maladaptation: the inappropriate use of coping mechanisms to deal with stressors

Stressors: demands that tax or exceed the resources of the individual

Death: cessation of an individual's life

Senescence, the time frame from 65 years of age until death, is when the individual evaluates past experiences and accomplishments and comes to terms with the final years of life. This time frame tends to encompass the death of one's spouse, numerous changes in bodily function, retirement, dealing with one's own imminent death, changes in socioeconomic status, and the psychosocial task of ego integrity versus despair (Erikson, 1963). Within the context of these developmental and psychosocial aspects, the following chapter will address family and individual tasks, personal stressors and coping mechanisms, and health alterations relevant to the senescent. How the nurse can intervene and appropriately deal with each of the aforementioned components will be discussed.

FAMILY TASKS

There are three major family tasks confronting the senescent. These tasks include: (1) maintenance of socioeconomic security, (2) review of family accomplishments, and (3) change in and maintenance of family relationships. Successful attainment of these three tasks requires the senescent to come to terms with the inevitable and systematic losses that occur during the twilight years of life.

Socioeconomic Security

Undoubtedly, one of the most difficult family tasks with which the aged family must contend is socioeconomic security. If the breadwinner has not retired before reaching 65 years of age (which is becoming increasingly more likely with the advancing longevity of today's society), he or she most likely will be forced to do so sometime early in the developmental stage of senescence. Retirement may become inevitable due to deteriorated health and/or the retirement age policies of the employer. Fortunately, an ever-increasing number of companies and institutions are re-evaluating their retirement policies and are no longer encouraging or demanding retirement at a given time.

The senescent family that has adequately planned for the retirement years will have ensured that they have the necessary credits for Social Security payments and available resources, such as savings bonds, annuities, and redeemable life insurance policies, for potential financial emergencies. For many elderly, however, retirement benefits may be minimal. Social Security, once regarded as supplemental income for the elderly, has become the main financial resource for many senescents. Approximately 46% of the total income of single elderly and nearly 33% of the total income of aged couples comes from Social Security payments (Annual Statistical Supplement, 1983).

Retirement often imposes the necessity of living on a fixed income, which may force the aged family to do away with expenditures related to recreation or socialization. Since the senescent family no longer has the flexibility of contending with an increase in the cost of living or with unexpected needs, such as health care costs, they are likely to be forced into a standard of living well below that which they have maintained throughout life. If financial planning has been inadequate or has not taken into account the needs of the aged family, when retirement takes place, the family may be forced to seek welfare in order to survive. It is important to remember that the elderly of today grew up with a strong work ethic and maintain pride in being able to provide for themselves and their families. Having to turn to others for financial assistance can prove emotionally devastating for members of an aged family, because it represents an inability to leave behind a family inheritance.

Family Accomplishments

The second task confronting the senescent family is the review of family accomplishments. In other words, the family reviews what it has achieved over the past years as a family unit. These achievements can include economic stability, success of one's children, attainment of the grandparent role, and preparation for leaving a family inheritance.

The aged family that believes it has achieved perceived goals will manifest a sense of accomplishment and satisfaction. If economic resources are available to enjoy retirement and the family does not have to rely on others for subsistence, they may identify themselves as being successful and having accomplished their goals as a family.

A sense of dissatisfaction or failure as a family may prevail, if the family feels, for example, that their offspring have not lived up to their expectations or provided them with desired grandchildren, and/or that they are unable to leave a respectable inheritance. As a result, the family unit is likely to view their past experiences with despair instead of manifesting a strong sense of ego integrity (Erikson, 1963).

Family Relationships

The third major task confronting the senescent family is change in and maintenance of family relationships. As the individual ages, roles and relationships within the family structure change. It is during senescence that: (1) the role of grandparent tends to be actualized: (2) one's spouse or one's self becomes dependent upon others for assistance; (3) one takes up residence in a retirement village or nursing home; and/or (4) one loses roles, such as child, brother, sister, or spouse, due to death. These changes require alterations in relationships that exist in the aged family.

The grandparent role is more likely, initially, to be assumed during middle age; however, for some individuals it may not become a reality until senescence. Although limited research exists on the grandparent role, from observations one can note that grandparents are less likely to be actively involved in rearing activities and more likely to be involved in leisure activities with their grandchildren. It is quite common to observe grandparents taking their grandchildren on picnics or trips, playing games with them, and sharing pictures and tales about their grandchildren with anyone who will listen.

Due to failing health, the senescent may become dependent upon others for carrying out his or her activities of daily living. This increased dependence can alter family relationships and place stress on all members involved. In some situations the spouse of the dependent senescent is capable of caring for the individual within the home environment. The spouse may note, however, that the ability to freely meet personal needs will be altered. For example, simply going to the grocery store, the barber or beauty shop, or house of worship may require a sitter for the dependent senescent. If extended family members are not readily available to assume the role of sitter, the aged family may have to pay another person to assume such a role. This requirement can place a financial burden on the aged family.

Living with children may become a necessity for members of an aged family, either due to financial conditions or due to the inability to independently care for one's self. When such a situation occurs, the aged family member takes on a dependent role in regard to his or her children. In the past, the senescent had been the provider and protector of the children. Now that the aged family member resides with children, the roles of the past are reversed. The children become the providers and protectors, while the elderly parent becomes the dependent member of the family. For some aged individuals, having to rely upon children for assistance can be extremely devastating and demoralizing.

In the event that a member of an aged family is unable to be cared for at home by a spouse or in the home of children, the individual may require care in a nursing home. Such a change in residence can alter a number of the roles within the family structure. If an aged spouse is left in the home while the dependent elderly spouse is placed in a nursing home, the typical roles of husband and wife will be altered. The ability to relate to each other on a personal or intimate level may be changed, due to lack of privacy or geographical inaccessibility. Time together will have to be planned in advance and may be limited if the individual left residing in the home environment has difficulty obtaining adequate transportation. The elderly individual in the nursing home will, no doubt, begin to establish new relationships with other residents in the nursing home. These new relationships will be foreign to the spouse, and he or she may encounter difficulty in understanding or accepting these new-found friends. By the same token, the elderly individual living at home may be able to continue long-time friendships. These well-established friendships eventually may become foreign to the elderly spouse residing in the nursing home if he or she has limited interaction with long-time friends. Feeling as though one is not a part of an old friendship which existed in one's home neighborhood is not uncommon for the elderly individual residing in a nursing home.

An alternate pattern of living, which many elderly couples prefer, is residing in a retirement village that offers independent living as well as graded forms of dependent living. If the senescent family is capable of caring for themselves, they have the option of living independently in their own apartment or modular home. Should the necessity arise for assisted living, nursing homes are on the retirement village grounds, which have graded forms of nursing care. Easy access to the nursing home from one's own independent living accommodations facilitates the maintenance of spousal relationships when one spousal member requires care in a nursing home.

Changes in family roles also occur within an elderly family, due to death. Senescence is the only life stage that encounters systematic loss of relationships with child, brother, sister, and/or spouse. All other life stages are marked by a steady growth of relationships, either through marriage, jobs, or the birth of children. Such losses often are difficult for the senescent to accept because these relationships frequently have lasted a major portion of the senescent's life. Undoubtedly one of the most difficult relationship losses with which the elderly individual must contend is the loss of the spouse. Coping with the loss of one with whom you have shared many of life's experiences can be devastating. Not only has the senescent lost a significant other, but he or she also has lost the significant role of spouse. In addition to losing one's spouse, the loss of other elderly family members, such as brothers and sisters, is not uncommon. The senescent literally sees the world of family relationships dwindling before his or her eyes.

INDIVIDUAL TASKS

Along with family tasks, the adult in senescence is faced with five specific individual tasks. These tasks can be categorized as physical changes in the body, personality development, interpersonal relationships, competencies and achievements, and societal and cultural endeavors. These tasks may or may not occur simultaneously; however, they all exist and must be dealt with during the senescent years.

Physical Changes

Physical changes that occur in the body during senescence are related to use, regression, growth, and hyperplasia (Rossman, 1977). These aging changes are normal, inevitable, progressive, irreversible, and lead to a decrease in one's ability to adapt to the environment and, therefore, to an increase in mortality rate. Although inevitable, the physical changes that occur as a result of aging take place at different rates in different individuals, depending upon such factors as genetic background, environment, nutritional status, and activity patterns (Gioiella & Bevil, 1985).

The cardinal feature of age-related physical changes is a progressive decrease in the number of cells in most organs. Loss of cells has been confirmed by changes in organ weights, total cell counts, and the amount of potassium, DNA, intracellular water, and nitrogen found in the senescent as compared to the young adult (Goldman, 1979). The decrease in cell number that occurs in the aged is believed to be due to the cessation of cellular function and cell division capacity (Latham & Johnson, 1979). The reasons for these cellular changes are unknown, but are the focus of extensive and intensive research (Hayflick, 1977).

A number of changes occur in the musculoskeletal system of the senescent. One is a decrease in height anywhere from 1/2 to 2 inches. Loss of height, however, is more pronounced in females and is the result of a loss of height in individual vertebrae and the narrowing of the fibroelastic disks between the vertebrae (Rossman, 1979). In addition to a decrease in height, a reduction in shoulder width and size occurs due to a decrease in the deltoid muscle and the acromion, the lateral extension of the spine of the scapula that forms the highest point of the shoulder (Rossman, 1977).

A decrease in lean muscle mass occurs in the senescent. The loss of muscle fiber leads to a decrease in muscle strength and function (Gutmann, 1977). Due to demineralization, the bones lose their density and become more prone to fracture. The joints become less mobile, with the large weight-bearing joints showing the greatest wear, friction, and stiffness. By age 50, nearly 25% of the population have osteoarthritic changes, but by age 70, over 75% exhibit some type of osteoarthritic change (Rossman, 1977).

With aging also comes a redistribution in major body components. There is an overall increase in the percentage of body fat, with a decrease in bone matrix and minerals, intracellular water, and tissue cell mass (Rossman, 1977). Such changes lead to porous bones, a decrease in total body water, and a steady decline in weight. The weight decline that occurs during senescence is more pronounced in men than in women. After age 55, males tend to experience a steady decline in weight of more than 20 pounds. In females, weight tends to increase until the sixth decade, plateau, and then gradually decrease. The weight decline that takes place in women, however, is proportionately less than it is for men (Rossman, 1977; Rossman, 1979).

The integumentary system undergoes alterations during senescence, with the size and shape of the individual's head appearing to change due to alterations in hair distribution and texture. Common baldness, hair loss that normally accompanies aging, may occur. A progressive decrease in the deep dermal blood vessels of the scalp may take place, along with a decrease in the size of the hair follicles. The result is the production of fine, short, nonpigmented hairs, which are lighter, thinner, and less numerous than when the individual was younger (Selmanowitz, Rizer, & Orentreich, 1977). Sex-linked baldness also may occur but is not the result of aging. Such baldness affects men, is inherited from the mother, involves several different patterns of hair loss, may begin as early as 20 years of age, and is effectuated in the presence of testosterone.

Graying of the hair tends to precede hair loss in the senescent. It occurs due to a reduction in the number of melanocytes at the base of the hair follicles. The melanocytes that remain are less productive of pigment, and as a result graying occurs (Selmanowitz, et al., 1977). In addition to color changes in the hair, the senescent also will experience a decrease in the secretion of sebaceous oil in the scalp. The results will be scalp dryness, lack of luster to the hair, and a decrease in the curling of the hair (Spollett, 1984).

Dry, wrinkled, and inelastic skin due to a decrease in the number of sweat glands, a decrease in the function of sebaceous glands in the skin, and the loss of subcutaneous fat will be experienced by the elderly individual (Selmanowitz, et al., 1977). Wrinkles, which normally begin on the forehead early in the second decade, will become particularly evident on the face and neck. Individuals past 60 years of age tend to develop multiple fine wrinkles on the upper and lower lips. In addition, the neck undergoes shrinking and wrinkling, which may prove to be more marked than facial wrinkling (Rossman, 1979).

Liver spots (lentigines), skin tags (ichthyosis), and small reddish areas on the skin caused by enlargement and dilation of capillaries (senile telangiectasis) commonly occur on the head and neck region of the elderly individual. Caucasian elderly may appear more white with age, due to the loss of skin ruddiness. Fragility of the blood vessels is common, so bruising may result even from a minor trauma (Spollett, 1984).

Changes that started in the cardiovascular system during middlescence begin to present symptoms during senescence. The elasticity of the blood vessels diminishes, and cardiac output decreases as the cardiac muscle begins to lose its strength. As a result, the heart in the senescent must work harder to provide adequate oxygenation for the body. Diminished perfusion to some organs, along with arteriosclerosis and atherosclerosis, may lead to ischemia and eventual death of the tissue in one or more organ systems (Kohn, 1977).

Peripheral resistance increases with age, due to diminished vascular flexibility. As a result of the increase in peripheral resistance, both the systolic and disatolic blood pressure may increase. The effects of these changes make the dynamics of the circulatory system less efficient. The senescent's circulation time lengthens and, when the heart rate increases to meet necessary demands, it requires a longer period of time to return to its resting rate (Kohn, 1977).

Like the arteries, the veins in the senescent undergo change. The valves of the large leg veins become inefficient, resulting in inadequate venous return. An increase in the tortuosity of veins is so common that it is considered a normal aging change (Syzek, 1976; Kohn, 1977).

Despite a number of age-related changes in the structure and function of the respiratory system, the senescent tends to retain the ability to maintain adequate oxygenation under conditions of health and moderate exercise. The structures of the respiratory system undergo changes that lead to a decrease in elasticity and an increase in rigidity (Klocke, 1977). The chest wall stiffens due to the increased calcification of costal cartilage and the decreased strength of intercostal and accessory muscles and the diaphragm. Chest wall stiffness, combined with a reduction in elasticity and recoil pressure of the lungs, results in an increase in residual volume and a decrease in forced expiratory volume. Residual volume increases by 100% and results in partial inflation of the lungs at rest (Klocke, 1977). Arterial oxygen decreases, while arterial carbon dioxide and pH remain unchanged. There is an increased susceptibility to lung congestion and infection, due to a decrease in the efficiency of airway clearance mechanisms such as ciliary action and the cough reflex (Gioiella & Bevil, 1985).

Aging changes in the nervous system involve gradual degeneration and atrophy, which leads to lessened acuity in the nerves and impaired sensation. There is a generalized loss of neurons and a progressive decrease in the weight of the brain (Brody & Vijayashander, 1977). Due to impairment in sensation, the senescent may be unaware of thermal injuries or pressure on soft tissue.

Acuity of the senses declines with age. Sensitivity to sound decreases, as well as some selective loss of hearing of the higher pitches. This age-related decline in hearing is called *presbycusis* and, in general, affects men to a greater degree than women (Botwinick, 1978). Visual acuity, especially for close reading, is decreased as a result of the aging process. The crystalline lens becomes hardened and opaque, and the ciliary muscles are less effective in dealing with changes in light intensity. An intolerance to glare and a delayed adaptive pupil response to darkness results.

Changes in the threshold of each of the tastes (salty, sweet, sour, and bitter) appear to be insignificant until after age 50. The decline in taste sensation is due to a decline in the average number of taste buds per papilla (Goldman, 1979). Data on the sense of smell in the elderly are sparse, and the results are conflicting. One study suggests that smell sensitivity does not decline with age, especially in healthy senescents (Engen, 1977). There tends, however, to be a general dulling of the sensations of touch, pressure, pain, and vibration with age. This is brought about by the decreased number and sensitivity of sensory receptors, dermatomes, and neurons in the central nervous system (Carter, 1979; Botwinick, 1978). According to Selmanowitz and associates (1977), these changes are a reliable indication of advancing age.

The physiological controls of fluid and electrolytes provided by the genitourinary system are altered due to aging. There is a decline in the glomerular filtration rate, which primarily is due to a decrease in renal plasma flow. By 80 years of age the glomerular filtration rate has declined by as much as 53% (Wesson, 1969). One major consequence of the age change is the potentiation of the half-life of many drugs that are excreted by the kidneys. Thickening of the basement membrane of Bowman's capsule and impaired permeability occur, which alter excretion and reabsorption. Bladder capacity may be decreased by as much as 50%. If the bladder is filled beyond capacity, there is either leakage or uninhibited bladder contractions that lead to an urgent demand to urinate (Goldman, 1977).

A number of changes occur in the gastrointestinal system, which compromise both ingestion and digestion. Inspection of the oral cavity will reveal that in the elderly there is a decrease in salivary gland secretion, engorgement of the oral mucosal vessels, loose teeth, tooth loss, and recession of the gingiva. Tooth loss generally will be the result of osteoporosis, inflammatory bone absorption around the teeth. The enamel on the teeth will be worn, and yellowish dentin will be visible

(Zack, 1979). In addition, the teeth will tend to have a glassy appearance and, as a result of exposure to temperature extremes over time, the incisors may have vertical cracks in the enamel (Spollett, 1984). A decrease in esophageal mobility may also be noted, along with atrophic changes in the mucosa and musculature of the remaining portions of the gastrointestinal tract. A decrease in digestive enzymes occurs, which may result in an increase in hypoacidity and achlorhydria (Spollett, 1984). Decreased sphincter control of the anus and relaxation of the perineal musculature may be noted when the senescent is asked to bear down.

The reproductive system undergoes change for both the male and female senescent. In the female, the vaginal barrel becomes shorter, narrower, and less elastic, while the epithelium of the vagina thins, giving it a pale appearance and making it susceptible to bleeding. There is a decrease in vaginal lubrication, which makes the canal susceptible to irritation and pain during intercourse. The fallopian tubes become increasingly atrophied until they are nonpalpable, and follicular activity becomes rare in women past 50 years of age (Talbert, 1977; Hogan, 1985). After menopause there is a marked decrease in the size and weight of the uterus. It must be kept in mind that changes that occur in the female genitalia stem from a decrease in estrogen production rather than from aging per se (Spollett, 1984).

In the male senescent the testes and penis decrease in size and the individual experiences fewer sustained erections. There is a decrease in testosterone levels and in the production of spermatozoa; however, reproduction is possible at least into the ninth decade (Gioiella & Bevil, 1985). The scrotal rugae diminish, and vasocongestion of the scrotum lessens during sexual excitement and stimulation. The prostate becomes enlarged, but tends to remain smooth and symmetrical. The seminal vesicles also undergo cellular change, but the aging changes that occur in the epididymis, which plays a major part in the maturation of sperm, remain unclear (Talbert, 1977).

Aging affects a number of aspects of the endocrine system, but it influences different organs in different ways. Increases in serum concentrations of gonadotropins (postmenopausal in females) and thyrotropin tend to occur. On the other hand, decreases in serum concentrations tend to occur in adrenal androgens, aldosterone, female estrogens, and testosterone (in males over 60 years of age). Hormones that tend to remain constant include antidiuretic hormone, growth hormone, thyronine, triiodothyronine, cortisol, insulin, glucagon, and male estrogens (Gregerman & Bierman, 1981). Research on normal endocrine function in the senescent has been hampered since it is frequently altered by the multiple chronic illnesses present in a large proportion of the aged population. As a result, there are many conflicting research findings.

Personality Development

Personality development during senescence involves stability in intellectual functioning and the maintenance of certain personality traits in relationship to the task of integrity (the need to look back at life's experiences and perceive them as purposeful, meaningful, and fulfilling) versus disgust or despair. Over the past 20 years, intellectual functioning of the elderly has been of interest to a number of researchers. These researchers have found that an individual's general intelligence tends to improve until approximately 50 years of age, at which time it stabilizes until shortly before death (Kimmel, 1974; Zarit, 1980; Schaie & Labouvie-Vief, 1974). The drop in various cognitive tests shortly before death has been identified as the *terminal decline* (Riegel & Riegel, 1973). Jarvik (1975) found that elderly subjects who had experienced declines in such cognitive test results as vocabulary, block design, and digit symbols were not likely to survive the next 5 years.

Changes that may occur in cognitive ability in the elderly include reaction time, memory, and problem solving. Speed of responses tend to decline with age on almost any performance measure (Welford, 1974). A slowing of reaction time is a manifestation of neurological aging, which is related to the slowing in the conduction of electrical impulses in the central nervous system (Birren, 1974). Slowed responses, however, can be exaggerated by social deprivation, yet improved by positive reinforcement. Hoyer, Labouvie-Vief, & Baltes (1973) found that the speed with which the elderly perform on ability tests can be increased markedly when rewards such as trading stamps are given.

The ability to maintain primary memory (the amount of information that can be held for active processing) appears to be stable as one's age increases. For example, an elderly individual who is asked to process and remember digits generally will not encounter any difficulty. However, if the senescent is asked to recall the digits in reverse order (reorganize the material), the elderly person undoubtedly will encounter problems remembering the digits (Craik, 1977). Secondary memory (primary memory that is transferred into a storage system and retrieved at a later time) also has been studied in the elderly. It remains unclear as to whether the elderly can perform at the same level as their younger counterparts on tests involving recognition and recall. Schoenfield's (1965) work indicates that the elderly can do as well as younger individuals, while Gordon and Clark (1974) and Perlmutter (1978) report that decreases in both recognition and recall occur in the elderly.

Problem-solving skills tend to be maintained in the elderly. If difficulties do arise, they seem to be the result of a combination of cognitive changes such as memory, learning, attention, and perceptual integration (Rabbitt, 1977). From the sixties to mid-seventies there may be a normal decline on some problem-solving abilities for some but not all individuals. This again attests to the remarkable diversity and individuality of the senescent population. According to Schaie (1980), beyond the age of 80, a decrease in problem solving is, however, the rule for most persons.

Personality traits, by in large, are the same in the senescent as when the individual was younger. Although some personality traits such as cautiousness, rigidity, dependence, and conservatism may intensify with the aging process, the senescent tends to be much as he or she was at earlier developmental stages.

Cautiousness, one of the personality traits, has been found to increase in the elderly (Botwinick, 1978). The senescent tends to be less willing than younger counterparts to take risks unless there is a high certainty of success. Birkhill and Schaie (1975) found that elderly individuals are least cautious when the conditions involve low risk and low anxiety.

Rigidity, another personality trait, has been found to increase with age (Schaie

& Labouvie-Vief, 1974). Senescents tend to have more difficulty shifting from one activity to another, adjusting to new surroundings, and changing daily habits than cohorts in younger age categories.

Dependence and conservatism become more prominent in later life. The elderly person tends to rely upon others more readily and to be preoccupied more with self in regards to bodily function, wants, and past reminiscences (Goldfarb, 1969; Lancaster, 1981). This inner-directedness or introversion tends to be consistent with the general desire of the elderly to avoid change.

The senescent who is capable of demonstrating integrity through the utilization of his or her intellectual functioning and positive personality traits has the ability to look back on life's experiences and perceive them as purposeful, meaningful, and fulfilling. The senescent who believes that life has been rich and rewarding will experience a sense of satisfaction and contentment with the remaining years. However, if the aged person does not evaluate life as such, he or she will face the final years with despair and disgust. As a result, the senescent is likely to become depressed and to manifest a low sense of self-worth, with an outcome of interpersonal impoverishment and self-absorption.

Interpersonal Relationships

One of the greatest changes that occurs during senescence is the realignment of interpersonal relationships. Senescence is a time when roles related to the job are lost and roles associated with family structure change. This is brought about by retirement, by death of family members and friends, and by the addition of grandchildren.

With retirement comes the loss not only of one's gainful employment, but also the loss of important relationships that occur outside of the family structure. Often work associates are individuals with whom one engages in social functions and activities that are not necessarily related to work setting. Retirement decreases the accessibility of individuals with whom the senescent has shared important past life experiences and events. If the senescent has not successfully disengaged from work associates and found alternate relationships through activities in such organizations as the church, senior centers, or social clubs, he or she may experience a sense of personal isolation.

Family roles change during senescence due to loss of one's spouse and/or the addition of grandchildren. The loss of the spousal role is one of the most profound relationship changes that can occur with aging. Loss of the individual with whom one has shared many intimate moments can be overwhelming. This loss is further compounded by the fact that many significant cohorts, who could aid in comforting the widow or widower during the bereavement process, are being lost due to death or confining illnesses. The number of cohorts that one has tends to diminish by the age of 65, with a marked decrease in number by 75 (Gioella & Bevil, 1985).

Research has found that with the death of the spouse, women have the capacity to transfer their need for intimacy to women friends, while men find it difficult to develop intimate friendships and, instead, tend to remarry (Lowenthal, 1975). Both elderly men and elderly women state, however, that the most frequent reason for remarriage is the desire for companionship.

The addition of grandchildren to the family structure creates a new role for the senescent, which tends to be perceived in a positive light. The displaying of a bumper sticker that reads "Ask Me About My Grandchildren" is one testament to such a fact. The grandparent role allows for enjoyment of the younger generation without the responsibilities of childrearing. It is not uncommon to see the grandparent taking part in a variety of recreational or leisure activities with grandchildren. Having grandchildren also allows for an avenue for general conversation among cohorts. The sharing among cohorts of pictures and/or accomplishment of one's grandchildren attests to the existence of such a phenomenon.

Competencies and Achievements

It is during senescence that one takes time to review and evaluate past life experiences and events. Reminiscing alone or with others about one's accomplishments over the years can positively influence a sense of self-worth. Talking and thinking about past events assists the senescent in dealing with regrets and guilt, as well as focusing on those experiences and events that brought happiness and joy.

The senescent who feels a sense of satisfaction and contentment with the past will freely *shift* his or her emphasis from the work role to a broader scene of activities. These activities can include involvement in social clubs, civic organizations, religious organizations, or hospital volunteer work, or being a provider of child care for family members and friends. The senescent may even opt to pursue a second or third career by learning a new skill or by refining an existing one such as carpentry or sewing. The senescent who has a sense of self-worth will become involved in establishing and maintaining satisfying relationships and in valuing the fact that the contributions that he or she has made to children, friends, and society will remain long after his or her death.

Societal and Cultural Endeavors

A disagreement between health care providers who practice Western medicine and the ethnic senescent may occur over conflicting beliefs and practices regarding health care. To overcome cultural barriers, the use of ethnic health care providers such as the *curandero* or the medicine man, ethnic organizations, and native foods should be incorporated into the senescent's health care plan whenever possible. In addition, understanding the role that the senescent plays in his or her culture is extremely important because some cultures, such as the Chinese-American and Native American, highly regard their elderly and look upon them as great sources of wisdom.

It is not uncommon for the elderly individual to retain folk health practices in an effort to maintain his or her cultural identity. Some of the more common ethnic groups that the nurse will find in the United States include Black Americans, Hispanics, Chinese-Americans, and Native Americans.

For Black Americans, in urban ghettos and in rural sections of the South, folk medicine has remained important. It is not uncommon that elderly individuals go through a lay referral system before seeking care from a physician at a clinic or hospital. In other words, the senescent may ask the advice of friends and relatives about his or her illness, as well as attempting to deal personally with the symptoms before seeking care (Bullough & Bullough, 1982). Black Americans also tend to equate health or wellness with the ability to work productively.

Certain segments of the population perceive illness as being the result of disharmony with nature. The presence of demons or bad spirits is thought by the individual to be the cause of this disharmony (Branch & Paxton, 1976). To deal with this disharmony, healers, prayer cloths, voodoo, and the wearing of amulets may be used.

Some *Hispanics*—the ethic group which includes Mexican-Americans and Puerto-Ricans—view wellness as a holistic balance between the person and the environment. Illness, on the other hand, is seen as having social, spiritual, and physical origins and as being due to fright, punishment, or supernatural influences (Clark, 1970). To deal with illness, the Hispanic senescent may resort to using foods classified as either *hot* or *cold*, to massages, and to using herbs or magical cures (Bullough & Bullough, 1982).

Elderly Chinese-Americans often adhere to health practices that incorporate prevention and the maintenance of a balance between energy systems (the yin and the yang). Intrusive procedures, such as the drawing of blood, are avoided if possible, because they are believed to affect the wholeness of the system. To deal with illness, the senescent Chinese-American may resort to the use of herbs, acupuncture, meditation, massage, and certain diets (Bullough & Bullough, 1982).

Native Americans vary in their health beliefs and practices depending upon the tribe. In general, the elderly Native American believes that health is God-given and reflects harmony with the universe. To deal with illness, the Native American may use herbs, drugs, or some supernatural article or agency that is believed to aid in the curing of a disease. In the hospital setting this article may be herbs or mixtures contained in a small cloth that is hung on the bed, placed on the nightstand, or worn around the neck (Bullough & Bullough, 1982).

POTENTIAL STRESSORS

Three major categories of potential stressors exist for the adult facing senescence. These include physical stressors, social and emotional stressors, and stressors related to conflict with family tasks. Understanding what role each potential stressor plays during senescence aids in preparing one to determine appropriate interventions to deal with each stressor.

Physical Stressors

Physical stressors facing the senescent include dealing with changes in bodily function due to the aging process and adjusting to the development of certain chronic illnesses.

Changes in bodily function due to aging currently are considered natural phenomena. However, the changes that do occur can and often do create stress for the elderly individual. For example, alterations in physical appearance and function related to normal aging may influence the person's perception of his or her body image. Body image is the perception or mental picture that one has of his or her physical appearance and/or function (Lambert & Lambert, 1985). When the older individual takes note of bodily appearance and function, he or she may find the presence of wrinkles and pigment changes in the skin, gray sparse hair, eyeglasses, hearing aids, dentures, a decrease in height, weight loss, dry skin, diminished sensitivity to tactile stimulation, a sunken appearance in the eyes, increased nasal hairs, a diminished sense of smell, a relaxation of facial musculature, and enlarged joints of the hands and feet (Kehril & Spenser, 1984). The aged individual, whose body image perception is one of youthful vigor and appearance and whose self-concept is closely linked with this perception, may encounter periods of anxiety when faced with ongoing changes in physical appearance brought on by the normal aging process.

A decrease in mobility due to normal physiological changes brought on by the aging process and/or the existence of arthritis is another major physical stressor for the elderly individual. Such a change often impedes the elderly individual's ability to carry out a wide variety of activities. Activities that involve very vigorous sports, the use of public transportation (particularly during rush-hour traffic), climbing stairs, bending, carrying heavy objects, and engaging in functions that require fine motor movements may need to be curtailed or disbanded. Not being able to do physical activities that once were a part of everyday life may prove frustrating for the elderly individual. Some alteration in life-style may be required by the elderly person in order to adjust to the decrease in mobility. If radical changes in activity are required, undue stress may be experienced. In most situations, radical changes are not needed.

Like the middlescent, the senescent is faced with the increased likelihood of having to deal with a chronic illness (Strauss, et al., 1984). Elderly individuals are more likely to have chronic conditions (and more of them) than their younger counterparts. As the body ages, a decline in integrated body function occurs, which in turn leads to a greater possibility of the development of a chronic health care problem.

Social-Emotional Stressors

The four major social-emotional stessors facing the senescent include dealing with one's imminent death, contending with loss of a significant other, living in a state of isolation, and facing a sense of powerlessness.

Without a doubt, the most profound social and emotional stressor facing the elderly individual is dealing with one's own imminent death. Death, a universal phenomenon, is not unique to the aged, but the chances of its occurrence are more likely than for other age groups. Death tends to be viewed as the ultimate loss, because it involves not only the loss of all significant relationships, but also the loss of oneself. Therefore dying may be seen by some individuals as the final developmental step in the human life experience.

Attitudes held by both society and members of the health care team can greatly influence the senescent's acceptance of the dying process. As members of society, we tend to fear death so much that we have resorted to institutionalizing its existence. People no longer die at home surrounded by family and friends, but tend to spend their final days and hours in hospitals and, particularly for the elderly, in nursing homes. All too often this means that the person may experience death alone. Health care professionals often view death as the antithesis of everything they believe and practice in their profession. Such an attitude does not facilitate the elderly person's acceptance of his or her imminent death.

Preparing for one's death involves a variety of activities. Some of these activities may include finalizing a will, achieving a long-desired goal, resolving interpersonal relationships, and bidding farewell to significant others. The senescent who is least likely to encounter difficulty with imminent death is the individual who is able to place value on his or her past life experiences. Such an individual finds meaning and understanding in life's final developmental task, death.

Loss of a significant other, the second social and emotional stressor with which the sensecent must deal, can be brought on not only by death, but also by geographical relocation. Although death of a loved one may be the primary means by which the elderly individual loses someone of personal importance, loss of a significant other also can occur when the elderly individual or the significant other is placed in a nursing home or moves in with children. If the significant other is the spouse, a great personal void will most likely be experienced. Coping with bereavement for one with whom one has shared many life experiences, memories, and plans can be extremely devastating. Like other individuals dealing with a loss, the senescent will experience a period of repudiation when he or she will not believe that loss of the loved one has occurred. Once the reality of the loss is acknowledged, the senescent will begin the stage of loss recognition (Lambert & Lambert, 1985). It is during this time that anger will be elicited and projected upon other individuals or circumstances in the environment, or directed toward the self in the form of depression (Engel, 1964). Following the expressed anger, the senescent may spend time being preoccupied with thoughts of the lost significant other. This preoccupation often is demonstrated by repetitive verbalization about the positive attributes of the deceased. The elderly individual begins to resolve the loss when he or she becomes less preoccupied with thoughts about the loved one and begins to become interested in new relationships and new activities. If the loss of a significant other is not effectively resolved, it is likely that the senescent's level of wellness will be affected. The incidence of health care problems have been shown to be higher in those who are recently bereaved when compared to those who have not suffered the recent loss of a loved one (Maddison & Viola, 1968; Parkes & Brown, 1972). The goal for the senescent is to develop a satisfactory single-person image and to function independently.

A sense of isolation, the third social and emotional stressor for the senescent, results when there is a lack of readily available peers for personal interaction. The presence of isolation may be the result of retirement, loss of friends and relatives due to death or relocation, decreased mobility, and social interactions that involve association with individuals who have more contemporary life-styles. Some elderly persons experience very little discomfort with a sense of isolation, especially if they tended to be isolates during their younger years. For other senescents, isolation can be very stress-provoking with responses of loneliness, boredom, depression, low morale, or any variety of physical symptoms. Even anger and hostility can develop, which may lead to increased withdrawal (Weiss, 1973) and a deepended sense of isolation. Reciprocal withdrawal will interfere with one's ability to find and make new social contacts. Sensory deprivation may result, which in turn deepens even further the senescent's sense of isolation. The senescent who actively seeks interactions with others through retirement centers, religious groups, social organizations, and civic groups will be less likely to contend with a sense of isolation than the senescent who openly guards against having to deal with the presence of others.

As a result of the aging process the individual may have to contend with the fourth social and emotional stressor of senescence, powerlessness. This stressor may occur as a result of prejudices or lack of resources. Negative views toward aging and disparaging attitudes about the elderly are not uncommon in Western society, with the outcome being rejection and neglect. Since the elderly have fewer resources than much of the rest of society, they often are viewed as less valued and less powerful. Therefore, their opinions and concerns may be ignored by society's decision-making bodies. Regardless of the impetus for the sense of powerlessness, being powerless places elderly individuals at risk (Lambert & Lambert, 1981). These risks include being unable to exercise control over one's life, having limited or no voice in issues that concern one, and being vulnerable to many of society's crimes.

Stressors Related to Conflict with Family Tasks

Contending with the ramifications of retirement and dealing with possible poverty are the major stressors related to conflict with family tasks. Both of these situations can create alterations in existing family relationships and may force the senescent to evaluate and potentially establish new and/or different role relationships.

Retirement is a significant life event for most men and for an increasing number of women in the Western world. One's occupation tends to confer status and social prominence in society. When retirement occurs, some individuals feel that they have lost their social role and status. With a decrease in income, a reduced standard of living also may occur. If social contacts were established and maintained by way of employment, the senescent may view retirement as a mechanism whereby he or she has lost meaningful relationships and important social interactions. For other elderly individuals, retirement is perceived as a reward, the beginning of the leisure years, a time of increased freedom to complete one's life's goals, and a time for discovery of new and different experiences. In other words, retirement is a major social shift for the senescent and involves a process of adjustment. The meaning of retirement, however, will depend upon the individual's unique life situation and his or her perceptions of the social significance of the situation.

Preparation for retirement can enhance the senescent's adjustment to this new developmental task. Financial planning for the retirement years and developing a realistic life-style are important issues that must be addressed in preparation for the years when one is living on a fixed income. Anticipating the possible loss of work associates and work-related friends by early involvement in groups not associated with one's employment may aid in dealing with the social ramifications of retirement. Slowly disengaging oneself from the work setting is another strategy that can prove useful in adjusting to the absence of activities of employment. While carrying out the act of disengagement, the senescent can begin to develop concrete plans for the use of forthcoming leisure time.

The amount of available time that married couples can spend together often increases when retirement occurs. This increased time together can be stress-provoking for either member of the marital relationships, because it can increase the intensity of the relationship and/or change the family role that each plays. Working together to develop alternate daily routines and daily work tasks may prove beneficial for the couple as they learn to adjust to each others' increased presence.

As a result of retirement, poverty, the second stressor related to family tasks, may occur. This may be due to inflationary effects on retirement income or the inability to have built adequate savings for the retirement years. This is not to say that some elderly have not lived at the poverty level their entire lives. However, once retirement occurs and a decrease in income results, many elderly find, for the first time in their lives, that they are living at a financial level far below their usual standard.

The consequence of being at a poverty level often will force the elderly individual to live in substandard housing. Hazards in this type of housing include fire, lack of heat, lack of refrigeration, lack of air conditioning, unsafe stairways and elevators, the presence of vermin and garbage, and a higher rate of crime. Even if the elderly individual owns his or her own home, due to lack of sufficient funds the home may be maintained inadequately, resulting in the occurrence of many of the afore-mentioned hazards.

Poor nutrition also tends to occur as a result of poverty. Insufficient funds forces the senescent to purchase inadequate quantities of reasonably nourishing food. Some senescents have resorted to eating canned dog or cat food in an attempt to obtain sufficient nourishment at a low cost. Such elderly are prime candidates for congregate meal plans and food services offered by senior centers.

With aging comes the increased incidence of chronic illness (National Center for Health Statistics, 1982) and, in turn, an increase in needed health care expenditures. Being at a poverty level ultimately will prevent one from obtaining adequate health care at will. Although Medicare has facilitated the elderly in securing needed health care, it in no way frees the individual of concerns about health-related expenses. For example, should the elderly individual require the services of an extended care facility, he or she must demonstrate the need for *skilled* nursing care before Medicare benefits can be used. If the senescent meets the appropriate criteria, the first 20 days of skilled nursing care are fully funded. Thereafter, some expenditure is required. Health care providers need to be sensitive to the stress of poverty and serve as advocates for the elderly so that they can readily access available services and so that society becomes increasingly aware of their financial plight.

COPING MECHANISMS

Health Beliefs and Behaviors

The senescent's perception of health tends to be associated with the ability to function. The elderly individual tends to enter the health care system when he or she believes that the body will not allow for participation in life's activities. To be healthy and, therefore, capable of actively engaging in life's processes is considered by many senescents to be a cherished gift. No doubt, this is because death and illness are an integral part of the daily existence of so many aged individuals. According to Alford (1982), the well senescent is one who participates in life's activities with zest, has no time to be ill, and enjoys life.

As in all other age groups, the elderly individual's daily health practices influence his or her current level of wellness. If the senescent has poor health habits that he or she has engaged in throughout life, it may be difficult to alter some of these habits. However, elderly individuals can be convinced of the necessity for change. The senescent who practices good health habits is more likely to exhibit better physical health than those who do not carry out good health practices.

An elderly individual's cultural background may facilitate or impede the carrying out of certain health practices. The senescent will more likely respond to a health care provider's guidance and instruction if he or she is from the same cultural background as the elderly individual. Should the senescent and the health care provider be from different cultural backgrounds, extreme care should be exercised to prevent miscommunication. An elderly individual unfamiliar with the health values and practices espoused by the health care provider may be resistive to change. If the health care provider is insensitive to the senescent's health beliefs or practices, then disregard for health advisement will occur. It is important for the health care provider to obtain a detailed account of the senescent's health practices. It is not uncommon to find the elderly individual utilizing self-treatment by way of over-the-counter drugs, discussing and diagnosing common complaints with neighbors and friends, and exchanging medications and home remedies with family and friends.

Responses to Stressors

Living with the bodily changes brought on by the aging process, contending with chronic illness, dealing with one's own imminent death, facing the loss of a significant other, struggling with a sense of isolation, feeling powerless, facing retirement, and living in poverty are examples of potential stressors for the senescent. When coping with these stressors, the senescent may respond in an adaptive or in a maladaptive manner. How the senescent deals with stressors will depend upon his or her ego strength and ability to exercise coping mechanisms.

Adaptive Responses. The senescent who has adaptive responses to the stressors of old age demonstrates awareness of his or her achievements and failures; is tolerant, flexible, and self-assertive; and manifests a high self-esteem as he or she looks back on life with approval and few regrets while looking forward with excitement to what is yet to come. Giving up activities that are too difficult to carry out, but engaging in new alternative activities; allowing more time to accomplish tasks; planning appointments and travel at times when crowding is low; maintaining a well-kept physical appearance; being truthful about age; and being involved in personal and social activities are examples of effective coping with the physical stressors of senescence. Adaptive responses to the social and emotional stressors of senescence include: preparing for one's death by putting business and personal affairs in order, such as finalizing a will and purchasing a cemetery lot; establishing new relationships after the loss of a significant other; becoming involved in new and different activities to prevent a sense of isolation; and maintaining and exercising control over one's life in order to prevent a sense of powerlessness. Behaviors of effective coping with the stressors related to conflict with family tasks include successful disengagement from the work setting, which is replaced with active involvement in leisure activities, social activities, and civic events. In addition, the senescent redefines his or her new role and successfully takes on its incumbent responsibilities.

Maladaptive Responses. Maladaptive responses to senescence can be exhibited in different ways. For example, the individual may manifest passivity and dependence rather than activity and self-sufficiency. Such an individual will be reluctant to venture out to meet new people or engage in new and different experiences. Unrealistic demands to meet personal needs will be placed by the senescent upon family members and friends. The senescent will retreat into self-pity and expect those around him or her to fight off the everyday stressors of life.

By comparison,the senescent may respond to old age with hostility and anger. Such individuals will be aggressive and complain about their dealings with other people. Due to a decrease in standard of living as a result of retirement, old age may be viewed in terms of starvation and poverty. It is not uncommon to see such a senescent be habit-bound, inflexible in attitudes, critical and contemptuous of the life that he or she has led, afraid of death, and envious of others. Such senescents see nothing good about old age and are not reconciled to its existence. Whether the senescent is dependent and passive or hostile and angry, both responses to old age are ineffective and maladaptive.

NURSING ASSESSMENT

Significant changes occur in an individual's life during senescence. In order to determine the impact that each of these changes impose, a comprehensive assessment of the senescent and his or her family needs to be conducted. See Table 11–1 for considerations that must be addressed when assessing the senescent and his or her family.

TABLE 11–1. ASSESSING THE FAMILY WITH A SENESCENT

	Environmental Data
Living conditions	Is the living area clean? Is there adequate temperature control? Does the living area provide adequate space for the occupants? How many people reside in the living area? Are unsafe conditions present in and around the living area? Is there adequate available nourishment in the living area? What mechanism exists for obtaining emergency assistance? How available are food, health care, safety, and transportation resources?
Family size	Is a spouse or significant other present? How many people comprise the family? Who comprises the family?
	Communication Patterns
Within the family	What types of verbal and nonverbal communications are used? Who speaks to whom and about what?
With members of society	What types of verbal and nonverbal communications are used? Who speaks to whom and about what?
	Problem-solving Skills
Decision-making abilities	Who makes the decisions? Is a systematic approach used to make decisions? How much time is taken in making a decision? What resources are used to help in decisions? What is the individual and family response to the decision made?
Use of the health care system	Is there recognition of the need for use of the health care system? Do the individual and the family know how to access the health care system? How frequently do they use the health care system? Are there available modes of transportation and finances to aid in accessing the health care system? For what reasons do they use the health care system? Do they adhere to prescribed health care regimens?
	Life-Style
Role within the family	What is the senescent's role within the family structure? How does the senescent view his or her role within the family?
Socioeconomic status	Who is the head of the household? Who contributes to the family income? What role does the senescent play in the socioeconomic status of the family? What is the socioeconomic status of the senescent? What is the income level of the family?
Recreational patterns	With whom does the senescent engage in recreational activities? What forms of recreation are used by the senescent and by the family? Do the family members and the senescent engage in recreational activities on a regular basis?
	Potential Stressors
Income level	What are the sources of income? Is the income level sufficient to meet the needs of the senescent and/or the family? What financial considerations are used in making a decision? Who makes the financial decisions? Is there a recognition of the consequences of the financial decisions made and of the resources available to the senescent and/or the family? What available financial resources exist, and is the senescent using them?

TABLE 11–1. ASSESSING THE FAMILY WITH A SENESCENT (continued)

Health status	What is the health status of the family and of the senescent? Has there been a recent change in the status of health in the family and/or the senescent? Is the senescent on a prescribed health care regimen? Is there anyone with an acute and/or chronic illness in the family?
Family structure changes	What changes have occurred in the family structure in the past year? What effect have the family structure changes had on the senescent?
Family Response Patterns	
Goal evaluation	How have the goals of the family and of the senescent changed? If they have changed, how have the family and the senescent adapted to the changes?
Counseling	Has the senescent or the family ever sought counseling? If so, for what reasons and where?

ALTERATIONS IN HEALTH

During the aging process, structure and function at all levels, from cells to organ systems, are affected. Each level is influenced in a different way at a different rate of change. However, the most significant changes that occur are those that influence complex, intersystem processes that are responsible for maintaining normal homeodynamics when the body is presented with stress. Since normal aging impairs the senescent's ability to adapt to stress at an optimal level, there is a slowing of recuperative power, with the senescent becoming more prone to actue and chronic illnesses.

The presence of illness during senescence can have devastating effects. Illness can interefere with the individual's sense of integrity, lead to undue economic strain, alter individual and family roles, and lead to death. For a list of the most prevalent acute and chronic illnesses that occur during senescence, refer to Table 11–2.

TABLE 11–2. HEALTH ALTERATIONS DURING SENESCENCE

Type	Definition
Acute	
Depression	A mental state characterized by dejection, lack of hope, and absence of cheerfulness.
Constipation	A condition in which waste matter in the bowel is too hard to pass easily or in which bowel movements are so infrequent that abdominal discomfort results.
Pulmonary edema	An abnormal accumulation of fluid in the air vesicles and interstitial tissue of the lungs.
Pneumonia	An acute inflammation or infection of the lung.
Urinary incontinence	The inability to refrain from yielding to the normal impulses of urination.

TABLE 11–2. HEALTH ALTERATIONS DURING SENESCENCE *(continued)*

Fractures	A break in the continuity of the bone caused by trauma, by twisting due to muscle spasms or indirect loss of leverage, or by disease that results in declacification of the bone.

Chronic

Cardiovascular disease	A pathological condition of the heart and/or blood vessels resulting in inadequate perfusion to the body's tissues.
Cancer	A neoplastic disease in which there is new growth of abnormal cells.
Diabetes mellitus	A disorder of carbohydrate metabolism characterized by an elevated blood sugar and an increased sugar content in the urine, resulting from inadequate production or utilization of insulin.
Renal calculi	A stone formation consisting of a crystallization of minerals found in the urinary system.
Pyelonephritis	A bacterial infection of the kidney tissue, which usually begins in the lower urinary tract, ascends into the kidney, and is brought on by an obstruction in the urinary tract.
Rheumatoid arthritis	A chronic, systemic connective tissue disorder of unknown cause that involves inflammatory changes, primarily in the small peripheral joints of the hands and feet.
Osteoarthritis	A degenerative disease of the joints, especially those bearing weight like the hips and the knees; characterized by destruction of articular cartilage, overgrowth of bone, and impairment of function.
Osteoporosis	A metabolic bone disease in which there is a failure of osteoblasts to lay down bone matrix, leading to thinning of the skeleton.
Chronic obstructive pulmonary disease	A disease process where obstruction of the small airways occurs, which leads to a decreased ability of the lungs to perform their function of ventilation.
Renal failure	Inability of the kidney to remove the end products of metabolism and to regulate the water, electrolyte and acid base content of the blood.
Diverticular disease	A disease where small mucosal outpouchings or sacs occur through defects in the muscular wall of the colon and which is thought to be due to a low intake of foods high in fiber.
Parkinson's disease	A progressive disease, characterized by stiffness of muscles and by tremors, which are due to lesions in the basal ganglia of the brain.
Alzheimer's disease	A disorder of unknown cause that results in degeneration of the neurofibrils and in the occurrence of plaques in the brain, which leads to impairment in intellectual functioning.
Dementia	A chronic brain disorder, due to generalized atrophy of the brain, which is characterized by deterioration in intellectual functioning.

NURSING RESPONSIBILITIES

The responsibility of the nurse is to assist the senescent in identifying and dealing with the positive and negative aspects of health and in becoming more actively involved in the maintenance and promotion of present and future health. The nurse, following a comprehensive assessment of the senescent and his or her family, can plan nursing interventions under three major categories. These categories include health maintenance, health promotion, and preventive measures.

Health Maintenance

To facilitate the senescent's maintenance of a high level of wellness, the nurse needs to assist the individual and his or her family in an overall assessment of the accomplishment of both individual and family tasks. For example, has the senescent family and/or the senescent obtained adequate financial security for the retirement years; accepted family accomplishments; become comfortable with the grandparent role; dealt with the loss of significant others; coped with the physical changes brought on by the aging process; achieved age-related personality development; established and maintained appropriate interpersonal relationships; been satisfied with past life experiences and events; and successfully incorporated, into activities of daily living, societal and cultural practices? If the aforementioned are true, the nurse should foster the manner in which these tasks have been achieved by providing positive feedback regarding accomplishments, providing information concerning pertinent federal and community resources that can assist with the accomplishment of family and individual tasks, and encouraging continued recognition of and adaptation to stressors. On the other hand, if these tasks have not been accomplished, health-promotion and health-prevention modalities need to be provided.

Health Promotion

The purpose of health promotion is to facilitate the senescent's optimal level of functioning. An optimal level of functioning can be promoted when certain basic health practices are carried out. These basic health practices include: (1) eating nutritious meals at regular times, instead of snacking, while maintaining appropriate body weight; (2) engaging in a regular schedule of moderate exercise; (3) obtaining 7 to 8 hours of sleep in a 24-hour period; (4) abstaining from smoking; (5) engaging in a variety of interesting activities; (6) taking some time each day to meet personal needs; (7) abstaining from or restricting the use of alcohol; (8) adhering to prescribed medical regimens. The senescent who practices most of these health habits is more likely to exhibit better physical health than those who practice only a few of these health habits.

Nutritional practices of the elderly may be one of the most important factors affecting health status that the nurse can directly influence. Changes associated with the normal aging process require some alterations in dietary requirements. Enhancing the senescent's consumption of nutritious meals, at regular times, while maintaining appropriate body weight, can be achieved if the nurse works with the individual on how to make effective changes.

A decrease in basal metabolism as well as mobility occurs with aging. As a result, the senescent needs to decrease his or her caloric consumption. The average male (5 feet, 9 inches tall) needs 2400 kcal per day, while the average female (5 feet, 5 inches) requires 1800 kcal per day (Townsend, 1980). The senescent may need considerably less than this requirement in order to prevent obesity. Stare (1977) has suggested that most individuals should decrease their caloric consumption by as much as 24% between the ages of 25 and 70 years. To enhance control of caloric consumption while enhancing appropriate nutritional intake, the senescent should be encouraged to use low-fat milk and cheese, food dense in nutritional value, and frequent small meals.

Tooth loss, a decrease in the secretion of saliva, and changes in the senses of taste and smell may affect the nutritional status of the senescent. Foods that are difficult to chew need to be cut into small pieces. Using moist foods and taking sips of water with foods helps with swallowing. To prevent the overuse of sugar and salt, due to the decrease in taste acuity, the senescent should be encouraged to use lemon juice, pepper, and spices for seasoning.

Decreased motility of the gastrointestinal tract may contribute to constipation in the elderly. Overuse of laxatives to counteract the problem may lead to vitamin deficiency, most notably vitamin A if mineral oil is used. Increasing roughage, fiber, and fluid intake (6 to 8 glasses) on a daily basis will help solve the problem more effectively.

A decrease in insulin production in many senescents leads to a decrease in glucose tolerance. Adult-onset diabetes mellitus (Type II) is a common health alteration in later life. Therefore, the senescent should be encouraged to limit the use of sugar and other concentrated sweets even before changes in glucose tolerance are noted.

The senescent should be instructed that different foods from each food group (fruits and vegetables, meats, bread and cereals, and milk) need to be included each day in the diet to assure that adequate vitamin and mineral intake is occurring. Purchasing frozen main dishes, small cans of food, and small quantities of fresh fruits and vegetables are strategies for assisting with the ease of nutritious food preparation. Should the elderly individual be unable to provide himself or herself with an adequate diet, Meals on Wheels or going to a senior center for meals may be an acceptable alternative.

Decreased mobility due to diminished muscle strength, joint stiffness, and arthritic changes can occur in the senescent. Engaging in a regular schedule of moderate exercise, however, can help reduce some of the debilitating effects of aging. According to Birren and Sloane (1980), lack of regular exercise can lead to premature aging. Activity stimulates and maintains bone tissue, muscle strength and endurance, joint flexibility, and work capacity. In addition, activity enhances gastrointes-tinal, cardiovascular, and nervous system function (DeCarlo, Castiglione, & Caousoglu, 1977).

Engaging in a regular schedule of exercise will not be a problem for senescents who have exercised regularly throughout life. They, however, may find that as they get older they need to decrease the intensity of their exercise program. Senescents new to exercise should obtain clearance from their physician before beginning a high-intensity program of exercise such as jogging, swimming, or tennis. However, most senescents can engage in walking and exercise that involves stretching, bend-ing, and moving all joints at least three times a week. Some elderly have enjoyed joining exercise and jazzercise programs designed especially for the senescent at the YMCA/YWCA or at the local senior center. According to a recent study, anxiety tends to decrease in the elderly when they engage in a program of regular exercise (Wiswell, 1980).

Sleep patterns tend to change with age by becoming shorter and shallower. Waking up at night is common as well as napping during the day. The senescent needs to be made aware of the fact that these changes in sleep pattern are normal. The senescent should, however, be encouraged to obtain at least 7 to 8 hours of sleep in a 24-hour period. To enhance sleep, the individual should be encouraged to avoid caffeine (i.e., coffee, cola, tea) and to engage in a relaxing activity (i.e. reading, listening to soft music, or taking a warm bath) prior to sleep. Sedatives should be avoided unless insomnia is undermining the senescent's state of health.

The incidence of pneumonia and chronic obstructive pulmonary disease in-creases in the senescent population. The senescent who smokes will have a greater likelihood of contracting these illnesses. Therefore, it is advantageous to assist the senescent in stopping the smoking habit if he or she is a smoker. It may prove difficult for the senescent to abstain from smoking if he or she has engaged in the habit for a number of years. It is possible to stop smoking, however, and the following maneuv-ers may prove helpful:

1. Place cigarettes or cigars in an inconvenient location.
2. Hide ashtrays.
3. Buy one pack of cigarettes or one cigar at a time.
4. Do not carry matches or a cigarette lighter.
5. If the urge to smoke occurs, wait a few minutes and then immediately change the activities or thoughts being pursued.
6. Try to go longer each day without a cigarette or cigar.
7. Slowly stop smoke-linked habits, such as a cup of coffee and a cigarette/cigar, a meal and a cigarette/cigar, or a party and a cigarette/cigar.
8. Have a friend stop smoking at the same time.
9. Attend a smoking cessation course.
10. Utilize a replacement for the oral gratification obtained from smoking, such as chewing sugar-free gum.

Above all, the senescent requires encouragement from family, friends, and members of the health care team as he or she attempts to alter the smoking habit.

With retirement comes the opportunity for engagement in a variety of interesting activities beyond the work role. The senescent who has, throughout his or her life, taken part in various activities will not encounter difficulty in shifting emphasis from the work environment to social, civic, and/or recreational activities. However, the senescent whose sources of entertainment have been linked in some way with the work role may encounter difficulties in finding things to do once retirement has occurred. Senior centers, YMCA/YWCAs, continuing education programs sponsored by local high schools and colleges, and senior citizen religious groups are rich arenas for providing activities and available new acquaintances. The senescent also may need to be encouraged to invest time and energy into the role of grandparent. Making toys, clothes, dolls, or scrapbooks for grandchildren can prove stimulating for the senescent, as well as providing a new avenue of communication with the grandchild.

Taking some time each day to meet personal needs is especially important for the senescent who is responsible for caring for an ailing spouse. When financial and personal resources are limited, the senescent may find that caring for an ailing loved one requires a considerable amount of time. Intentionally planning for some personal time each day is important not only for one's physical well-being, but also for one's psychological well-being. During the planned personal time the individual should engage in some activity which he or she enjoys, such as reading, carving, sewing, making flies for fishing, watching TV, talking on the telephone, doing fingernails, or simply soaking in the bathtub. Knowing that one can take some time for himself or herself each day without feeling guilt about it can aid in enhancing the senescent's ability to contend with the stressors of caring for a dependent spouse.

The incidence of alcoholism among the elderly is much higher than most professionals realize (Mishara & Kastenbaum, 1980). It is not uncommon for the lonely and depressed senescent to turn to alcohol for solace. Abstaining from or restricting the use of alcohol is advisable for the senescent, because the aging process results in declining kidney and liver function, which in turn leads to a slower process of alcohol and drug detoxification within the body. The senescent who has resorted to alcohol abuse for a period of time will find it difficult to change the habit. Referring the individual to Alcoholics Anonymous or to a local drug rehabilitation center is advisable. Above all, the nurse must be alert to the fact that, like other age groups, the elderly encounter difficulties with alcohol abuse and require specific intense therapy.

Adhering to prescribed medical regimens may not always occur in the elderly population. Use of over-the-counter medications or of someone else's prescribed medications, not following a required dietary regimen, or using home or ethnic remedies is not uncommon in the senescent population. Before reacting to the individual's health care practices, the nurse needs to find out why the senescent is carrying out activities that are perceived by the nurse to be unsafe. It is quite possible that the senescent may be using over-the-counter medications and/or someone else's prescribed medications because of lack of access to the health care system. This lack of access may be due to finances, inaccessible transportation, or inadequate knowledge about how to obtain entry into the health care system. After assessing the situation, the nurse needs to identify and activate the resources that are available to the senescent (i.e., Medicaid benefits, transportation buses for the elderly, telephone numbers and names of health care providers for the senescent to contact when in need of care). Being able to readily access the health care system often changes the senescent's health behavior.

Not following required dietary regimens often can be resolved by providing information about the reasons for the dietary restrictions and how the senescent can go about adhering to those restrictions. For example, a diabetic senescent may believe that it is necessary to purchase special dietetic foods, which are too expensive for his or her budget. Planning meals for one week with the senescent with the types of foods that he or she tends to purchase often aids in alleviating the problem. Also, the nurse can point out to the senescent that the food that is cooked for the diabetic can be eaten by the rest of the family.

The use of home or ethnic health care remedies is not an uncommon practice in the elderly population. However, before the nurse instructs the senescent that he or she must abstain from using such remedies, it is advisable to determine whether the remedy is unsafe. Home and ethnic remedies may play an important part in the senescent's life. If the remedy is deemed safe, it would be inadvisable to request that the senescent abstain from using it. Allowing the individual to use his or her remedies along with prescribed health care regimens often will prove more effective. For example, an arthritic Chinese-American woman who finds accupuncture helpful in controlling her pain should be encouraged to use this form of therapy along with her prescribed gold salts. If her use of accupuncture is acknowledged, she will adhere, more likely, to the use of gold salts.

Preventive Measures

Changes such as diminished visual acuity, decreased muscle mass and strength, osteoporosis, decreased coordination, alterations in gait, decreased attention span, and postural hypotension place the senescent at a high risk for falls. The most common fracture sites in the elderly include the vertebral bodies, the upper end of the femur, the distal end of the radius, and the proximal end of the humerus. Of all of these, fractures of the upper end of the femur (hip fractures) are the most common and potentially the most disabling (Devas, 1976; Vallarino & Sherman, 1981).

To prevent fractures, the nurse can assist the senescent by teaching him or her to remain alert for hazards in the environment and for behavior patterns that promote accidents and falls. A great deal can be done to modify the senescent's living area (see Table 11–3); however, it is imperative that the changes made are done with the cooperation of the individual. Above all, the senescent should be instructed on having emergency telephone numbers readily available at each telephone and printed large enough so that he or she can read them.

TABLE 11–3. MEASURES FOR PREVENTING FRACTURES

Remove unneccesary obstacles
Arrange furniture in an orderly fashion, with wide traffic paths
Avoid the use of extension cords, or tape them down to prevent tripping
Remove throw rugs
Tack down carpets
Build bannisters on stairways
Paint walls and stairways different colors for purposes of differentiation
Keep staircases well lighted and place nonslip treads on stairs
Install grab bars and bath mats in the bathroom
Install a nightlight to ensure safe passage between the bedroom and the bathroom at night
Wear sturdy, well-fitting shoes with substantial soles
Avoid wearing long, flowing nightgowns or robes and thongs
Use extreme caution when going out in snowy or icy weather
Clean up spills and pick up fallen objects immediately
Do not keep floors highly polished
Check out the environment by turning the head and scanning with the eyes
Check mobility aids, such as canes or walkers, for any malfunctioning parts

The senescent is at risk for infection even when relatively small amounts of infectious agents are present. The elderly individual's ability to resist infection is compromised by poor nutrition, poor metabolic function, decreased defense mechanisms, medications, and disease. Therefore, it is imperative that measures be taken to prevent infection.

One site for an infectious process is the respiratory tract, due to the decreased efficiency of the airway clearance mechanisms (i.e., ciliary action and the cough reflex). To decrease the incidence of a respiratory infection, the senescent should be encouraged to obtain flu shots on a regular basis, stay away from highly congested areas during flu and cold season, and avoid close contact with people who are experiencing an upper respiratory infection. In addition, the senescent should be encouraged to dress warmly during cold weather and stay indoors when smog alerts are reported.

The skin is another potential site for an infectious process, due to fragility, poor circulation, and the increased incidence of diabetes mellitus. The potential for dry, cracked skin is great. To prevent an opening in the skin, the senescent should be encouraged to apply emollients to the skin and to bathe in water that contains bath oils. In some situations it may be advisable for the senescent to bathe every other or every third day, since soaps tend to dry the skin. If the senescent is a diabetic, he or she should carry out foot care every day even if a complete bath is not taken on a daily basis. In addition, any cuts or breaks in the skin should be washed, treated with an antiseptic, and covered with a sterile bandage.

Dealing with vast fluctuations in the environmental temperature can create serious problems for the elderly. Since the elderly often live on fixed incomes and may try to curb their expenditures by not adequately heating or cooling their residence, it is not uncommon to find them suffering from frostbite, heat stroke, or even dying. To prevent frostbite and heat stroke, the nurse needs to advise the elderly individual of the availability of community shelters where he or she can go for refuge during severe environmental temperature fluctuations. In addition, the nurse needs to instruct the elderly individual on how to dress appropriately during the different seasons of the year, as well as how to eat and drink during times of severe temperature change.

The elderly are not immune to fires, and they must be instructed on how to prevent their occurrence. It is not uncommon to find an array of wires plugged into a single outlet in the home of a senescent. Overloading old circuitry, especially with heating appliances, can be a serious hazard in older buildings and homes. With diminished visual acuity the hazards of frayed electrical cords on lamps and appliances may go unnoticed. To prevent the occurrence of fires the senescent's home should be checked for unsafe electrical appliances, overloaded circuitry, and combustibles such as paints, kerosene or gas, and unnecessary newspapers. In addition, the senescent should be warned about the hazards of extra heating devices, kerosene stoves, gas heaters, and exposed steam pipes. All senescents should be encouraged to install smoke alarms in their living quarters and be instructed on how to rapidly evacuate the premises should a fire occur.

With the increasing crime rate, senescents are becoming frequent victims. A major consideration in the safety of the elderly is to prevent intruders. As a precaution, the elderly may need to install extra locks on doors, locks on windows, alarm systems, and gates on windows. However, gates on windows should be designed to open from the inside of the home. Gates that cannot be opened or that require keys are illegal and extremely hazardous in the event of a fire. Above all, the senescent should have the phone number of the police readily accessible and should set up some type of checking-in procedure with family members or friends.

Elderly individuals often are victims of one or more chronic illnesses that may require emergency care. If the individual is living alone or has no one readily accessible who can communicate his or her specific health care needs, delayed or inappropriate emergency health care may be given. To prevent this, the nurse should instruct the senescent on how to obtain and how to fill in the appropriate information for the "Vial-of-Life," a plastic container that encloses a brief health history of the individual, including diagnosis, medications, name of physician, and persons to call in case of an emergency. The vial is stored in the top right shelf of the refrigerator, and a Vial-of-Life sticker is posted on the refrigerator door. In addition, the chronically ill senescent should be encouraged to wear specially designed jewelry that contains information about the individual's health care problems. Such jewelry can be worn in the form of a bracelet or a necklace and alerts emergency health care providers of the needs of the senescent when he or she is not in the home environment.

Acute Caregiver

When assessing the acute health alterations of the senescent, the nurse must keep in mind that: (1) an age-related decline in immune function results in less rapid and less effective responses to infections, (2) stress situations (physiological and psychosocial) produce more profound reactions in the elderly and require a longer period of time for readjustment, (3) complex functions that require multisystem coordination show the most obvious decline and require the greatest compensation and support, (4) the elderly frequently have an atypical presentation of illness, and (5) the most prevalent acute illnesses in later life are acute respiratory conditions such as pneumonia and pulmonary edema. Thus obscure and unexplained changes in health status should not be accepted as signs of normal aging, but should be carefully evaluated.

The nurse in the acute care situation should be cognizant of the fact that the senescent who becomes acutely ill is likely to be apprehensive and worried, because his or her security is more profoundly influenced by illness than is the security of a younger individual. In addition to illness and the depleted physical energy that almost always accompanies it, the senescent may have no family and few friends. Thus, fears about helplessness and physical dependence upon others may become prominent. The nurse can be most helpful in assisting the senescent and the family by offering a variety of options and resources that may help in meeting their specific needs. To be successful in meeting the needs of the senescent dealing with an acute health alteration, the nurse needs to be knowledgeable about all aspects of aging and incorporate this knowledge into nursing care modalities.

SUMMARY

Senescence, the time frame from 65 years of age until death, is when the individual evaluates past experiences and accomplishments and comes to terms with the final years of life, deals with retirement, contends with living on a fixed income, takes on the grandparent role, deals with the loss of a spouse, contends with the normal physical changes of aging, and copes with chronic illness. To facilitate the senescent's optimal level of health, the nurse needs to thoroughly assess the developmental and psychosocial aspects of the individual and his or her family, and initiate and foster appropriate health maintenance, health promotion, and preventive measures.

CARE PLAN FOR THE FAMILY WITH THE SENESCENT WITH OSTEOARTHRITIS

Situation

Mrs. Brown is a 72-year-old, alert, obese, sedentary lady who lives with her 75-year-old husband in a two-story home that they purchased over 40 years ago. Their three offspring are married and live approximately 500 miles away. For economic support, the Browns rely solely upon Mr. Brown's monthly Social Security checks. Over the past 6 months, Mrs. Brown has encountered increasing pain in her right knee after climbing the staircase in her home. Although Mrs. Brown has noted the knee pain for the past six months, she has put off seeing a physician since she believes that her knee problems are not "all that serious." When Mrs. Brown finally did see a physician, she was diagnosed as having osteoarthritis, which is to be treated with weight loss, limited physical activity involving the affected joint, and acetylsalicylic acid (aspirin). Mrs. Brown is being visited twice a week by the community health nurse because she has encountered some difficulty in complying with her prescribed health care regimens. During the nurse's first visit, the following nursing diagnoses were identified. Following the nursing diagnoses is a care plan developed by the nurse, which addresses Mrs. Brown's most prominent diagnosis, noncompliance to prescribed health care regimens related to lack of perceived seriousness of osteoarthritis.

Nursing Diagnoses

1. Noncompliance to prescribed health care regimes related to lack of perceived seriousness of osteoarthritis.
2. Alteration in comfort (pain) related to joint disease.
3. Activity intolerance related to joint disease.
4. Alteration in nutrition, more than body requirements, related to decreased physical activity at home.

SAMPLE CARE PLAN

Nursing Diagnosis	Goals	Nursing Intervention	Evaulation
Noncompliance to prescribed health care regimens related to lack of perceived seriousness of osteoarthritis.	Mrs. Brown will follow her diet, activity, and analgesic plan at least 50% of the time for 1 week.	The nurse will review with Mrs. Brown the reasons for and importance of limiting her caloric intake, of limiting physical activity involving her right knee, and of taking her medication	Mrs. Brown will follow her diet, activity, and analgesic plan at least 50% of the time for 1 week.

Review Questions

1. Discuss the major areas of concern for the senescent in regard to the accomplishment of family developmental tasks.
2. Discuss the major areas of concern for the senescent in regard to the accomplishment of individual developmental tasks.
3. Discuss the role that the nurse plays in assisting the senescent in accomplishing his or her family and individual developmental tasks.
4. Identify major stressors confronting the senescent, and describe how the nurse can facilitate the individual's coping process.

5. Define eight major chronic illnesses that can occur during senescence.
6. Discuss what role the nurse plays in providing health maintenance, health promotion, and preventive measures to the senescent.

REFERENCES

Alford, D. (1982). Expanding older persons' belief systems. *Topics in Clinical Nursing, 3*(4), 35–45.

Annual Statistical Supplement. (1983). Shares of money income from earnings and other sources for aged and nonaged households. *Social Security Bulletin*, 67.

Birkhill, W., & Schaie, K. (1975). The effect of differential reinforcement of cautiousness in intellectual performances among the elderly. *Journal of Gerontology, 30* 578–583.

Birren, J. (1974). Translations in gerontology—from lab to life: Psychophysiology and speed of response. *American Psychologist, 11* 808–815.

Birren, J. & Sloane, R. (Eds.) (1980). *Handbook of mental health and aging.* Englewood Cliffs, NJ: Prentice-Hall.

Botwinick, J. (1978). *Aging and behavior: A comprehensive integration of research findings.* New York: Springer-Verlag.

Branch, M., & Paxton, P. (1976) *Providing safe nursing care for ethnic people of color.* New York: Appleton-Century-Crofts.

Brody, H., & Vijayashander, N. (1977). Anatomical changes in the nervous system. In C. Finch & L. Hayflick (Eds.), *Handbook of the biology of aging.* New York: Van Nostrand Reinhold.

Bullough, V., & Bullough, B. (1982). *Health care for the other American* New York: Appleton-Century-Crofts.

Carter, A. (1979). The neurologic aspects of aging. In I. Rossman (Ed.), *Clinical geriatrics.* Philadelphia: Lippincott.

Clark, M., (1970). *Health in the Mexican-American culture: A community study.* Berkeley: University of California Press.

Craik, F. (1977). Age differences in human memory. In J. Birren & K. Schaie (Eds.), *Handbook of the psychology of aging.* New York: Van Nostrand Reinhold.

DeCarlo, T., Castiglione, L., & Caousoglu, M. (1977). A program of balanced fitness in the preventive care of elderly ambulatory patients. *Journal of the American Geriatrics Society, 25,*331–334.

Devas, M. (1976). Orthopedics. In F. Steinberg (Ed.), *Cowdry's: The care of the geriatric patient.* St. Louis: Mosby.

Engel, G. (1964). Grief and grieving. *American Journal of Nursing, 3*(4), 35–45.

Engen, T. (1977). Taste and smell. In J. Birren & K. Schaie (Eds.), *Handbook of the psychology of aging.* New York: Van Nostrand Reinhold.

Erikson, E. (1963). *Childhood and society.* New York: Norton.

Gioiella, E., & Bevil, C. (1985). *Nursing care of the aging client: Promoting health adaptation.* E. Norwalk, CT: Appleton-Century-Crofts.

Goldfarb, A. (1969). The psychodynamic of dependency and the search for aid. In R. Kalish (Ed.), *The dependencies of old people.* Ann Arbor, MI: Institute of Gerontology.

Goldman, R. (1977). Aging and the excretory system: Kidney and bladder. In C. Finch & L. Hayflick (Eds.), *Handbook of the biology of aging*. New York: Van Nostrand Reinhold.

Goldman, R. (1979). Decline in organ function with aging. In I. Rossman (Ed.), *Clincial geriatrics*. Philadelphia: Lippincott.

Gordon, S., & Clark, W. (1974). Application of signal detection theory to prose recall and recognition in elderly and young adults. *Journal of Gerontology, 29*, 64–72.

Gregerman, R., & Bierman, E. (1981). Hormones and aging. In R. William (Ed.), *Textbook of endocrinology*. Philadelphia: Saunders.

Gutmann, E. (1977). Muscle. In C. Finch & L. Hayflick (Eds.), *Handbook of the biology of aging*. New York: Van Nostrand Reinhold.

Hayflick, L. (1977). The cellular basis for biological aging. In C.Finch & L. Hayflick (Eds.), *Handbook of the biology of aging*. New York: Van Nostrand Reinhold.

Hogan, R. (1985). *Human sexuality: A nursing perspective*. E. Norwalk, CT: Appleton-Century-Crofts.

Hoyer, W., Labouvie-Vief, G., & Baltes, P. (1973). Modifications of response speed deficits and intellectual performance in the elderly. *Human Development, 16*, 233–242.

Jarvik, L. (1975). Thoughts on the psychobiology of aging. *American Psychologist, 30*, 567-583.

Kehril, N., & Spencer, M. (1984). Aging. In D. Jones, M. Lepley, & B. Baker (Eds.), *Health assessment across the life span*. New York: McGraw-Hill.

Kimmel, D. (1974). *Adulthood and aging*. New York: Wiley.

Kocke, R. (1977). Influence of aging on the lung. In C. Finch & L. Hayflick (Eds.) *Handbook of the biology of aging*. New York: Van Nostrand Reinhold.

Kohn, R. (1977). Heart and cardiovascular system. In C. Finch & L. Hayflick (Eds.), *Handbook of the biology of aging*. New York: Van Nostrand Reinhold.

Lambert, V., & Lambert, C. (1985). *Psychosocial care of the physically ill: What every nurse should know*. Englewood Cliffs, NJ: Prentice-Hall.

Lambert, V., & Lambert, C. (1981). Role theory and the concept of powerlessness. *Journal of Psychosocial Nursing and Mental Health Services, 19*(9), 11–14.

Lancaster, J. (1981). Maximizing psychological adaptation in an aging population. *Topics in Clinical Nursing, 3*(1), 31–43.

Latham, I., & Johnson, L. (1979). Aging at the cellular level. In I. Rossman (Ed.), *Clinical geriatrics*. Philadelphia: Lippincott.

Lowenthal, M. (1975). Psychosocial variations across the adult life course: Frontiers for research and policy. *Gerontologist, 15*(1), 6–12.

Maddison, D., & Viola, A. (1968). The health of widows in the year following bereavement. *Journal of Psychosomatic Research, 12*, 297–306.

Mishara, B., & Kastenbaum, R. (1980). *Alcohol and old age: Seminars in psychiatry*. New York: Grune & Stratton.

National Center for Health Statistics, Health Interview Survey, U.S. Department of Health and Human Services, (1977). Unpublished data, and *Vital and Health Statistics* (1982, October). (Current estimates from the National Health Interview Survey, Series 10, No. 141).

Parkes, C., & Brown, R. (1972). Health after bereavement: A controlled study of young Boston widows and widowers. *Psychosomatic Medicine, 34*, 449–461.

Perlmutter, M. (1978). What is memory aging the aging of? *Developmental Psychology, 14*, 330–345.

Rabbitt, P. (1977). Changes in problem solving ability in old age. In J. Birren & K. Schaie (Eds.), *Handbook of the psychology of aging*. New York: Van Nostrand Reinhold.

Riegel, K., & Riegel, R. (1973). Development, drop and death. *Developmental Psychology, 6*, 306–319.

Rossman, I. (1977). Anatomic and body composition changes with aging. In C. Finch & L. Hayflick (Eds.), *Handbook of the biology of aging*. New York: Van Nostrand Reinhold.

Rossman, I. (1979). The anatomy of aging. In I. Rossman (Ed.), *Clinical geriatrics*. Philadelphia: Lippincott.

Schaie, K. (1980). Intelligence and problem solving. In J. Birren & R. Sloane (Eds.), *Handbook of mental health and aging*. Englewood Cliffs, NJ: Prentice-Hall.

Schaie, K., & Labouvie-Vief, G. (1974). Generational versus ontogenetic components of change in adult cognitive behavior: A fourteen-year cross-sequential study. *Developmental Psychology, 10*, 305–320.

Schoenfield, D. (1965). Memory changes with age. *Nature, 208*, 918.

Selmanowitz, V. Rizer, R., & Orentriech, N. (1977). Aging of the skin and its appendages. In C. Finch & L. Hayflick (Eds.), *Handbook of the biology of aging*. New York: Van Nostrand Reinhold.

Spollett, G. (1984). Physical examination of the aging. In D. Jones, M. Lepley, & B. Baker (Eds.), *Health assessment across the life span*. New York: McGraw-Hill.

Stare, F. (1977). Three score and ten plus more. *Journal of the American Geriatric Society, 25*, 529–533.

Strauss, A., Corbin, J., Fagerhaugh, D., Glaser, B., Maines, D., Suczek, B., & Weiner, C. (1984). *Chronic illness and the quality of life*. St. Louis: Mosby.

Syzek, B. (1976). Cardiovascular changes in aging: Implication for nursing. *Journal of Gerontological Nusring, 2*(1), 28–32.

Talbert, G. (1977). Aging of the reproductive system. In Finch & L. Hayflick (Eds.), *Handbook of the biology of aging.*. New York: Van Nostrand Reinhold.

Townsend, C. (1980). *Nutrition and diet modifications*. Albany, NY: Delmar.

Vallarino, A., & Sherman, F. (1981). Principles of rehabilitation treatment. In L. Libow & F. Sherman (Eds.), *The core of geriatric medicine: A guide for students and practitioners*. St. Louis: Mosby.

Weiss, R. (1973). *Loneliness: The experience of emotional and social isolation*. Cambridge, MA: MIT Press.

Welford, A. (1974). Motor performance. In J. Birren & K. Schaie (Eds.), *Handbook of the psychology of aging*. New York: Van Nostrand Reinhold.

Wesson, L. (1969). *Physiology of the human kidney*. New York: Grune & Stratton.

Wiswell, R. (1980). Relaxation, exercise, and aging. In J. Birren & R. Sloane (Eds.), *Handbook of mental health and aging*. Englewood Cliffs, NJ: Prentice-Hall.

Zack, L. (1979). The oral cavity. In I. Rossman (Ed.), *Clinical Geriatrics*. Philadelphia: Lippincott.

Zarit, S. (1980). *Aging and mental disorder: Psychological approaches to assessment and treatment*. New York: Free Press.

Appendices

Name	Source	Age Group	Concepts	Remarks
E. Duvall	*Marriage and Family Development* (5th Ed.). Philadelphia: J. B. Lippincott.	Childbearing years	Family life cycle, family developmental tasks, the expectant phase	Just as individuals go through successive stages of growth and development, so do families. Each stage of family development has its own specific developmental tasks. *Family developmental tasks* refer to growth responsibilities that must be achieved by a family during each stage of development so as to meet (1) its biological requirements, (2) its cultural imperatives and (3) its own aspirations and values
A. D. Colman & L. L. Colman	Colman, A. D., & Colman, L. L. *Pregnancy: The Psychological Experience.* New York: Hearder & Hearder.	Reproductive years	Fundamental tasks of pregnancy: 1. Pregnancy validation 2. Fetal embodiment	Pregnancy has subtasks to be accomplished in order for the experience to be integrated into the total life process.

APPENDIX 1. MAJOR THEORISTS APPEARING IN TEXT *(continued)*

Name	Source	Age Group	Concepts	Remarks
			3. Fetal distinction 4. Role transition	Successful resolution of each task prepares one for coping with future tasks
Alexander Thomas & Stella Chess	Thomas, A., & Chess, S. Dynamics of Psychologic Development.	Infant	Infant temperament	Temperament is a reaction pattern inherent in all infants. Type of temperament can strongly affect relationship with major caretaker
Erik Erikson	Erikson, E. (1963). *Childhood and Society,* (2nd Ed.). New York: W. W. Norton.	Infant	Trust vs. mistrust	Establishment of trust is foundation for all other relationships
Jean Piaget	Wolff, P. H. (1960). The developmental psychology of Jean Piaget and psychoanalysis. *Psychological Issues Monograph,* 2(1).	Infant	Sensorimotor phase	Intellectual organization is begun through adaptation to the environment. This adaptation is done through learning and development
Erik Erikson	Erikson, E. (1963). *Childhood and Society* (2nd Ed.). New York: W. W. Norton.	Toddler (early childhood and the will to be oneself)	Autonomy versus shame and doubt	Achievement or mastery of one level facilitates mastery of next level. Family relationships are very important in helping child to develop.
Jean Piaget	Wolff, P. H. (1960). The developmental psychology of Jean Piaget and psychoanalysis. *Psychological Issues Monograph,* 2(1).	Preschool child (childhood and the anticipation of roles) Sensorimotor Stage (birth to 24 months)	Initiative versus guilt; sex role identification Assimilation Accommodation	Development occurs in a sequential, predictable order. Each phase challenges child's existing thinking patterns, changes them and levels off.
		Preoperational State (2–7 yr)	Symbolism Animistic thought	
Erik Erikson	Erikson, E. (1963). *Childhood and*	School-age child 6–12 yr	Industry vs. Inferiority	Theory of personality

APPENDIX 1. MAJOR THEORISTS APPEARING IN TEXT *(continued)*

Name	Source	Age Group	Concepts	Remarks
	Society (2nd Ed.). New York: W. W. Norton.	Adolescence 13–19 yr	Identity vs. Role Confusion	development with each stage having 2 opposing components, a favorable and an unfavorable, termed a "crisis." Progression to each successful stage is dependent on the resolution of the crisis of the present stage.
Erik Erikson	Erikson, E. (1968). *Identity: Youth and Crisis.* New York: W. W. Norton.	School-age child	Latency stage	Belief that underlying motivation of human behavior is sexuality or sexual energy (libido)
		Adolescence	Genital stage	Drives are dormant during latency stage. Psychic energy is centered upon a specific body region which is the primary source of pleasure for the person.
Lawrence Kohlberg	Kohlberg, L. (1969). *Stages in Development and Moral Thought and Action.* New York: Holt, Rinehart, & Winston.	Ages 7–11. Conventional stage	Good boy/good girl Law and order	Theory of moral development seeing it as being closely related to cognitive development
Jean Piaget	Wolf, P. H. (1960). The developmental psychology of Jean Piaget and psychoanalysis. *Psychological Issues Monograph,* 2(1).	Ages 12 and up. Post conventional stage Schoolf-age child. Period of concrete operations	Social contract individual conscience. Inductive to deductive logic Classification Sorting Ordering Conservation	Theory of cognitive development with belief that reaching intellectual potential is dependent on environmental stimulation. Experiences, and not simply maturation, are the foundation of a child's cognitive development
Gail Sheehy	Sheehy, G. (1974). *Passages.* New York:	Adolescence; period of formal operations	Abstract logic Scientific reasoning	From popular press Studies adult

APPENDIX 1. MAJOR THEORISTS APPEARING IN TEXT (continued)

Name	Source	Age Group	Concepts	Remarks
	E. P. Dutton.	Young adult: 20–44 yr.	Pulling up roots	development
			All you need is. . .	Believes there are predictables
			Catch-30	Crises that are the
	Sheehy, G. (1981). Pathfinders. New York: Morrow.		Individuals are unique	same for both sexes but the rhythms are
			Deadline decade	different
Erik Erikson	Erikson, E. (1963). Childhood and Society (2nd Ed.) New York: W. W. Norton	Young adult	Intimacy versus isolation	Search for intimacy is a basic human motive
Erik Erikson	Erikson, E. (1963). Childhood and Society (2nd Ed.). New York: W. W. Norton.	Middlescent: 45–65 yr	Generativity versus stagnation	This time frame in one's life encompasses the launching-center stage and the middle-aged-parent stage of the family life cycle. During this time frame a vital interest outside the home occurs with a major focus on establishing and guiding future generations with an optimistic hope of bettering society
Erik Erikson	Erikson, E. (1963). Childhood and Society (2nd Ed.). New York: W. W. Norton.	Senescent: 65 yr of age until death	Ego integrity versus despair	This time frame in one's life tends to encompass death of one's spouse, numerous changes in bodily function, retirement, dealing with one's own imminent death, and changes in socioeconomic status. If the mature adult has developed a strong sense of self-worth and is able to place value on his or her past life experiences, feelings of despair will be overcome

APPENDIX 2. KOHLBERG'S STAGES OF MORAL DEVELOPMENT

Level I—Preconventional

Age 4–7

(1) Punishment	*(2) Hedonism*
This involves a punishment-and-obedience orientation, with rules obeyed in order to avoid punishment.	This involves a "What's in it for me" attitude. Feelings of loyal gratitude or justice are not incorporated. Doing what is right is viewed in terms of satisfying one's own needs.

Level II—Conventional

Age 7–11

(3) Good boy/good girl label	*(4) Law and order*
The child seeks approval by being nice. There is a beginning orientation to interpersonal relations, valuing conformity, loyalty, and active maintenance of social order.	Moral judgments are beginning to be based on laws and rules. Doing one's duty and showing respect for authority come into focus. Many adults never reach past this stage.

Level III—Postconventional

Age 12 and upward

(5) Social contract	*(6) Individual conscience*
This involves a social-contract orientation. Decisions are made on one's own, but based on the needs and viewpoints of society. There is a beginning internationalization of conscience, but it is without clear, rational, and universal principles.	This involves a universal moral principle orientation. Individual conscience guides decisions; no other rationale is needed. Respect for the dignity of others as individuals and concepts of justice and ethics are integrated into moral decisions.

Adapted from Kohlberg, L. (1969). Stages in Development of Moral Thought and Action. New York: Holt, Rinehart, & Winston.

INDEX